FOUNDATIONS IN
Behavioral Pharmacology

An Introduction to the Neuroscience of
Drug Addiction and Mental Disorders

Third Edition

Mark Stanford, Ph.D.

Foundations in Behavioral Pharmacology:
An Introduction to the Neuroscience of Drug Addiction and Mental Disorders
 (3rd Edition)

Lightway Centre Publishers
P.O. Box 7902
Santa Cruz, CA 95061

Dedicated To Sidney Cohen, M.D.

About the Author

Mark Stanford, Ph.D. is the Senior Manager of Medical and Clinical Services for a large County's Health & Hospital System Department of Alcohol & Drug Services - Addiction Medicine and Therapy Division. He has direct clinical experience working in every modality of addictions treatment including inpatient, residential, day treatment, outpatient and medication-assisted treatment programs.

Dr. Stanford is also a clinical research educator in the behavioral neurosciences. He has taught psychopharmacology throughout the Bay Area of California including a 20-year history with U.C. Berkeley Extension Department of Biological and Behavioral Sciences and Mathematics, and as a lecturer at Stanford University Department of Family and Community Medicine. He also teaches Treatment and Clinical Considerations of Substance Abuse Disorders for LCSW's, MFT's and Psychologists for their CEU licensing requirements.

Dr. Stanford has authored numerous materials in the behavioral neurosciences including serving as the chief editor of the "Professional Perspectives on Addiction Medicine" series, which includes the books, "Understanding Opioid Addiction and the Function of Methadone Treatment" and "Beyond Medical Marijuana: Toward Cannabinoid-Base Medicines".

CONTENTS

CHAPTER 3. THE ELECTROCHEMICAL NEURON

CHAPTER 4. THE CHEMISTRY OF BEHAVIOR

SECTION II: BEHAVIORAL PHARMACOLOGY OF SUBSTANCE ABUSE

CHAPTER 5. NEUROBIOLOGICAL ASPECTS OF SUBSTANCE ABUSE

CHAPTER 9. MARIJUANA, CANNABINOIDS AND CANNABINOID-BASED MEDICINES

CHAPTER 10. HALLUCINOGENIC DRUGS

CHAPTER 11. INHALANTS

CHAPTER 12. STEROIDS

CHAPTER 13: METHODS OF DRUG TESTING

SECTION III: BEHAVIORAL PHARMACOLOGY OF PSYCHIATRIC MEDICATIONS

CHAPTER 14. MEDICATIONS FOR MENTAL HEALTH

CHAPTER 15. A REVIEW OF CO-OCCURRING DISORDERS

APPENDIX SECTION

SECTION I: BASIC CONCEPTS IN PHARMACOLOGY AND NEUROPHYSIOLOGY

SECTION INTRODUCTION

The overall objective of this book is to help the healthcare provider gain a working understanding of the neurobiological and pharmacological factors which contribute to substance abuse and mental health disorders. Over the last decade, an enormous amount of data began pouring in from the various findings of long-term neuroscience research that started in the late 1970s and 1980s. This research focused on discovering the biogenetic, neurobiological, biochemical and pharmacological determinants that are significant in substance abuse and mental health disorders.

From this information, virtually every discipline within the helping profession experienced a dramatic influence as a result of these discoveries. This ultimately led to the incorporation of the information, in varying degrees, into their given disciplines, and changed the traditional psychodynamic viewpoint considerably. Take for example, the evolution of the Diagnostics and Statistics Manual (DSM), where yesterday it was largely psychodynamic, but today includes a significant amount of the neurobiological aspects of behavior.

Previous to this occurrence, therapists and providers could exist within their own philosophical domains without having to peer out and experience different perspectives from other behavioral health areas. Now however, the profession as a whole has incorporated many research findings across various disciplines including social work, psychology, psychotherapy, counseling and rehabilitation therapy. Indeed most providers view behavior from a biopsychosocial perspective as a result of the impact research had made. The "bio" aspect of the biopsychosocial perspective brings a critical component into the health care mix, providing therapists with important tools that would not be available otherwise.

As the behavioral health care industry continues its mysterious journey of on-going change, case management now requires a multidisciplinary treatment team to provide for their patients as a single unit. This requires a much greater degree of cross-communication between medical and non-medical providers. The healthcare industry also continues to expect social workers, psychologists, counselors and therapists to monitor acute behavioral signs of substance abuse and side effects of medications used in mental health. For providers who work with dual diagnosis, it has been critical to assist the patient with medication and treatment compliance, along with their chemical dependency recovery program. Regardless of patient focus, providers have had to embrace the multidisciplinary approach to treatment, not simply because of changing healthcare, but in response to the dramatic impact neuroscience has made on understanding behavioral problems.

Therefore, while all health care professionals do not have a background in biochemistry, neurobiology and pharmacology, they should have a basic and practical knowledge of these perspectives as they pertain to behavioral health – a foundation in behavioral pharmacology. This book will help enhance the reader's understanding about the "bio" part of the biopsychosocial aspects of behavior.

Toward this end, there are five objectives I sincerely hope the reader will achieve:

1. To better understand the pharmacological and neurobiological factors that influence drug abuse involvement and patterns of substance abuse.

2. To improve awareness and understanding of the chemical and pharmacological aspects of any given substance of abuse, which in turn, determine who, how, when, where and why a specific drug is abused.

3. To gain a working knowledge of the specific chemicals of abuse concerning:
   - sources of the abused substances
   - chemical identity of active components
   - typical behavioral patterns of abuse
   - routes of drug administration
   - influence of other drugs in combination
   - salient pharmacological effects and mechanisms of action
   - major toxicological effects
   - drug/disease interactions
   - treatment modalities

4. To competently and confidently respond to questions frequently asked in a community setting regarding drug abuse and mental health disorders.

5. To comprehend the biological basis for behavioral problems and be able to articulate the pharmacological rationale for current medical and psychiatric treatment interventions

Dynamics of Brain Chemistry and Behavior
Behavior has no clear beginning or end. The analysis of behavior starts out innocently enough to describe the interactions of the organism with the environment. More specifically, it is the interaction of the organism's brain with the environment. The environment includes not only the outside world, but also the organism's internal environment. Of course, the brain is a part of that internal environment and the behavior itself becomes a part of the environment. Lest we become tempted to pursue the logical proof that the universe is made up of behavior, let us return to some more direct issues to illustrate that these considerations are not just idle philosophical musings--we must understand the implications of these interactions in order to

appreciate the dynamics of brain chemistry and behavior. These interactions are presented as six principles for understanding behavioral pharmacology

Principle 1. *Changes in brain chemistry produce changes in behavior.*
This is perhaps the most straightforward principle and the one that has guided most of the research in behavioral pharmacology. Manipulation of the chemical system that controls behavior will change behavior.

Principle 2. *Changes in behavior produce changes in brain chemistry.*
This principle is a bit more subtle and offers the opportunity to confuse cause and correlation. The fact that behavioral change is correlated with the chemical changes that produced it is simply a restatement of Principle 1. The important point here is that behavioral change can actually produce changes in brain chemistry. One type of change is an increase in the efficiency of the chemical system that produces the behavior (analogous to increased muscle efficiency with exercise). This change may, in turn, produce changes in related chemical systems that were not directly involved in the first bit of behavior.

Principle 3. *Changes in the environment produce changes in behavior.*
This principle is the simple definition of behavior and requires little in the way of explanation. The major point that needs to be made is that the environment is quite extensive. It includes not only the relationships and contingencies of the external world, but also the internal milieu--blood pressure, gastrointestinal activity, level of energy stores, memory of past experiences, etc.

Principle 4. *Changes in behavior produce changes in the environment.*
In some sense, the only role of behavior is to change the environment. In the simplest case, the behavior is operant and results in opened doors, captured prey, warmed cockles and the like. But just as the environment was expanded in the preceding paragraph, so must our notions of the effects of behavior be expanded to include, for example, changes in the internal environment either directly (as in the case of autonomic responses to a fear arousing situation) or indirectly (as in the case of nutritional changes).

Principle 5. *Changes in the environment produce changes in brain chemistry.*
We begin to complete the circuit through brain, behavior and environment by noting that environmental changes can produce changes in brain chemistry. In some cases, the environment has tonic influences on brain chemistry as exemplified by responses to seasonal changes, temperature fluctuations, lighting changes and so forth. Other environmental changes are more closely interactive with behavior, and include responses to crowding, members of the opposite sex, complexity of the physical and behavioral environment, etc. These and many other types of environmental manipulations have been shown to alter the status of the neurochemical transmitter systems.

Principle 6. *Changes in brain chemistry produce changes in the environment.*
On the surface, this seems to be the least likely of the principles. Changes in brain chemistry obviously cannot directly perform operants like opening doors. It can, however, produce significant changes in the internal environment and set the stage for such operants to occur.

The listing of these six principles is a formal way of stating the major considerations that must accompany our study of behavioral pharmacology. Drugs indeed change behavior. But the effect of a drug can be altered by the organism's behavior, which in turn has been produced by current and past changes in the environment. Drugs do not possess some essence that magically induces a change in behavior. They act through the normal channels of our physiological response to the environment. As human organisms in a complex environment, we are fortunate that these interactions are complicated.

In the spirit of research, and to introduce this work, I offer the following questions as a general outline. Periodically, as you are reading through the chapters, you may wish to revisit some of these questions and see if your response to them might have changed.

General
- What behavioral processes control patterns of drug-seeking behavior?
- How are pharmacological processes important in abuse of specific drugs (half-life, absorption, distribution and route of administration)?

CNS Depressants (Alcohol)
- Know the basic pharmacology of alcohol.
- What CNS neurotransmitters and their receptors have been implicated to explain the addictive effects of alcohol and the sedative-hypnotics?
- CNS Stimulants (Amphetamines, Cocaine)
- Describe the behavioral manifestations that accompany administration of stimulants. How does the form of the drug and the route of administration alter behavioral effects?
- Describe the psychiatric features of chronic amphetamine or cocaine abuse of as well as symptoms of the withdrawal syndromes.

Hallucinogens
- What are the consequences of long-term marijuana use on higher CNS function, the hypothalamic-pituitary axis and the pulmonary system? Does tolerance develop? Is there a withdrawal syndrome associated with abstinence?
- What are the predominant effects of hallucinogens (d-lysergic acid diethylamide)?
- What are the unique physical signs and symptoms of PCP intoxication?

4

Nicotine
- Is there a commonality between nicotine and alcohol abusers?
- Is nicotine a truly addicting substance?

Psychiatric Medications
- Describe the advantages/disadvantages of the newer antipsychotics and antidepressants over the more traditional medications.
- Describe current theories on the biological aspects of depressive disorders and schizophrenia.
- What is behavioral toxicity and how can it be identified from a primary illness?
- Where does it seem the future of medications for mental health is headed?

As you will discover, there are three sections to this book. The first section emphasizes the function of the nervous system. Since the brain is the target organ for psychoactive drugs, it is important to build an understanding of how the brain and the rest of the nervous system work. After the first section builds a foundation of the basic understanding of the nervous system, the second section then covers the behavioral pharmacology of drugs of abuse. Finally, the third section provides a review of the pharmacological foundations for the principal psychiatric medications used in the treatment of mental illness.

There are several excellent books that provide a rich and detailed account of the historical perspective of drug abuse and mental illness, but that is not the purpose of this work. There are even more great books written on the many psychosocial theories and dynamics about substance abuse and mental health disorders, but these also are not the focus of this book. Rather, the principal focus here is to provide an accurate yet understandable, current and practical account of the biological aspects which add to the biopsychosocial perspective of human behavior, with an emphasis on behavioral pharmacology of substance abuse and mental health disorders.

CHAPTER 1: VOCABULARY LIST

Absorption   *The process of how the target system absorbs the drug.*

Administration   *The process of how a drug enters the body.*

Behavioral tolerance   *Behavioral changes that reduce drug potency.*

Bioavailability   *After administration, the rate ay which a drug is absorbed and available to the body*

Biotransformation   *Rendering a drug less active by specialized enzymes in the liver.*

Blood-brain-barrier   *A membrane that impedes the distribution of certain molecules into the brain.*

Cellular tolerance   *Decreasing drug effects as a result of decreasing receptor sites due to repeated drug exposure.*

Chemical name   *The name of the chemical composition of a drug.*

Conjugation   *One of several ways the liver metabolizes adding a substance to a drug to change it to a form that cannot reabsorb well.*

Cross tolerance   *Reduced potency of one drug because of repeated exposure of another drug of the same category (i.e. alcohol-Valium)*

Cytochrome P-450   *Specialized set of liver enzymes versatile in their metabolizing capacity*

Direct-acting agonist   *A drug that resembles a neurotransmitter and mimics its normal action*

Direct-acting antagonist   *A drug that can bind to a receptor site but inhibits any response.*

Dose-response   *The effects of a drug at varying dosages*

Down regulation   *Decrease in neuron sensitivity due to excessive activity causing over stimulation.*

Drug fate   *How a drug is deactivated and eliminated by the body.*

Drug half-life	The amount of time the body requires to eliminate half of the total drug present in the system. There is an algorithm of the number of half lives needed prior to achieving steady state.
ED50	The median effective dose that is effective in 50% of the individuals studied.
Enteral	The route of administration by way of the intestine
Enzyme competition	*Multiple drugs taken simultaneously compete for a limited number of enzymes.*
Generic drug name	*A shorter more convenient label to avoid long or complicated chemical names.*
Indirect-acting agonist	*Augments neurotransmitter activity by extending the time they remain in synapse.*
Indirect-acting antagonist	*Reduces neurotransmitter actions by inhibiting their effects.*
Ion	*A charged drug molecule which is not lipid soluble and does not absorb well*
Ischemia	*A restriction in blood supply, generally due to factors in the blood vessels, with resultant damage or dysfunction of tissue.*
LD	*The lethal dose range that causes death in a percent of the studied population*
Metabolic tolerance	*Drug-induced elevated liver enzyme activity and increased drug metabolism.*
Metabolism	*The process of how a drug is deactivated or broken down (biotransformed) by the liver.*
Oxidation	*The most common metabolism process where liver enzymes directly involve oxygen.*
Pharmacon	*(Greek) medicine or "poison", depending on the context in which it is used.*
Placebo effect	*Drug effects that have nothing to do with its pharmacological aspects.*

Potency   *A drug's ability to produce an intended effect at the lowest dose possible (different than a drug's purity).*

Tachyphylaxis   *The rapid onset of tolerance to a drug's effects - perhaps as soon as after a first dose.*

Therapeutic index   *The range between minimum effective dose and the maximum dose without toxicity.*

Trade name   *The label given by a drug's manufacture (ie. Bayer for aspirin).*

CHAPTER 1: PHARMACOLOGY BASICS

Pharmacology, in its most fundamental definition is the science of studying the chemical effects on biological systems. Behavioral pharmacology, a specialized area of the pharmacological sciences, is the study of drug effects on the nervous system and how the effects alter behavior. The primary objective of this science is to discover a drug's selective toxicity. That is, how a drug can produce only the desired effect and no others.

The word pharmacology comes from the Greek word, *pharmacon,* which can mean both medicine or "poison", depending on the context in which it is used. The primary effect of a drug is usually its desired effect, or the effect that is intended. A drug's side effects are those effects that are not intended, but take place nonetheless.

Drugs Have Multiple Effects
It is almost a truism that every drug has multiple effects. Ideally, a drug would have only one effect, which could be used for a specific therapeutic purpose. More commonly, any given drug may have several major effects and several minor effects. As an example, a particular drug may be given as a muscle relaxant, but have a side effect of producing drowsiness. The same compound may be prescribed for another patient for the purpose of producing drowsiness and lowered anxiety, with a side effect of muscle relaxation. Along with these major effects, several minor side-effects might be common to both prescriptions and include cardiovascular problems, gastrointestinal upset, skin rashes, and so forth. In general, the higher the dosage, the greater the number of different drug effects.

Low doses of epinephrine produce a slight drop in blood pressure, whereas high doses produce a large increase in blood pressure. This curious reversal of effects can be explained as follows: The molecular structure of epinephrine allows it to interact with both alpha and beta receptors. The beta receptors, although fewer in number, are more sensitive than the alpha receptors. With *low* dosages of epinephrine, the *beta* receptors are the only ones effected and they inhibit the smooth muscles of the blood vessels causing a decrease in the pressure through vasodilation.

High doses of epinephrine stimulate *alpha* receptors, which cause the constriction of blood vessels and a corresponding increase in blood pressure. The beta receptors are also stimulated, but their influence is overpowered by the effects of the alpha receptors.

Almost exactly the same type of change in blood pressure can be observed with low and high doses of acetylcholine, but for different reasons. *Low* doses of acetylcholine reduce the blood pressure by acting on the muscarinic receptors which inhibit the smooth muscles of the blood vessels to cause vasodilation. *High* doses of acetylcholine produce a large increase in blood pressure by stimulating the nicotinic receptors of the autonomic ganglia. These nicotinic receptors are much less sensitive to circulating levels of acetylcholine, but once stimulated, their effects are much more potent than those of the muscarinic stimulation. Under these conditions, the sympathetic ganglia predominate, and the resulting stimulation of the adrenal gland and release of norepinephrine from the sympathetic fibers cause an increase in blood pressure. Thus, the large dose of acetylcholine increases blood pressure indirectly via sympathetic arousal.

In these examples, we see the essence of dose-response interactions. Two completely different drugs (epinephrine and acetylcholine) produce identical profiles of change in blood pressure (a decrease at low doses and an increase at high doses.) In each instance, the reversal occurs because low doses influence one type of receptor while high doses influence a different type of receptor. Furthermore, in the case of acetylcholine, the final effect is actually due to the indirect activation of an opposing system. This particular set of results makes sense because the underlying mechanisms have already been determined. In many cases of drug and behavior interactions we do not yet enjoy this luxury.

Individual Differences in Drug Effects
The effectiveness of specific drugs can also be influenced by a wide range of organismic variables such as species, age, sex, disease status and behavioral history. In many cases, the specific origin of these differences in drug response cannot be identified, but some general comments can be made in relation to the dosage considerations discussed above. The notation of such variables as age, sex, species, and so forth does not describe the underlying cause of differences in drug response, but is rather used as a convenient label for sub-populations that may share some common physiological variable.

One of the most important physiological differences that interact with the behavioral effects of drugs is the neurochemical status of the brain. There are well documented changes in brain chemistry during the course of development and continuing through senescence. The presence or absence of sex hormones, the environment of the organism, and the behavior that the organism engages in can all modulate these neurochemical changes.

Since most of the behaviorally active drugs produce their effects through interaction with these chemical substrates, the variables that alter neurochemistry interact with drug response. It is simply easier and more convenient to specify some external variable such as age or sex, rather than attempting to outline the more directly relevant neurochemical factors.

Differences in drug response can also occur in the absence of any important differences in the neurochemical substrates. All of the ports of entry into and exit from the bloodstream vary as a function of these external variables. For example, liver function is not fully developed in the very young and no longer fully efficient in the very old. Differences in behavioral and dietary history will alter liver function, gastrointestinal function, cardiovascular efficiency and general metabolism. Body fat levels vary in response to a wide range of variables. Each of these changes has the capacity to alter the drug response through a simple shift in the time course of effective drug concentration in the bloodstream. The same relative quantity of drug might produce an increase in the behavior of a young organism, no change in adult females, and an impairment of behavior in aging males.

Generic Drugs

Generic drugs are chemically identical to the original drug and have similar biological characteristics such as the rate and extent of absorption and elimination. Drugs that are marketed in the United States as generic equivalent are equivalent to the original product and represent an opportunity to save substantial amounts of money compared to the trademarked original product.

In many cases, the generic products are from the same production lines as the original product. There may be many generic versions of a specific drug. Each of them must be similar to the prototype product, but are never tested against each other. This situation can allow one generic to differ from another by more than the accepted tolerance limits. Switching generic brands should be avoided. It is always best to start with one specific brand and not switch to another brand with every refill from the pharmacy. When a change of generic manufacturers cannot be avoided, closer monitoring for adverse effects and loss of efficacy will allow the small dosage adjustments needed to compensate for ay clinically significant differences.

Pharmaceutical Names

All drugs have a chemical name that denotes the chemical make-up or composition of the drug. Because chemical names can be quite long and complicated, the drug is usually given a shorter generic name. Also, the drug's manufacturer will typically give the drug a trade name as well. Trade names are always identified by the ® (registered) symbol following the name of the drug, and the first letter is always capitalized. Thus, it is possible for a substance to be known by several different names.

A drug might have slang or street names by what addicts may call it when distributed and used illegally. A good example of how a single drug will have numerous names is found in the case of amphetamines: the chemical name is *alphamethylphenylethylamine,* the generic name is amphetamine, the trade name is Dexedrine, and the street name is "speed".

Adverse Effects

Adverse effects are the unwanted side effects that are caused by the drug that is intended to produce therapeutic benefits. Generally, the more recently developed drugs tend to have fewer and milder adverse effects than older ones. However, it is usually true that any effective intervention will have some adverse effects, even if mild and well tolerated.

The goal of selecting a medication is to achieve high efficacy with minimal adverse effects. Some adverse effects are dose-related and are less common or less severe at lower doses, other adverse effects are not and may be present at any dose. It is important to realize that adverse effects are pharmacologically similar to the therapeutic effects and have a unique dose-effect curve. Use of the lowest possible dose that is effective is the best strategy to minimize adverse effects.

The graph below shows three hypothetical dose-effect curves. Effect A is the desired profile for a drug's therapeutic effect. Between doses of 1 and 10, the effect increases proportional to the dose and approaches the maximum possible effect. Effect B is an example of a dose-limiting adverse effect. In this case, the benefits of the drug (as shown in Effect A) are limited by adverse effects above doses of 5. Finally, Effect C shows a threshold effect at a dose of 10 that appears so rapidly that there does not appear to be any relationship between dose and the size of the effect. Every drug and effect would have a unique curve in each individual.

The basis of our use of drugs is based on population responses and adverse effects. The inability to predict the exact effect curves in an individual is what causes a lack of response and adverse effects.

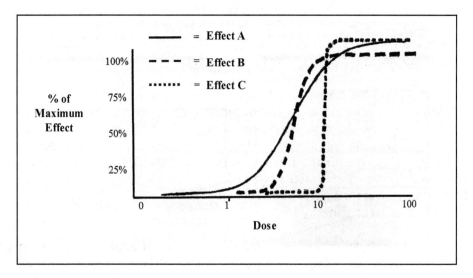

Dosage Titration
Unfortunately, drug therapy does not work rapidly. This is because of several factors: pharmacokinetics and pharmacodynamics. These cause a delay between a dose adjustment and arriving at the final amount of the drug in then patient's body. After this steady state amount of drug is present, then the effect of the drug can exert its effect. The action of the drug may be indirect and require an intermediate response before the clinical effect can be seen.

An example of this can bee seen in the use of an antidepressant. It can take up to two weeks for a clinical response after a dose adjustment. An important consequence of this is that doses are frequently adjusted far too rapidly and may be substantially higher than are needed for the clinical response. The higher dose may increase the chance of the patient having an adverse effect that reduces the clinical benefit. More rapid dose titration has not been shown to increase the rate of response in replicated studies. In general, dosage adjustments should not be made more often than weekly and possibly as infrequently as monthly.

When would the physician make a dose increase? When the adverse effects after reaching pharmacokinetic steady state are acceptable to the patient and physician and the response is still inadequate then the dose might be increased. If the patient has had any improvement at all, it is usually best to wait and see if the improvement will continue without a dose increase. If the adverse effects worsen after a dosage increase, then it may be desirable to decrease the dose to its previous level. Usually the adverse effect will subside and the dose may again be increased if needed for increased response.

It may be possible to increase the dose without unacceptable adverse effects if the dose increment is half of the previous increment and the interval between subsequent increases is twice what it was.

Drug Interactions Are Not All Bad
Drug interactions are an important and growing area of research and patient care because more drugs are being used at the same time. There is a common misconception that a drug interaction is inherently bad. Actually, the only bad interactions are those that are not understood and go undetected until a bad outcome occurs. Understanding the mechanism of drug interaction and close monitoring can prevent most bad outcomes. Lack of knowledge about the patient's total medication and diet regimen can lead to problems, but usually problems occur slowly enough that permanent harm is avoided. Also, if an interaction is well understood, it can actually be used to intentionally to improve the patient. An example would be the addition of a diuretic to a patient on Lithium to decrease urine volume. For the most part, however, drug interactions should be avoided. The easiest way to avoid them is to reduce the number of drugs that a patient is taking and carefully selecting the drugs that they need to take.

Pharmacology has long noted that all psychoactive drugs, legal or otherwise, produce side effects. However, in pharmacology, the noted side effects are not simply unintended aspects to be avoided or minimized. In some cases, a drug's side effects might even be the primary or intended effect. For example, antihistamines might be used to relieve allergies and may produce side effects of drowsiness and sedation. The same drugs may also be prescribed by a physician to treat anxiety which, when used in this context, would have side effects of allergy suppression. A drug's known side effects can be utilized for various situations, so primary effects have a relative distinction from side effects. It is possible to administer a drug at such a small dosage that no effect occurs. A larger dosage might bring about the intended effect, while an even larger dose might be toxic.

The range between the minimum effective dosage and the maximum dosage where no toxic symptoms occur is the therapeutic index: Psychoactive drugs also have a dose-response relationship. That is, some drugs produce different effects at different dosages. For example, diazepam (Valium) at low doses is a sedative, and at higher doses it induces sleep. Still at higher doses, Valium becomes an anti-convulsant, and with higher levels yet, it can be an anesthetic.

The potency of a drug is its ability to produce an intended effect at the lowest dose possible. Many people mistake the word potency for purity levels. However, potency is the specific dose-response relationship the drug can produce. For example, heroin is more "potent" than morphine because it takes less heroin to produce the same level of analgesia as morphine. The route of administration can also produce effects that have nothing to do with its pharmacological aspects; this is called the placebo effect.

Pharmacokinetics: Mechanism of Action
Pharmacokinetics is the aspect of pharmacology that seeks to understand how a drug acts after it had been introduced into the body: the drug's *mechanism of action.* It is the study of how a drug is delivered into the body, how it moves throughout the body and brain, and how it eventually gets eliminated.

The single most important objective in pharmacology is to understand a drug produces its overall effects. In other words, how does morphine suppress pain? How does Cymbalta treat depression? What is the mechanism of action of antipsychotic drugs that produce the side effects of impaired movement coordination? Why is it that chemicals like amphetamines or cocaine produce effects of euphoria and inhibit sleep? What are the effects when several drugs are taken in combination (polypharmacy), such as THC and chemotherapy, alcohol and Valium, or morphine and cocaine? What are the mechanisms of action where drug molecules can produce effects and side effects? And how do they work in the brain and body? These are all questions related to a drug's pharmacokinetics.

These and other questions are the areas where pharmacology seeks answers. Pharmacokinetics is the investigative process of understanding a drug's mechanism of action. When a drug is delivered into any biological system, there are some fundamental processes that have a tremendous influence on the amount of the drug reaching its target area. These processes can be divided into five dynamics:

Administration

Administration of a drug includes the various ways a drug is delivered and released into the body. There are several means by which a drug enters the body. Each route of administration has great bearing on the drug's overall effects.

> 1. *Administration:* how a drug enters the body,
> 2. *Absorption:* how the target system absorbs the drug,
> 3. *Distribution:* how a drug moves throughout the target system,
> 4. *Metabolism:* how a drug is deactivated or broken down (biotransformed), and
> 5. *Elimination:* how a drug exits the target system (excretion).

It is important to understand that drugs do not produce an effect on all body tissues. Most drugs effect only target systems that are fairly specific and limited in their area of influence. This area is referred to as the drug's *site of action.* A drug can enter into the body but unless it reaches its site of action, it will not produce its primary effect.

Thus, it is important to understand how drugs move from their initial route of administration to the final site of action. Some nutritional supplements, foods and medicines may contain large amounts nourishment and healing, but simply putting them into the body (i.e., orally *per os)* is no guarantee that they will produce a desired effect. The route of administration determines whether the drug reaches the site of action and how fast or how much of it gets there.

The major routes of drug administration are enteral (through the intestines) or parental (outside of the intestines), and include several paths into the body where they will enter the bloodstream. The following list details these pathways:

Enteral: Taken into the body by way of the intestine
- Oral *(per os):* by way of the mouth, swallowing
- Sublingual: beneath the tongue, sucking
- Rectal: by way of the anus (suppository)

Parenteral: Taken into the body or administered in a manner other than through the intestines, as by intravenous or intramuscular injection or inhalation.
- Intracutaneous (IC): within the skin
- Subcutaneous (SC): beneath the skin
- Intramuscular (IM): within the muscles

- Intravenous (IV): within a vein, injection
- Intraperitoneal (IP): within the peritoneal cavity (containing the visceral organs: the liver, the intestines and the spleen)
- Intracardiac: within the heart
- Pulmonary: within the lungs, inhalation
- Transcutaneous: through the skin (patch)

Drugs come in many forms, and the same drugs may be prepared as a pill, a liquid, a suppository, an inhaler, or even an I.V. (injectable) solution. For a drug to produce an effect, it has to enter the bloodstream in a way for it to be distributed to its specific target system within the body or brain.

The liver prepares substances for elimination by the kidneys by chemically altering them and changing them into what are called metabolites. An important factor of oral (per os) route of drug administration is that when the substance has been absorbed into the blood from the gastrointestinal tract, it moves through the liver where a portion of the drug molecule is metabolized or broken down.

Absorption
Regardless of the route of administration, once a drug has been ingested it must be absorbed by its target system. Following *enteral* administration, the drug must move from the gastrointestinal tract into the circulatory system, where it then is distributed throughout the body. *Parenteral* administration often stimulates faster absorption because of quicker access to the bloodstream.

Membranes are usually made of *lipid* (or fatty) material. For a drug to pass through a wall of cells, such as the lining of the intestines, there must be holes or pores large enough to allow drug molecules to diffuse through. Several factors influence absorption rates, but the primary dynamic is the drug's ability to absorb into fatty tissue. This rate, called solubility, is a central factor in absorption dynamics. In general, the more lipid soluble a drug is, the easier it will absorb into tissue. The figure below illustrates the various absorption areas through two different routes of administration.

For enteral administration, absorption is most efficient in the intestines, since intestine walls are lined with capillaries that absorb nutrients from food; they readily absorb drugs as well. All body tissue is made of cells and each cell is surrounded by a membrane. To get to the capillaries, the drug must first pass through the membrane of the intestinal wall.

All drug molecules differ somewhat in their degree of lipid solubility, the ease of which drugs dissolve in and through fatty or lipid tissue. However, when a drug carries an electrical charge, its lipid solubility is significantly reduced. Such a charged molecule is called an *ion*. Ions are not lipid soluble and do not dissolve well in fatty tissue.

When a drug is dissolved in a fluid, some or all of its molecules become ionized. The percentage of ionized molecules in a solution determines its *pH,* which describes the degree to which a solution is either an acid or a base, or its *pKa,* meaning the pH at which half of its molecules are ionized. The percentage of non-ionized molecules is available for absorption at any given period of time, and therefore determines the rate of absorption.

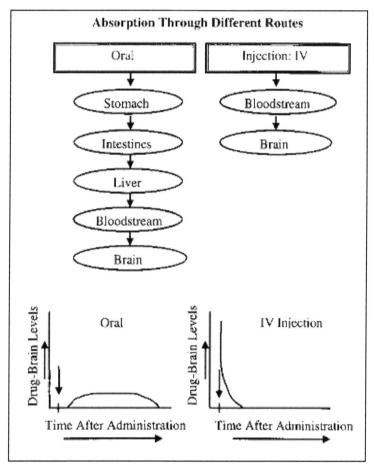

Non-ionized molecules of various drugs have varying degrees of lipid solubility. These ranges of lipid solubility are expressed in terms of the *oil: water partition coefficients,* since testing for solubility involves using olive oil in equal parts with water. The oil and water are put in a container, and a fixed amount of a drug is mixed in. After some time the oil and water separate, and the amount of drug dissolved in each is measured. Drugs that are more lipid soluble have a higher concentration in the oil, and drugs that water soluble concentrate in the water. This test can somewhat predict the degree to which a drug will dissolve in lipid material (fatty tissue) within the body.

The amount of a drug that reaches circulation is called its bioavailability, the percentage of the drug dosage available to the body. Thus, drugs taken intravenously are 100% bioavailable, whereas drugs that are administered by other routes are less bioavailable.

A drug must absorb into a targeted system to produce an effect. In order for a drug to be absorbed and reach the nervous system, it must cross membranes. Drugs cross membranes in different ways, including facilitated diffusion, active transport or passive transport. Most drugs are absorbed by passive transport, where they move across a lipid membrane via a carrier or specialized molecule. A non-lipid soluble drug molecule attaches itself to a "carrier" molecule that diffuses across the membrane, releasing the drug molecule on the other side. In this way, a drug can move from high to low concentration on either side of a membrane.

The Blood Brain Barrier
The brain is one of the most richly vascularized organs of the body. The two internal carotids and two vertebral arteries (which supply all the blood to the brain) branch out into an extremely dense system of capillaries. Consequently, the brain is responsible for nearly twenty percent of the body's total oxygen consumption, even though it accounts for less than two percent of the body mass. Neurons are particularly vulnerable to ischemia and such a lack of blood flow for as little as four to five minutes can lead to serious brain damage.

The dense capillary system of the brain is very selective in terms of the molecules that will pass through into the surrounding tissue space. Water, oxygen, carbon dioxide pass freely through the endothelial walls. Glucose, which supplies virtually all of the nutritive requirements of brain tissue, also passes through relatively freely. Thus, there is an efficient exchange of molecules that are essential for the high metabolic demands of neural tissue.

The capillaries of the brain have two special features that tend to prevent the passage of molecules into the adjacent tissue space. The endothelial cells that form the walls of the capillaries are densely packed, such that only small molecules can pass through the junctions. Additionally, glial cells called astrocytes surround about 85% of the surface of the capillaries, adding a lipid barrier to the system. Thus, large molecules and molecules that are not lipid soluble do not easily penetrate the brain. These special features of the cerebral vascular system have been termed the blood-brain barrier.

Another special feature of the central nervous system is the cerebrospinal fluid (CSF) that fills the ventricles of the brain and central canal of the spinal cord. The CSF is formed by blood vessels within the ventricular system, most notably the concentrated groups in the lateral ventricles which are termed the choroids plexus. The CSF excreted by these vessels is similar to blood plasma, except for very low levels of proteins and cholesterol. It is the extracellular fluid of the brain, which is formed continuously and absorbed at a rate of about 10% per hour. Thus there is a continual flow of the fluid which bathes the brain cells. The capillary walls of the choroid plexus have the same dense epithelial structure as those within the brain tissue proper, hence provide an extension of the blood-brain barrier.

The blood-brain barrier should not be viewed as a system which isolates the brain, but rather as one which buffers it from the changing conditions of the remainder of the body. The critically important ions that determine the electrical excitability of neurons (Na+, K+, Ca+, and Cl-) equilibrate with the brain fluids very slowly, requiring as much as 30 times longer than in other tissues. Relatively small molecules such as urea are exchanged rather freely with muscle tissue and other body organs, but enter the brain very slowly over a period of several hours. Larger molecules such as bile salts and circulating catecholamines (from the adrenal glands and peripheral autonomic nervous system) are essentially blocked from entering the brain.   Thus, the brain is protected from fluctuations of chemicals in the plasma compartment, allowing homeostatic processes a considerable margin of time to correct any deviations while the brain's environment remains relatively constant.

The nature of the blood brain barrier poses a number of problems in terms of the behavioral response to drugs. In the most extreme cases, some compounds simply do not enter the brain in significant concentrations. In other cases (e.g., neurotransmitters like dopamine or serotonin), the relevant compound per se does not enter, but the precursor molecules can be administered to facilitate the synthesis of the active form within the brain. The compounds can also be injected directly into the brain or CSF, physically bypassing the barrier, but several compounds have so called paradoxical effects on brain tissue. For example, penicillin produces convulsions, epinephrine in the ventricles leads to somnolence, and curare can lead to seizures. Aside from some general guidelines relating to molecular size and lipid solubility, it is difficult to predict with accuracy how easily a drug will penetrate the brain and what the effect will be. In many cases, it is necessary to make an empirical determination.

A more subtle aspect of the blood brain barrier is that it is differentially effective in different areas of the brain. The white regions of the brain are composed mainly of fibers, which are surrounded by glial cells to form the myelin sheaths. As a result of this additional lipid barrier, these regions of the brain reach equilibrium with certain drugs much more slowly than the cellular regions of grey cortex. To the extent that these different areas serve different behavioral functions or are differentially sensitive to the drug, the overall response to a drug dosage over time will become increasingly complicated.

Distribution
Distribution refers to the delivery of a drug to its site of action. Distribution is of

course, greatly influenced by blood flow, since drug molecules diffuse out of the bloodstream and into the targeted area. The blood-brain-barrier (BBB) impedes the distribution of some molecules into the brain. This is a barrier made of specialized cells called *glial cells* and *astrocytes* that form a tight-knit membrane or matrix that repels water-soluble molecules. The glial cells wrap tightly around capillaries and block pores that molecules would diffuse through. These provide a very strong lipid barrier so that non-lipid soluble molecules have great difficulty getting into the brain. Because of the BBB, the diffusion of a drug into the brain is inversely proportional to its water solubility. However, psychoactive drugs (which change thought, mood and movement) are lipid soluble and therefore, distribute through the BBB and into the brain quite easily.

Metabolism and Drug Fate
When discussing drug ingestion, the primary agent involved is the liver, a large organ located under the diaphragm, up in the abdomen. Its two main functions are to chemically alter substances into forms that are more beneficial to the body (biotransformation), and reduce toxic substances into safer ones (detoxification). These processes are called metabolism. Drug metabolism usually refers to chemical breakdown, but metabolism actually describes several biological processes including synthesizing chemicals (anabolism), and producing energy for the body.

Drug fate is how a drug's action is deactivated, so the drug can ultimately be eliminated. In behavioral pharmacology, *biotransformation* is mostly used in describing drug fate. Most drugs are biotransformed and thus rendered less active by specialized enzymes in the endoplasmic reticulum of the liver, a system usually referred to as the microsomal system.

The microsomal system is also called the mixed-function enzymatic oxidizing system *(MEOS),* and the primary enzyme is Cytochrome P-450. The enzymes in the MEOS are "mixed-function" because they are versatile in what types of substances they act on. Mostly through its specialized P-450 enzymes, the liver transforms substances from one state to another by reducing the drug molecules' lipid solubility so that they cannot absorb well or circulate. P-450 enzymes had probably evolved to digest environmental toxins that might otherwise threaten the body. In general however, biotransformation reduces the effects of many drugs, especially when drugs are ingested orally *(per os).*

One of the main functions of biotransformation is related to solubility. As a general rule, lipid-soluble drugs dissolve and absorb easily into membranes and tissue, whereas water soluble drugs do not. For biotransformation, the liver will reduce the lipid solubility and change the drug into a form that is more water soluble, and hence it will not reabsorb well.

The process of changing a drug molecule's solubility is called metabolism, and the byproducts of metabolism are called metabolites (these are usually water soluble). Through biotransformation, the liver essentially alters the potency of a drug by changing its degree of lipid solubility. In this way, a drug will not be able to reabsorb since its lipid solubility is reduced, and in its more water soluble state, it gets trapped by the kidneys and prepared for elimination. Metabolites are usually inactive, but sometimes, the metabolite will have toxic effects on the body as well. Just because a drug gets metabolized does not mean it is necessarily rendered inactive or non-toxic. Drugs such as alcohol, THC and polycyclic hydrocarbons (Benzpyrene and benzanthracene), have active and toxic metabolites that will produce an additive effect with the parent compound. But, metabolites are more likely to get ionized, become unable to reabsorb into the blood, and their action is ended.

The liver utilizes four types of biotransformation to metabolize chemicals; *oxidation, conjugation, reduction, and hydrolysis.* Oxidation is the most common form of biotransformation. This is where liver enzymes involve oxygen directly in the metabolism process. A metabolite of oxidation becomes ionized and therefore is unable to reabsorb into the system and will become excreted.

Conjugation is where the liver adds a substance to the chemical being metabolized and, as a result, deactivates the chemical or changes it to a form that is too large to reabsorb. *Reduction* is a process where the liver enzymes separate the chemical being metabolized into smaller parts where each part is a simpler compound unable to reabsorb. Since the chemical structure of the substance being metabolized has been "reduced" by this process, it is called reduction.

Finally, *hydrolysis* is where the liver modifies a chemical by adding a water molecule to it. The modification then renders the chemical being metabolized inactive, and is another way to increase water solubility.

Most biotransformation involves oxidation and conjugation. *Cytochrome P-450* is the principal mixed-function oxidase in the liver. P-450 is the key MEOS responsible for the metabolism of many different drugs including alcohol, anti-anxiety drugs, antidepressants, and a variety of other drugs.

Several factors influence drug metabolism in the liver and as such, affect each drug's intensity and duration of action. One factor is *liver enzyme induction*, which is an increase in enzyme function from previous exposure to a drug that used that same enzyme for deactivation. Continued exposure to any substance that is oxidized by P-450, for example, will cause the smooth surface of the liver's endoplasmic reticulum to enlarge, and increase production of even more P-450. Remember, it is the liver enzymes that deactivate a drug and render the effects inactive. Thus, the more liver enzymes induced, the more a drug will get deactivated.

When liver enzymes are increased through induction, metabolic tolerance takes place. That is, more of the drug is deactivated by increased liver enzymes which means that less of the drug gets into the brain to produce its effects.

For example, alcoholics will accumulate massive amounts of enzymes, induced by repeated alcohol intake. In the liver, alcohol causes the release of the enzyme alcohol dehydrogenase, which begins the breakdown process of alcohol into alcohol metabolites. Since alcohol induces much more enzyme activity, and since increased enzyme activity means increased metabolism of alcohol, alcoholics build a tolerance to the drug's effects, and are more resistant to intoxication than non-alcoholics. Unfortunately, since more alcohol is deactivated by the liver and therefore never gets to the brain, the person will consume even more in an attempt to stay above the increased enzymes. This can have debilitating effects as we will see in the chapter on alcohol.

Mixed-function oxidases, such as P-450, metabolize many different substances including various drugs, air-born pollutants, pesticides, food preservatives, insecticides and some carcinogens. The concept of *competition* is where molecules from multiple drugs taken simultaneously compete for a limited number of available liver enzymes for their deactivation. While liver enzyme induction will trigger deactivation of a drug, there are only so many liver enzymes able to be induced. Therefore, when multiple drugs are consumed, they have to compete for available enzymes. If one drug is working on most of the available P-450 then the other substances are forced to wait and will remain active in the bloodstream for a longer period of time than usual.

For example, if an alcoholic who had been drinking the day of an automobile accident requires a tranquilizer to treat the trauma, the medication will produce its effects too fast, perhaps even fatally. The reason for this is that the alcohol has induced P-450 and there is very little enzyme left to deactivate the tranquilizer. Thus, when the tranquilizer is administered, more of it moves through the liver unchanged and a greater amount reaches the brain.

An opposite example is when a drug has induced liver enzyme activity, but the drug has since left the system while the increase in liver function remains. In our example with the alcoholic, if that person had not been drinking the day of the accident, the liver still has an increase in enzymes but with hardly any drug for those enzymes to work on. When tranquilizers are administered in this scenario, the medication's therapeutic index would be difficult to obtain.

This is due to an abundance of P-450 enzymes with hardly any alcohol to breakdown. When the tranquilizer is administered, much of the drug is readily deactivated by the massive amount of alcohol-induced enzymes, and not enough can get into the brain to produce its sedative effects.

Another factor that influences metabolism is a person's age. Enzyme systems are not fully developed at birth and require time to develop properly to where they are functional for metabolism. Thus, children metabolize drugs much more slowly than their adult counterparts. There is also deficient liver function for elderly people as well. Liver functioning is less efficient in older people, and doses are generally reduced for this population to compensate for decreased liver capacity for drug metabolism.

Drug Half Life

Most drugs that are clinically useful have *linear*. The linear refers to dose proportionality where doubling the dose would double the blood level. The drug's pharmacokinetics are usually first-order processes where a fixed-fraction of the dose is processed - absorbed, distributed, metabolized, or eliminated – in a specific length of time which is described by the half-life. A drug's half-life describes the duration of action of psychoactive drugs in the body. Accordingly, a drug's half life is defined as the time for the plasma level of drug to fall by 50%. It is independent of the absolute level of drug in blood and, a varying amount of drug is metabolized with each half-life (fewer actual molecules). Half lives are measured in hours or in days (recovery from a drug may take a week or more).

It takes 4 half-lives for 94% of a drug to be eliminated and 6 half-lives for 98% of a drug to be eliminated. The drug persists in the body at low levels for at least 6 half-lives. For example, if 100 mg of a drug with a 4-hour half-life was administered at 12 noon, then, 50 mg of the drug would remain in the body at 4 pm. If an additional 100 mg of the drug was administered at 4 pm, then 75 mg of drug would remain in the body at 8 pm (25 mg of first dose and 50 mg of second dose). If this administration schedule were continued, the amount of the drug in the body would continue to increase until a plateau (*steady state*) concentration was reached.

Accumulation and Steady State

In one half-life, a drug reaches 50% of the concentration that will eventually be achieved. After 2 half-lives, the drug achieves 75% concentration (25% of first dose and 50% of the second dose). After 3 half-lives, the drug achieves 87.5% concentration (12.5 % of the first dose, 25% of the second dose and 50% of third dose. And, after 6 half-lives, the drug achieves 98.4% concentration, essentially at steady state.

If the half-life for a drug is known, you can calculate how much will be present at any later time, measured in half-lives. This can be seen in the following graph that shows the approach to steady state.

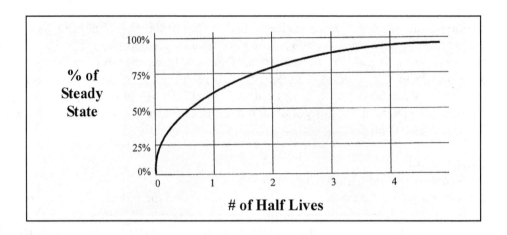

% of Steady State (y-axis)

# of Half Lives (x-axis)

Elimination (Excretion)

The primary organ for excreting a drug from the body is the kidney. However, drugs can also be eliminated from the body through the bowels, saliva, sweat glands (tearing), skin (perspiration) and lungs. The associated requirement for drug excretion is the drug's biotransformation into a more water soluble form. The main function of the kidneys is to maintain an optimal balance between water and salt in the body. The functional unit of the kidneys is called the *nephron,* and there are millions of nephrons which work together as a kind of filtering mechanism that physically eliminates certain substances from the body.

However, the kidneys do not just filter out impurities from the blood; they seem to filter <u>everything</u> out of the blood and then selectively reabsorb back those substances that are required or needed by the body. The excretion rates of a drug can be influenced by the pH of the urine. The pH directs the degree of ionization and therefore will influence the degree of reabsorption. Urine is largely acidic, whereas blood tends to be basic. The pH of the urine can be manipulated to be more acidic or more basic.

In general, the acids stay in the blood and the bases tend to stay in urine where they are excreted more easily. Acidifying the urine by administering IV ammonium chloride reduces urinary pH, and thus allows a greater percentage of a weak-base drug to exist in an ionized (excreatable) form. For example, acidifying the urine will increase the excretion rate of amphetamines and therefore reduce the duration of an otherwise toxic overdose.

In another example, weak acids like aspirin can be eliminated faster through the administration of sodium bicarbonate, which will alkalinize the urine and reduce the potential overdose of someone who has ingested too much aspirin. In general, the kidneys will excrete excess amount of water from the body (through the urine) and will also excrete molecules of toxins that have been biotransformed by the liver.

In terms of excretion rates, the other factor in determining a drug's fate is its *half-life*. The half-life of a drug is the amount of time the body requires to eliminate half of the total substance present (as measured by its concentration in the blood). Thus, the first half of the substance amount, whether metabolized or not, are then excreted, usually with the urine. Substances can also be excreted with the feces, sweat, saliva, tears, and breast milk. If they are gaseous, they can be excreted by the lungs as well.

Dosage and Behavior Considerations - Dose-Response Curves

One of the most important principles of behavioral pharmacology is the concept of the dose-response curve. The most general expectation would be that larger dosages produce larger effects. Indeed, this is almost always true within some range of the drug dosage, but there is usually some level of dosage beyond which this relationship breaks down, and larger dosages produce progressively less of an effect or even an opposite effect. An example of this type of dose-response relationship can be seen in the Figure below which shows a change in behavior as a function of various dosages of a drug. Using the same behavioral measure, other drugs would show differently shaped curves at different peak plasma levels. The main point is that the effect of a drug on a behavior cannot be stated in a simple manner: A particular drug may enhance the behavior at low dosages, have no observable effect at some higher dosage, and impair the behavior at still higher dosages.

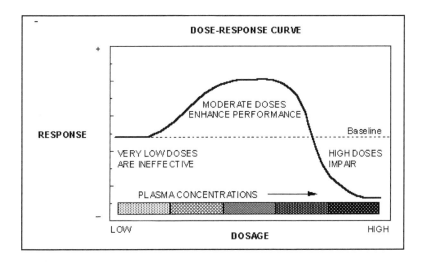

As shown in the Figure below, the plasma concentration of a drug changes continuously over time, as discussed in the previous section of this chapter.

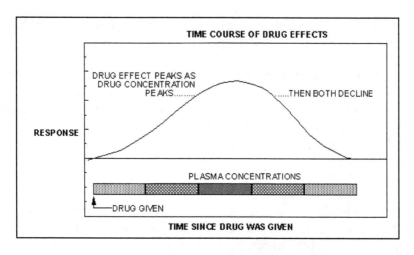

If one were to transfer sections of this changing concentration curve to the dose response curve in the Figure below, the behavioral effect at any given time would be changing in accordance with the changing concentration curve. In fact, with a single large dosage, it would be possible to show a gradual enhancement of behavior as the drug concentration was increasing, a decline and eventual impairment of behavior as the plasma concentration reached very high levels, a return to enhanced behavior as the drug concentration began to lower, and finally a return to baseline levels as the drug was cleared from the plasma compartment completely. Thus, the effect depends not only on the amount of drug administered, but on the amount of time that has elapsed since the administration.

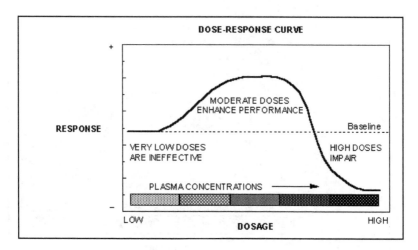

Given the interaction of behavior with drug dosage and the dynamic nature of the drug concentration, about the best one can hope for in terms of a stable effect is that shown in the Figure below. Properly spaced multiple dosages of a drug can lead to a more or less sinusoidal variation in plasma concentrations within the range of dosage that has the desired behavioral effect.

28

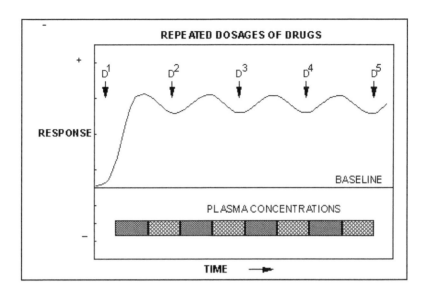

REPEATED DOSAGES OF DRUGS

+

D^1 D^2 D^3 D^4 D^5

RESPONSE

BASELINE

PLASMA CONCENTRATIONS

−

TIME

Forms of Tolerance

Chronic administration of a drug can change the drug's potency. As discussed, a drug's potency is defined as the minimal amount necessary to produce a specified effect. In general, tolerance is the decreased potency of a drug as a result of over-exposure. However, there are actually six different types of tolerance that result from different systems affected by repeat exposure to many drugs: *cellular tolerance, metabolic tolerance, cross tolerance, rapid tolerance* (tachyphylaxis), *behavioral tolerance,* and *reverse tolerance* (sensitization).

Cellular tolerance is when the potency of a drug is decreased as a result of a reduction in the drug's mechanism of action. The compromised action is caused by a reduced number of neurotransmitter receptors where the drug molecule binds. If a drug molecule requires binding at a neurotransmitter receptor site to produce its effects, and the system adapts to this activity by decreasing the number of available receptor sites, more drug will be required to produce the same level of effect.

Cellular tolerance is related to a process called *down regulation.* This is a condition where neurons have decreased their sensitivity to a drug when there is an excess of chemical activity causing over stimulation. For example, if a person over stimulates neurons with methamphetamine, the neurons might counter the response by decreasing the number of available receptor site "entry points" used for the stimulating effects. The reduction of receptor sites by neurons seems to act in a compensatory function for the system to exert some control on the level of its own sensitivity to stimulation.

Metabolic tolerance, described earlier, is where repeat drug exposure increases the liver function, causing an increase of available liver enzymes to deactivate a greater portion of the drug. Since more of the drug is deactivated prior to it getting into the brain, the drug's mechanism of action is reduced because of an increase in metabolism.

Cross tolerance is the reduction of potency of one drug because of chronic exposure to another one, usually in the same drug category. For example, tolerance to heroin produces cross tolerance to morphine or codeine. Tolerance to alcohol produces cross-tolerance to barbiturates and benzodiazepines. Following chronic use of diazepam (Valium) to induce sleep, a tolerance to the drug's sedative effects will develop. Switching to another benzodiazepine to produce sedation will not work because the person is equally as tolerant to that drug as well.

A rather interesting type of tolerance can develop very quickly (between 2 and 24 hours) with certain types of drugs. This is called rapid tolerance, commonly known as tachyphylaxis. The effects of drugs such as LSD can produce a fast reduction in potency even *after* the first dose.

Some drugs, which are normally not tachyphylactic produce rapid tolerance, when smoked or inhaled. Such drugs include crack cocaine and smokable methamphetamine. Second day administration of the drug requires a marked increase in dose to achieve an equivalent effect. For smokable cocaine and methamphetamine there is the rapid depletion of both norepinephrine and dopamine. The rapid tolerance produced by LSD is still unknown.

Behavioral tolerance is where a deliberate change in behavior offsets the potency of the drug. The behavioral change is usually a response to anticipated adverse consequences of being discovered by others for being under the influence. For example, heavy alcohol intake impairs motor coordination, so the alcoholic learns to behave in ways as to not draw attention to themselves, like not standing up too fast (to avoid falling down). Alcoholics will often walk close to stationary objects and use their hands to coordinate quick adjustments of vertical posture. Marijuana users avoid bending over due to orthostatic hypotension (dizziness and vertigo). Heroin addicts learn to inject their drug of choice in a comfortable location so they can sit or lie down during the initial drug "rush" which could cause them to lose their balance. In other words, addicts and alcoholics often adapt behaviors so that the effects of the drug are less pronounced.

As we are discussing, tolerance is where the potency of a drug is reduced as a result of chronic exposure. Reverse tolerance (sensitization) is the opposite, where there is an increase in potency as a result of continuous exposure to a drug. Cocaine, for example, will increase motor activity when administered to an animal. However, after several exposures to the drug, the original dose level actually produces a greater motor response. Drug dose-response studies of chronic cocaine exposure show that the same level of motor activity can be achieved with a lower dose of cocaine. The animal has, in a sense, been sensitized to the drug. This is somewhat different than "priming", which is where several exposures of a drug are required before a desired specific effect takes place.

Reverse tolerance can also be a sign of pathological development in target organs as a result of chronic exposure. For example, chronic alcoholics can show a marked decrease in their ability to metabolize alcohol, and so the effects of very small amounts will produce intoxication. In this case, potency has been radically altered. Reverse tolerance such as this is usually an indication that the liver is so damaged it can not induce sufficient levels of enzymes to metabolize alcohol. This can be an important medical concern because if the person's liver can no longer produce enough enzymes to deactivate alcohol, it will not be able to respond to a host of other toxins, since the same enzymes work on many different substances.

Dose Response Relationships
Science uses the metric system to describe amounts, specifically drug doses which are usually described in milligrams (mg). A milligram is 1/1000 of a gram, and there are over 28 grams in an ounce. In research, doses are generally illustrated in terms of the amount (mg) per body weight (kilograms or kg). A kilogram is equal to about 2.2 pounds. Even though the overall effects of a drug are certainly related to the amount ingested by an individual, the effects are also related to the drug's concentration in the body. Thus in research science, measuring a drug's effects is described in mg/kg (like the amount of the drug being studied in a specified body weight).

In order to determine the various effects of a drug, science needs to know the possible range of effects and their intensities. In this way, we can determine what dose level produces a predictable response in a given group of animals or humans. The range of responses can be observed, studied and plotted along a graph called a dose-response curve (DRC). There are many ways to show a DRC. One way generally used in pharmacology, is to plot the frequency distribution of certain responses to different drug doses, then chart the cumulative percentage of subjects who show the particular drug effects. This type of DRC will also show variance of responses to a drug in a given group of subjects.

In DRC's that use cumulative percentiles, it is common to describe curves and compare effectiveness of different drugs by using the ED50 notation. ED50 is the median effective dose, or the dose that is effective in 50% of the individuals studied. If, for example, a dose of a drug being tested produced an ED10, it would mean that the dose was deemed effective in 10% of the subjects being tested. If, in the continued DRC testing, a larger dose produced an ED85, it would mean that the dose was effective in 85% of the population being tested. This way of illustrating the DRC in populations is used to calculate the relative safety of drugs.

All psychoactive drugs produce side effects. Since drugs will produce multiple effects, DRC's can measure the side effects in determining a drug's safety as well. For instance, a drug being tested may have an ED95 for one effect and also show an ED10 for side effects. This would mean that the effective dose worked in 95% of the population studied and that about 10% showed side effects to the drug dose. Another factor in DRC's is the lethal dose range (expressed by the letters LD). So, a drug's LD50 would be the dose that causes death in 50% of the population being studied.

Obviously, in drug testing during clinical trials, the DRC range is important to know in order to stay in or above the ED90 range. And, of course, the further away the LD is from the ED, the safer the drug being studied. The relationship between the LD and the ED is reflected in the therapeutic index (TI). The TI is the ratio of the LD50 to the ED50 and can be expressed by the formula; TI = LD50/ED50. By utilizing the TI, scientists will note that the higher the index, the safer the drug will be. Drug safety can also be described as the ratio of ED99 and LD1.

Agonists and Antagonists

Drugs are administered for the effects they can produce as related to the drug's overall mechanism of action. Generally speaking, drugs can be divided into groups as to whether they cause an increase in neural activity (agonist) or cause a decrease in activity (antagonist). The drugs that affect receptor site systems can be classified into one of four groups which describe its overall mechanism of action: direct-acting agonists, indirect-acting agonists, direct-acting antagonists and indirect-acting antagonists.

Direct-Acting Agonists

A direct-acting agonist drug is one that resembles a chemical messenger on a receptor site and will mimic the normal chemical action by neurotransmitters at synapse. Heroin, for example, is a direct-acting agonist in that it binds directly at opioid receptor sites just like endorphins normally do.

Indirect-Acting Agonists

Indirect-acting agonists will augment the activity of neurotransmitters by extending the amount of time they remain in synapse. The antidepressant Effexor, for example, disallows the neurotransmitter from going back into the cell and therefore prolongs its activity in synapse. Note that indirect-acting drugs usually do not mimic a neurotransmitter by direct binding released at a receptor site.

Direct-Acting Antagonists

Direct-acting antagonist drugs can bind at a receptor site but disallow any response. As a receptor site blocker, for example, a direct-acting antagonist will inhibit neural activity. When such a drug blocks a receptor site, it will interfere with the neurotransmitter's ability to occupy the receptor and therefore reduce the effect. An example of such a drug is naloxone (Narcan) which blocks the effects of morphine-like drugs (including heroin) by taking up all of the receptor site entry points where the neurotransmitter or the drug itself would otherwise bind and stimulate.

Indirect-Acting Antagonists

An indirect-acting antagonist will reduce neurotransmitter actions usually by causing a depletion of neurotransmitter storage in presynpatic cells. Those are the cells that transmit chemical information to other cells.

Depleting the pre-released neurotransmitter results in the unavailability of enough substance to produce any action synaptically once it is released. A drug called Reserpine, for example, is an indirect-acting antagonist in that it works by causing stored neurotransmitters to get destroyed prior to their release into synapse.

In general, knowing about these different agonist and antagonist strategies can be very helpful in understanding the pharmacological actions of most drugs. A more detailed discussion on agonist and antagonist actions will be discussed in a later chapter.

CHAPTER 1: SELF STUDY TEST

TRUE/FALSE

1. *The primary objective in the science of behavioral pharmacology is to discover a drug's selective toxicity.*

2. *All psychoactive drugs, whether legal or otherwise, produce side effects.*

3. *The potency of a drug relates to its ability to be extremely pure in drug content.*

4. *One of the main functions of bio-transformation is related to the concept of solubility.*

5. *There are actually 7 different types of tolerance that can develop with repeated drug exposure.*

6. *Metabolic tolerance is where repeat drug exposure has increased liver function where the increase of available liver enzymes deactivates a greater portion of the drug.*

7. *Tachyphylaxis is a word used to describe the slow development of tolerance.*

8. *A drug that works as an agonist is, in general, is one that produces an increase in neural activity, whereas an antagonist drug decreases neural activity.*

9. *Direct-acting antagonist drugs include receptor site blockers such as the drug Narcan (naloxone), an opiate antagonist.*

10. *A direct-acting agonist drug is one that resembles a chemical messenger on a receptor site such as the drug heroin.*

* Answers to Self Study Tests are located on page 351

Chapter 1 Selected Reading

Altshuler, H.L. et al. Pharmacol. *Biochem. Behav.* **13** Suppl 1, 233–240 (1980).

Brunton, L, Lazo, J, and Parker, K. *Goodman & Gilman's The Pharmacological Basis of Therapeutics*. McGraw-Hill Professional. (2005).

Franklin, T.R. et al. *Biol. Psychiatry* **51**, 134–142 (2002).

Grusser, S.M. et al. *Psychopharmacology* (Berl.) **175**, 296–302 (2004

Hamilton, L. W. & Timmons, C. R. *Principles of behavioral pharmacology: a biopsychological perspective*. Englewood Cliffs, NJ: Prentice-Hall. (1990).

Harvey, RA, Champe, PC, Finkel, R, nd Cubeddu, L. *Lippincott's Illustrated Reviews: Pharmacology, 4th Edition)* Lippincott Williams & Wilkins. (2008).

Hitner, H, and Nagle, BT. *Pharmacology: An Introduction*. Career Education. (2004).

Kamienski, M, and Keogh, J. *Pharmacology Demystified*. McGraw-Hill Professional. (2005).

Katzung, BG. *Basic and Clinical Pharmacology*. McGraw-Hill Medical. 2006.
Golan, DE, et al. *Principles of Pharmacology: The Pathophysiologic Basis of Drug Therapy*. Lippincott Williams & Wilkins. (2007).

Martinez, D. et al. *Neuropsychopharmacology* **29**, 1190–1202 (2004).

Myrick, H. et al. *Neuropsychopharmacology* **29**, 393–402 (2004).

Roberts, A.J. et al. J. *Pharmacol. Exp. Ther.* **293**, 1002–1008 (2000).

Stringer, JL. Basic Concepts in Pharmacology. McGraw-Hill Professional. (2005).

Volkow, N.D., Fowler, J.S. & Wang, G.J. *Neuropharmacology* **47** (Suppl.) 3–13 (2004).

Woodrow, R, and George, D. *Essentials of Pharmacology for Health Occupations*. Thomson Delmar Learning. (2006).

CHAPTER 2: VOCABULARY LIST

Afferent nerves   *Specialized <u>sensory</u> fibers that carry information into the CNS from sense organs.*

Amygdala   *Located in the Limbic system, it is important for emotional or affective behaviors. Emotional memory seems to be stored there as well.*

ANS   *The autonomic nervous system (ANS) regulates unconscious rates and temperatures.*

Basal ganglia   *Coordinates muscle movement, and located on the left and right of the thalamus.*

Broca's area   *Located in the inferior frontal gyrus of the left frontal lobe, an area critical for human language production.*

Cerebellum   *Aka, "Little brain", is an important hind-brain section that coordinates movement and learning.*

Cerebral Cortex   *The most recently developed and most complicated area of the brain involved in higher functioning.*

CNS   *The central nervous system, including the brain and the spinal cord.*

Efferent nerves   *Specialized <u>motor</u> fibers that carry information away from the CNS to muscles.*

Fissures   *Large grooves or convolutions of the cerebral cortex.*

Frontal lobe   *The frontal lobes are considered our emotional control center and home to our personality. They are involved in the ability to recognize future consequences resulting from current actions, to choose between good and bad actions (or better and best), override and suppress unacceptable social responses, and determine similarities and differences between things or events.*

Ganglia   *The name for a collection of neurons specifically in the PNS.*

Gonads   *Sexual glands including the ovaries and testes, that secrete sex hormones.*

Gray matter	Cells that predominate and give the cerebral cortex a grayish brown color.
Hippocampus	The limbic structure that plays an important role in short-term, or recent memory.
Hypothalamus	Controls autonomic functions and the hormone system from the base of the brain.
Limbic system	Contains an interconnecting circular route between the cortex and hypothalamus.
Meninges	Three layers of special membranes that protect the brain and spinal cord.
Nucleus accumbens	A primary area of the reward circuitry involved in pleasure and reinforcing behaviors.
Occipital lobe	The main region where thalamus axons innervate from the visual pathways.
Parietal lobe	Monitors touch, stretch and joints from between occipital lobe and central sulcus.
Pituitary gland	Releases hormones into the bloodstream that regulate activities of other glands.
PNS	The peripheral nervous system, nerves that extend away from the CNS.
Pons	Meaning, "bridge", the Pons are large bulging structures in brain stem that regulate sleep or arousal.
Reticular formation	Receives sensory information and projects axons into the spinal cord.
Satiation point	The cutoff when behavioral release from tension is no longer rewarding.
Temporal lobes	Located near both temples, primary target for hearing .
Thalamus	Referred to as the "sensory way-station" of information on its way to the cortex.
Wernicke's area	The area responsible for the comprehension of language in the left temporal lobe.

White matter   *Large concentration of myelin that gives the sub-cortex an opaque appearance.*

CHAPTER 2: THE NERVOUS SYSTEM

The principal target organ for psychoactive drugs is the brain. As previously stated, psychoactive drugs are those substances that alter thought, affect (mood) and movement. Since psychoactive drugs alter behavior, and behaviors are facilitated by the nervous system, is important to understand the basics of how the human nervous system works.

The nervous system consists of two subdivisions: the central nervous system (CNS), which refers to the brain, and the spinal cord, and the peripheral nervous system (PNS) that part of the system outside of the CNS which consists of nerves that extend from the CNS. The PNS contains those nerves that link the periphery of the body, including the smooth muscles and internal organs, to the CNS. Notice in the chart below how the PNS and CNS contain various sub-systems, which they govern, to facilitate behavior.

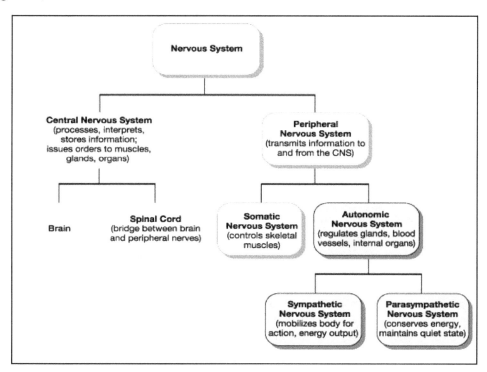

The Peripheral Nervous System (PNS)
The PNS is divided into two areas: the somatic nervous system facilitates voluntary muscle movement and allows conscious control over the skeletal muscles, and the autonomic nervous system (ANS) regulates all unconscious events such as heart rate, digestion, respiration, blood pressure and body temperature. The peripheral nervous system (PNS) consists of all the nerve fibers that transmit data to and from the central nervous system (CNS) as well as those

that lie outside of the CNS.

The illustration below shows the physical relationship between the CNS and PNS in the body.

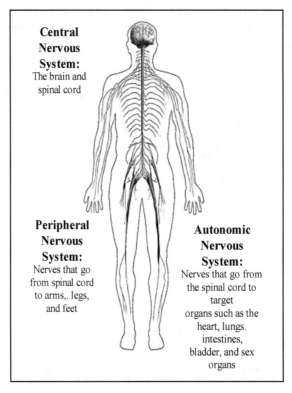

Central Nervous System:
The brain and spinal cord

Peripheral Nervous System:
Nerves that go from spinal cord to arms,. legs, and feet

Autonomic Nervous System:
Nerves that go from the spinal cord to target organs such as the heart, lungs. intestines, bladder, and sex organs

Specialized nerve fibers, called afferent (sensory) nerves, carry information into the CNS from the various sense organs and therefore aid sensations of pain, temperature and touch. Other specialized nerve fibers within the PNS, called efferent (motor) nerves, carry information away from the CNS for muscle control, movement and specific body functions. Efferent nerves are divided into two categories: somatic fibers that control the function of skeletal muscles, and autonomic fibers, which control activities of the viscera (smooth muscles), heart muscle and the exocrine (secretory) glands. Somatic nerve fibers leave the spinal cord as a continuous uninterrupted unit from their originating site (via a motor neuron) and attach to the skeletal muscles.

The ANS is again divided into three areas: the sympathetic nervous system (SNS), the parasympathetic nervous system (PNS) and the enteric nervous system (ENS). Sympathetic nerve fibers leave from the thoracic and lumbar sections in the middle of the spinal cord. The parasympathetic nerves leave from the upper cranium and lower sacral parts of the spinal cord. There is both a physiological and biochemical difference in these two divisions of the ANS.

The enteric nervous system, not discussed much, is a meshwork of nerve fibers that connects and coordinates actions of the viscera including the gastrointestinal tract, pancreas and gall bladder.

As you see in the chart below, the SNS activates the system for the fight-fright because it prepares the body for high level activity and rapid response. The PNS, which controls subconscious activity during periods of relaxation, activates those physiological factors related to the deceleration or slowing down of various bodily processes including heart rate. Since the PNS, when activated, increases food digestion, it is sometimes referred to as the "feed and breed" system.

Drugs act both centrally (within the CNS) and peripherally (within the PNS). For example, cocaine acts centrally by altering thought and mood, producing effects of euphoria, sleep and appetite suppression, perhaps causing paranoia and severe depression. Its peripheral actions affect target organs and peripheral muscles, including tachycardia (racing heart), arteriole constriction and elevated blood pressure.

Differences Between the SNS and PNS in Regulating Behaviors

Sympathetic System *(fight-flight response)*	**Parasympathetic System** *(feed-breed response)*
Pupil dilation	Pupil constriction
Heart acceleration	Heart deceleration
Arteriole constriction	Arteriole dilation
Bronchial dilation	Bronchial constriction
Adrenal gland secretion	Adrenal gland inhibition
Pancreas inhibition	Pancreas activation
Urinary bladder inhibition	Urinary bladder contraction
Digestive process inhibition	Digestive process stimulated
Tear gland stimulation	Tear gland inhibition
Salivary gland inhibition	Salivary stimulation
Glucose release	

NOTE: In the PNS, a collection of neurons is called ganglia, and axons are called nerves. In the CNS, a collection of neurons is called a nuclei, and axons are called tracts.

The Central Nervous System (CNS)

The brain receives signals rom both inside and outside the body. It maintains basic bodily functions like heart rate, breathing rate and body temperature without us having to be conscious of these behaviors happening. CNS also initiates conscious decisions to do things like running, walking, playing a musical instrument and many more complex motor tasks. Although the CNS creates our personalities, moods and emotions come from, the human brain only makes up about one-fiftieth (1/50) of the body's weight.

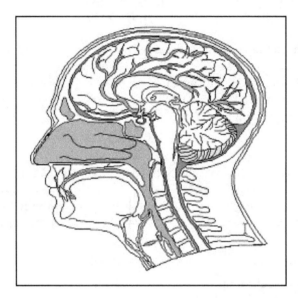

Three layers of special membranes called meninges cover the brain and spinal cord where they serve as a protective covering. The space between the middle and inner layers contains cerebrospinal fluid, a clear, watery solution similar to blood plasma. It circulates over the entire surface of the brain and spinal cord and provides a protective cushion as well as a source of nourishment for these structures. The cerebrospinal fluid is continuously being formed by a plexus (network) of blood vessels in the brain. As it forms, a like amount is continuously reabsorbed.

The human brain is thought to contain 100 billion neurons - about the same number as the stars in our Galaxy. Each neuron may be in contact with a thousand other cells, providing the possibility for over a trillion different types of communication routes. The human brain is truly an amazing organ. The major divisions of the brain are the **hindbrain, midbrain** and **forebrain,** resulting from its own evolutionary development. Each division, or region, contains some principal structures as described below.

HINDBRAIN STRUCTURES

Spinal Cord
The simplest part of the nervous system is the spinal cord. Many behaviors can be regulated within the spinal cord and signals do not have to travel into the brain for analysis and action commands. For example, the knee-jerk reflex, sneezing, and eye blink reflex are some reflex behaviors that originate in the spinal cord

The spinal cord is basically the "information super-highway" for nerve impulses traveling into and out of the brain. In fact, all communication with the brain travels through the spinal cord. The two principal functions of the spinal cord are to distribute motor fibers to effecter organs of the body (glands and muscles), and to collect sensory information to be processed by the brain.

The spinal cord, like the brain, consists of white and gray matter. Unlike the brain, its white matter (ascending and descending bundles of myelinated axons) is on the outside, and the gray matter (neural cell bodies and short unmyelinated axons) is on the inside. The spinal cord contains 31 pairs of spinal nerves, with both sensory and motor fibers, that lead from the cord to all parts of the body. The spinal cord is protected by the vertebrae structures.

Cerebellum (Balance and Coordination)
The *cerebellum* (meaning "little brain") plays an important role in coordination and movement. Complicated movements are initiated, coordinated and stored as fixed behavioral patterns within the cerebellum. The cerebellum is present even in primitive animals, and its importance increases along the evolutionary scale. The more complicated the motor activity of an animal, the larger the cerebellum. Damage to the cerebellum impairs standing, walking or performing coordinated movements. The cerebellum is also involved in learning.

Pons
The pons are large bulge-like structures in the brain stem. Pons, meaning "bridge", play a role in the regulation of sleep and arousal as well as coordination of movement patterns.

Medulla (Autonomic Reflexes)
The *medulla* is located just above the spinal cord and is involved in the regulation of respiration (breathing), cardiovascular function (heart rate), coughing, sneezing, salivation and other reflex behaviors.

Reticular Formation (Alertness)
The reticular formation receives the sensory information from neural pathways and projects axons into the cerebral cortex, thalamus and spinal cord. It plays an important role in the coordination of sleep and arousal (the sleep-wake cycle), attention, muscle tone, movement and various vital reflex

behaviors including the startle reaction.

MIDBRAIN STRUCTURES (Sight and Movement)

Tectum (Hearing and Vision)
The tectum contains two substructures involved with hearing and vision. The first substructure, called the inferior colliculus, is involved in the perception and conveying of auditory information. The other substructure within the tectum, called the superior colliculus, is a part of the visual system, and in mammals is primarily involved in visual reflexes and reactions to moving stimuli.

Tegmentum (Movement Coordination)
The tegmentum is located beneath the tectum and is part of the motor system that coordinates nerve signals down the spinal cord or up to the basal ganglia. The tegmentum contains two primary substructures involved in coordinating gross body movements; the substantia nigras and the ventral tegmental area (VTA).

The **substantia nigras** contains dopamine-secreting neurons and plays a critical role in movement and muscle coordination. Degeneration of neurons within the substantia nigras causes Parkinson's disease. The *VTA* also contains dopamine-secreting neurons that project to the basal forebrain and cerebral cortex and have been implicated in the behaviors of learning and motivation.

FOREBRAIN STRUCTURES

Limbic System (Emotion)
The limbic system contains interconnecting areas that run in a circular route between the cortex and hypothalamus. The limbic system actually includes parts of the frontal cortex, thalamus, hypothalamus, amygdala and hippocampus. Functioning together in a complex neural group, all of these areas contribute to the control of emotional behavior and memory. Substructures within the limbic system include the amygdala, hippocampus and the septum.

The amygdala is a structure that governs aggressive behaviors, fear and territoriality. In addition to aggression, the amygdala has some of the circuitry for sexual behavior. Studies have shown that stimulation of certain parts of the amygdala in primates will induce aggressive, assaultive behaviors, stimulation in adjacent areas can even produce fear responses and amnesia.

The hippocampus plays an important role in memory. One interesting case history that shows the effects of a damaged hippocampus is where a man had a severe form of viral encephalitis. This caused a destruction of brain hippocampal areas, and his ability to retain new information was greatly impaired. For example, each time he saw his wife, even after only a few minutes, his reaction was as if he had just seen her for after she had been gone for a long period of time. The man's condition did not allow him to retain new information for any longer than a few *minutes.* It was as if his memory storage could not hold any information. Every time he would turn away from an interaction, any memory of the event disappeared.

Interestingly in this case history of damage to the hippocampus, memories stored prior to the illness remained intact. In fact, this man was a rather popular musician and could retain his musical abilities both as a performer and conductor. However, when he was out of this context, his memory abilities were observably deteriorated. This case, as well as many others, has told us something about the hippocampus and its role in memory processing.

The septum is involved with inhibition. It seems that the septum is the "checks and balances" to the amygdala. That is, where the amygdala becomes active during times of fight-flight and is associated with immediate survival modes of behavior, the septum governs more nurturing behavioral aspects including mating rituals, grooming and hygiene, caring for offspring and sexual arousal.

Basal Ganglia (Posture and Movement)
The basal ganglia is located to the left and right of the thalamus and in general, coordinates muscle movement. However, the basal ganglia does not control movement directly, and there are no axons that extend directly into the medulla or spinal cord. Rather, they send signals to the thalamus and the midbrain, which in turn relay the information to the cerebral cortex which then sends messages to the medulla and spinal cord.

Thalamus (Sensory Processing)
Much of the surface of the cerebral cortex is divided into regions that receive neural projections from parts of the thalamus. Practically all sensory information projects first to the thalamus in the center of the forebrain, and then to the cerebral cortex, with the exception of the sense of smell which enters the olfactory bulb. The thalamus, based on its functioning, is sometimes referred to as the "sensory way-station" of information on its way to the cortex.

Hypothalamus (Neurohumors and Hormones)
The hypothalamus lies at the base of the brain beneath the thalamus. Although a small structure, its functions are enormous. Basically, the hypothalamus controls autonomic functions and the endocrine (hormone) system, through its connections with the pituitary gland. It also coordinates those behaviors related for the survival of the species — fighting, feeding and mating. The hypothalamus has wide-spread connections into the forebrain and midbrain areas and plays a critical role in the behaviors of eating, drinking (body water fluid level), body temperature regulation, sexual behavior, aggression and energy levels.

The hypothalamus has direct control over the pituitary gland and thus regulates the hormone secretion. The hypothalamus contains special receptors for specific hormones. In response to changes in the levels of certain hormones, the hypothalamus will signal chemical messages to the pituitary gland and stimulate it to release hormones. Damage to one of the hypothalamic nuclei causes abnormalities in eating, drinking, temperature, aggression and sexual arousal.

Pituitary and Endocrine Glands (Hormones)
Attached to the base of the hypothalamus is the pituitary gland, which is divided into two sections: the anterior and posterior. The anterior part of the pituitary gland releases hormones into the bloodstream that regulate the activities of the other glands. The hypothalamus actually only controls the anterior part of the pituitary gland. There is a chemical interplay between the hypothalamus and the anterior pituitary that regulates many of the body's hormonal levels. Basically this starts with the hypothalamus detecting some hormone level decrease which is beginning to adversely affect the system.

The hypothalamus releases a chemical known as a releasing factor, that acts on the anterior pituitary. The anterior pituitary, in response, releases a hormone that is delivered to the target gland and stimulates it to release more of its own hormone. Target glands are specialized cells that have the ability to produce and release various hormones. The target glands controlled by the anterior pituitary include the *thyroid, adrenal cortex* and the *gonads.* The thyroid releases the hormone called thyroxine, which regulates a substance called adenosine triphosphate (ATP) and has potential energy for behavior. ATP augments energy and distributes it through cells. A deficiency in thyroxine (hypothyroidism) includes symptoms of fatigue and energy drain.

The adrenal cortex produces over forty different hormones known collectively as steroids. Steroids generally have a four-fold function: they regulate metabolism and blood pressure, and control sexual appearance and sexual behavior. The gonads include the ovaries and testes and secrete steroidal sex hormones. In males they secrete testosterone, and in females they secrete estrogen and progesterone. These hormones control the development of sexual appearance and maintain reproductive organs as well as sexual behavior in adults. Not all hormones are controlled by the hypothalamus-pituitary axis (also called the hypax). Insulin is one example.

Medial Forebrain Bundle (Pleasure, Learning and Motivation)
Within the medial forebrain bundle (MFB) are the neural communication systems between the brain stem, the limbic system and the cerebral cortex. Of particular importance within this communication system is an area called the nucleus accumbens.

Nucleus Accumbens (Reward Circuitry)
Over the last twenty years, research has demonstrated the role of the nucleus

accumbens in brain stimulation-reward experiments. These widely published studies show convincingly that the brain's reward circuitry includes the nucleus accumbens as a major area involved in pleasure and reinforcement in learning behaviors. For example, laboratory animals with electrode implantations in the˙ nucleus accumbens will learn to press to gain pleasurable stimulation from the electrode. The animal will continue pressing the lever until it becomes exhausted. In fact, the reinforcing effects of brain stimulation-reward in the nucleus accumbens is so strong that the animal will prefer this type of brain stimulation over the intake of food and water.

Studies with humans have also shown that brain stimulation-reward in the nucleus accumbens reinforces those behaviors that had the effect on that brain area. It seems that the nucleus accumbens coordinates pleasure responses that normal reinforce behaviors of eating, sleeping and procreating, and the desire to repeat these behaviors is strengthened. Psychoactive drugs of abuse apparently act on this area of the brain and therefore can become powerfully reinforcing.

Indeed, all experiences of relief from biological tensions will include the activation of the nucleus accumbens. In terms of the normal tension-release patterns of hunger, thirst, and sexual drive, there is a *satiation point* when behavioral release from tension is no longer rewarding. It seems that for these types of sensations, animals will *satiate* and stop trying to relieve biological tension. The feeling of fullness or contentment will ultimately override the need or desire to reduce the biological tension. Animals will stops eating when full, stop drinking when no longer thirsty and stop sexual activity after orgasm.

Interestingly, for drug abuse behavior, there is no apparent satiation point. That is, animals will continue to act in ways to receive drug reward to the point of sheer exhaustion. One study showed that animals will even exceed pain thresholds for drug reward beyond those for food and water. In other words, the animal is apparently willing to pay a very high price with adverse consequences for drug induced brain stimulation.

Studies confirm the role of the nucleus accumbens in the brain's reward circuitry during drug abuse. When the nucleus accumbens is removed in animals that have become addicted to drugs, there no longer is any interest in pursuing those drugs through self administration. More will be discussed on the nucleus accumbens and its role within the brain-reward circuitry of the *mesocorticolimbic pathway* (MCLP) in the chapter on the neurobiology of reward and drug reinforcement. But for now, however, suffice it to say that if a drug has any potential for abuse, it is because it targets and acts on the brain's MCLP.

Cerebral Cortex (Higher Functioning)
The *cerebral cortex* is the most complicated region of the nervous system.

In humans, the cerebral cortex is greatly convoluted. These convolutions, consisting of sulci (small grooves), fissures (large grooves) and *gyri* (bulges between adjacent sulci or fissures), greatly enlarge the surface area of the cortex, compared with a smooth mass. The cerebral cortex is made of glial cells and neurons. Because cells predominate, giving the cerebral cortex a grayish brown color, it is referred to as gray matter.

Beneath the cerebral cortex are millions of neuronal axons that connect the neurons in the cerebral cortex with those located elsewhere in the brain. The large concentration of myelin gives this tissue an opaque white appearance and therefore the term white matter. The cerebral cortex is divided into four parts, called lobes, named after the bones of the skull that overlie them; the *parietal lobe,* the *temporal lobes,* the *occipital lobe* and the *frontal lobe.* All sensory perceptions are projected onto the cerebral cortex, and the outside world is represented by these projection fields.

The Parietal Lobe
The parietal lobe lies between the occipital lobe and the central sulcus, one of the deepest grooves in the surface of the cerebral cortex. The parietal lobe is specialized for dealing with the sensory information of touch, muscle-stretch and joint receptors. It is the brain's primary somatosensory area where the integration of many incoming sensations are processed and experienced. The parietal lobe is also important for relating visual information to spatial information. For example, you know you are looking at the same object even if you alter your perspective (i.e. looking at this page and then tilting your head to view it sideways, you know it is still the same page). Damage to the parietal lobes can result in symptoms where the person has great difficulty interpreting information from touch and using it to control movement. Such symptoms from damage to the parietal lobes might include: impairment of identifying objects by touch, lack of coordination on the opposite side of the body where the brain damage took place, inability to draw or use maps, difficulty giving directions, or problems recognizing different angles of view.

The Temporal Lobes
The temporal lobes are located in both left and right hemispheres near the temples, on each side of the head. They are the primary target for auditory information (hearing) and coordinate with the vestibular organs (the inner ear that deals with equilibrium and balance). The temporal lobes also contribute to the complexities of vision and perception, such as recognition of patterns that make up faces.

In humans, the left temporal lobe contain the area called Wernicke's area, which is the brain area responsible for the comprehension of language. The temporal lobes may also play a role in some emotional and motivational behaviors. Damage to the temporal lobes can lead to unprovoked laughter, joy, anxiety, depression or violent behaviors.

The Occipital Lobe

Located at the posterior (caudal) end of the cortex, the occipital lobe is the main region where axons from the thalamus innervate from the visual pathways. The very posterior pole of the occipital lobe is called the primary visual cortex. Complete destruction in this area can lead to blindness. In addition to vision, the occipital lobe is responsible for types of learning as well. For example, blind laboratory animals will show occipital lobe activity when learning maze directions. Also, damage to this area of the brain impaired maze-learning even in animals that were already blind.

The Frontal Lobe

The frontal lobe extends from the central sulcus to the anterior part of the brain. The posterior area of the frontal lobe controls fine movements, such as moving one finger at a time. The left frontal lobe, in humans, is an area critical for language production called *Broca's area.*

The anterior area of the frontal lobe is called the prefrontal cortex which is the only area of the cortex that receives input from all sensory modalities including olfaction (smell). The prefrontal cortex is critical for memory, emotional expression, and social inhibitions.

The illustration below provides a view of the relative location of the four lobes of the brain.

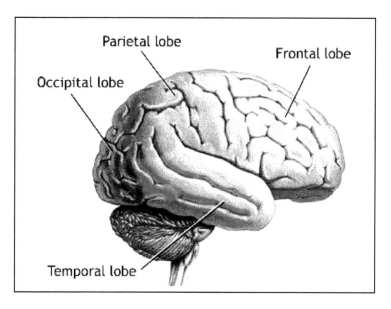

Fun Brain Facts!   Did you know . . .

- Your brain uses 20% of your body's energy, but it makes up only 2% of your body's weight
- The brain feels like a ripe avocado or a sponge and looks red because of the blood flowing through it
- Your brain weighs about 3 pounds (1,300-1,400g), is about the size of a cantaloupe, and wrinkled like a walnut
- The total surface area of the cerebral cortex is about 2500 sq. cm (~2.5 ft)
- The entire area of your skin weighs three times as much as your brain
- A newborn baby's brain grows almost 3 times in its first year of life
- Babies lose half their neurons at birth! It is estimated that a baby loses about half their neurons before they are born. This process is sometimes referred to as *pruning* and may eliminate neurons that do not receive sufficient input from other neurons.
- Early Brain Growth.   During the first month of life, the number of connections or synapses, dramatically increases from 50 trillion to 1 quadrillion. If an infant's body grew at a comparable rate, his weight would increase from 8.5 pounds at birth to 170 pounds at one month old.
- Reading aloud stimulates child development.   Reading aloud to children helps stimulate brain development, yet only 50% of infants and toddlers are routinely read to by their parents
- Working Memory Stores Seven Digits: It's no accident that telephone numbers in the United States are seven digits long. Our working memory, a very short-term form of memory which stores ideas just long enough for us to understand them, can hold on average a maximum of seven digits. This allows you to look up a phone number and remember it just long enough to dial.

CHAPTER 2: SELF-STUDY QUESTIONS
TRUE/FALSE

1. The principal target organ for psychoactive drugs is the kidneys.

2. The peripheral nervous system (PNS) is divided into three sub-divisions, the somatic nervous system, the autonomic nervous system and the empathetic nervous system.

3. The major divisions of the brain are the hindbrain, midbrain, forebrain and newbrain.

4. The simplest part of the nervous system is the spinal cord.

5. To date, it seems that drugs with abuse potential, among other things, act as agonists within the mesocorticolimbic pathway.

6. The cerebral cortex is the most complicated region of the nervous system.

7. The cerebral cortex is made of mostly glial cells and neurons – because these cells predominate, they give the cerebral cortex a grayish brown color, and it is thus referred to as gray matter.

8. The temporal lobe is the primary target for auditory information (hearing) and coordinates with the vestibular organs (the inner ear that deals with equilibrium and balance).

9. The occipital lobe is the main region where axons from the thalamus innervate from the auditory pathways.

10. The prefrontal cortex is critical for memory, emotional expression and social inhibition.

* Answers to Self Study Tests are located on page 351

Chapter 2 Selected Reading

Ashton, H., *Brain Function and Psychotropic Drugs,* Oxford Press, New York, 1992

Bear, MF, Connors, B, and Paradiso, M. *Neuroscience: Exploring the Brain.* Lippincott Williams & Wilkins. 2006.

Carvey, P.M., *Drug Action in the Central Nervous System,* OxfordUniversity Press, New York, 1998.

Diamond, MC, and Scheibel, AB. *The Human Brain Coloring Book.* Collins. 1985.

Herz, A., *Handbook of Experimental Pharmacology: Opioids I,* Springer-Verlag, Berlin.

Nolte, J. *The Human Brain: An Introduction to Its Functional* Anatomy. Mosby. 2002.

O'Shea, M. *The Brain: A Very Short Introduction.* Oxford University Press. 2003.

Simon, S. *The Brain: Our Nervous System.* Collins. 2006.

Thompson, RH. *The Brain: A Neuroscience Primer.* Worth Publishers. 2000.

CHAPTER 3: VOCABULARY LIST

Action potential   A change in electrical potential on the surface of a cell that occurs when it is stimulated, resulting in the transmission of an electrical impulse.

All-or-none law   Basic principal that states that the action potential either fully occurs or not.

Autoreceptors   Specialized to inform presynaptic neurons about the chemicallevels in synapse.

Axon   The part of the cell that transmits a signal away from the soma to the axon endings.

Dendrite   Greek for "tree", the part of the neuron that receives neurochemical info to the soma for potential processing.

Depolarization   An action potential, an impulse created by a neuron stimulatbeyond its threshold.

Glial cells   Forms a connective tissue which bind bundle of cells together.

Graded potential   Varied signal from dendrites in proportion to the magnitude of the stimulation.

Homeostasis   The ability or tendency to maintain internal balance by adjusting physiological processes.

Membrane   Cell wall that limits the flow of materials inside the cell to outside environments.

Mitochondria   The part of the cell that performs metabolic activities to make energy for other activities.

Myelin   Cells that wrap themselves around the axon to create directional flow during an action potential.

Nodes of Ranvier   Bare unmyelinated points along the axon that speed the signal transfer of information.

Nucleus   Inside the soma, a structure that converts amino acids into neurotransmitters needed for neural communication.

Polarization   *Also called resting potential, this is where neurons that have the potential for energy release are not activated and are" at rest" until a biochemical event causes an action potential.*

CHAPTER 3: THE ELECTROCHEMICAL NEURON

As you have seen, the anatomy of the brain is very complex. In fact, the exact functioning of the brain is still not yet entirely understood. Up to this point, we have been discussing large areas of the brain, from the hindbrain through the midbrain and finally to the forebrain structures. The fundamental unit of the nervous system that conducts signals from one area to another is the neuron. The ability of the neuron to transmit information is a function of both its ability to send electrical charges as well as its capacity to synthesize, store and release very specific chemicals from its axon endings.

The basic function of electrical activity within a neuron is to transfer signals to other nerve cells. The critical operation of the brain, processing sensory information, programming movement and emotions, learning and memory - all are carried out by individual neurons. To create a behavior, each sensory or motor neuron involved carries out a sequence of responses. For each neuron – regardless of size, shape, dedicated neurotransmitter substance or behavioral function – most neurons can be described functionally by four components; an integrative component *(signaling),* a local input component *(receiving),* a conductile component *(triggering)* and an output component *(chemical release).*

One or more of these four components can become impaired with drug abuse. Furthermore, behavioral neuroscience has discovered that imbalances in neural components contribute to many psychiatric disorders that will be discussed later. For now, it is important to understand how neurons communicate, since this is the common *lingua franca* of the neurobiology of behavior.

The brain is composed of two classes of cells: *nerve cells* (neuron) and *glial cells.* The glial cells are basically a connective tissue which bind bundle of cells together. Neurons, however, are cells that transfer information within the nervous system, and process it to form behavior. The network between neurons increases dramatically during the first years of life, when new connections are constantly developing. Neurons can alter their shape even after maturity.

An enriched environment can lead to longer and more widely branched dendrites which produce more routes that did not previously exist. However, adverse neural effects can be caused by deficient environments, including alcohol abuse which can shrink dendrites. Healthy and alert elderly people seem to have an increased proliferation of dendritic branches, whereas senile persons have slightly shrunken dendrites. Neurons come in many shapes and varieties according to the type of function they perform (see Figure below).

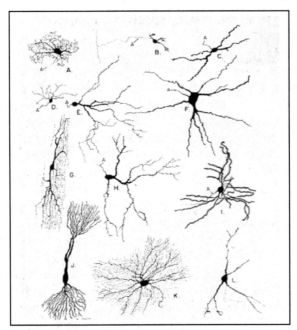

Different types of neurons

Regardless of the type of neuron, they all possess the same basic anatomy (see Figure below). The neuron is composed of four major structures: the soma (cell body), the dendrites, the axon and the axon endings (presynaptic terminals).

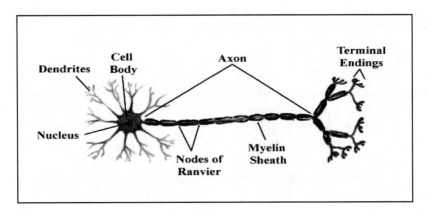

The Soma (Integrative Component / Signaling)

The *soma,* or cell body, is essentially the <u>heart</u> of the neuron. Inside the soma is the *nucleus,* a structure that contains the chromosomes. The nucleus is also the part of the neuron that makes specific neurotransmitters, chemicals that are used to convey information from cell to cell. The soma also contains much of the biological "machinery" that sustains and nurtures the cell as a whole. One of the "machines" in this regard is the *mitochondria,* where the cell performs all of its metabolic activities that provide energy for the cell's other activities, including transmitting data to other neurons.

The Dendrites (Local Input Component / Receiving)
Dendrites (Greek for "tree") carry neurological information to the soma for interpretation and potential processing. As neurons communicate with each other, the dendrites serve as important recipients of these messages. The dendrite's surface is lined with specialized junctions at which the dendrite receives information from other neurons. In general, the larger the surface area of the dendrite, the greater the amount of information it can receive.

The Axon (Conductile Component / Triggering)
The axon is a long slender tube that carries information away from the soma to the axon endings. The message is electrical in nature until it reaches the axon endings where the message is converted to a chemical one. Some neurons have very small axons, while others have axons that are very long. There are also some types of neurons with more than one axon.

The axon ending does not actually touch the next neuron. Thus, between each neuron there is a small space called the *synapse*. The neuron that transfers information into the synapse is called the *presynaptic neuron* and the neuron that is on the other end of the synapse, and receives information is called the *postsynaptic neuron.*

A difference between axons and dendrites is the material surrounding them. Most axons are covered with a fatty 'sheath, known as myelin, which gives axons a white appearance, but no such sheath surrounds dendrites. Myelin is made of special non-neural cells that literally wrap themselves around the axon in layers. In the peripheral nervous system, they are *Schwann cells,* and in the central nervous system they are called *oligodendrocytes.,* but both are neuroglial cells. They prevent nerve signals of adjacent neurons from interfering with one another.

Myelin also insures that nerve impulses during depolarization are directional. A disease related to the *demyelination* (destruction of myelin) is Multiple Sclerosis (MS). As one might imagine, symptoms of MS caused by poor coordination of nerve impulse result in tremors and postural rigidity. Myelin destruction eliminates the insulation between adjacent neurons and results in the scrambling of neural messages.

The myelin sheath itself is divided into segments that leave bare unmyelinated points along the surface. These points are the *nodes of Ranvier,* which speed the process of the myelin sheath conducting information through the nervous system. Nerve cell activity, called depolarization or "firing", is triggered at each node of Ranvier, and is passed along the myelinated area to the next node. This jumping from one node to the next is called saltatory conduction (from the Latin *saltare,* "to dance").

Axon Endings (Output Component / Chemical Release)
The axon divides and branches several times. At the ends of the axons are tiny bulbs, called axon endings (sometimes also called *terminal endings*) which have a specialized function. The axon endings release chemicals that cross through the synapse, the junction between each neuron. When a message is transmitted down the axon to the axon endings, a chemical messenger called a neurotransmitter is released.

There are over 200 different types of these chemicals which either excite or inhibit further action in the next receiving cell. Properties that determine what type of message the axon endings convey will be discussed later.

The Nerve Impulse
The nerve impulse is an electro-chemical event. That is, the information moves as an electrical pulse (from dendrite to the soma and along the axon) and then becomes transferred to a chemical transmission (the neurotransmitter that crosses the synapse and affects the postsynaptic neuron).

Every cell *is* surrounded by a *membrane* that *limits* the flow of materials between the inside of the cell and the outside environment. A few chemicals like water, oxygen and carbon dioxide, flow freely across the membrane, while other chemicals, such as large molecules, do not. The neuron's membrane is *selectively permeable* to chemical passage, which means it will allow some molecules to pass through but not others. Several important ions such as sodium, potassium and chloride enter the cell through pores or channels in special proteins that are embedded in the membrane.

The neuron, like an electrical wire, is a conductor of electricity. Neurons maintain a difference in electrical charge (measured in millivolts or mV) across their external membrane. This difference is the resting potential, also called *polarization* since positive and negative charges are polarized, and kept separate by the cell membrane. Thus, the difference in electrical charge is determined by the distribution of ions outside versus inside the neuron. The resting potential is caused by unequal distribution of sodium ($Na+$), potassium ($K+$), and chloride ($Cl-$) ions, and organic protein anions ($A-$) across the cell membrane. Changes in the neuron's membrane permeability to $Na+$ and $K+$ will produce the electrical message that will ultimately be transmitted down the axon.

During resting potential, there is an accumulation of $Na+$ ions outside the cell, producing a more positive charge than the inside negative charge created by the amount of organic anions ($A-$). The distribution of ions this way establishes the potential for energy release by the neuron, but unless an event happens to allow $Na+$ ions to permeate the membrane, the cell remains in a state of polarization.

It is important to remember that during resting potential, where there is the potential for energy release but none is taking place, the membrane permeability to K+ is high and to Na+ is low. Neurons are able to maintain a resting potential by means of a hypothetical energy driven sodium-potassium "pump" which controls the flow of ions in and out of the neuron in such a way as to keep the outside of neuron slightly more positive than inside. The resting potential will remain stable until the neuron is stimulated.

When the neuron is stimulated beyond a certain threshold, it will generate a nerve impulse, called the action potential. When an action potential occurs, its size (amplitude) is independent of the intensity of the stimulus that initiated it. This *all-or-none law* basically states that the action potential either occurs or it does not. Once triggered, it is transmitted down the axon to the axon endings. All action potentials take place in the axon and are equal in size. In contrast, dendrites will produce what are called *graded potentials* which will be proportional to the magnitude of the stimulation. So as the strength of the stimuli decreases, so will the intensity of the graded potential.

The action potential is related to the movement and distribution of ions across the cell membrane. When the stimulation reaches the threshold, it causes a change in the permeability of the membrane. The channels along the membrane previously too small to accommodate Na+ molecules are now opened wider. As Na+ now moves inside the cell, there is a reversal of charge to where the inside is more positive and the outside is more negatively charged. When this occurs, the neuron has depolarized or "fired", meaning that it has released energy for the neural communication process.

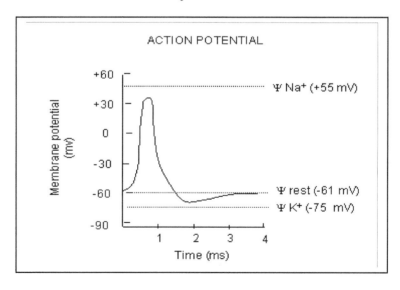

After depolarization, the neuron apparently requires a brief period when it is resistant to reexcitation. For 1 millisecond after an action potential, the cell is in a *refractory period.* The first part of this period is called the *absolute refractory period* because no matter how strong the intensity of a new stimulus is, the cell will not produce an action potential. The second part of the period is called the *relative refractory period,* during which a stimulus must exceed the usual threshold in order to produce an action potential. The time span during refraction is apparently required for the sodium channels to recover after depolarization.

As you have read, stimulation of the neuron inverses the membrane potential from negatively charged (at rest) to positive (action potential). This transformation occurs only at the point of stimulation. The positive charges inside the membrane attract neighboring negative charges and travel towards them. A similar process occurs outside the membrane as well. This results in positive charges transferring along the axon towards the synapse, and negative charges towards the soma. Sodium channels open when the membrane potential is positive. Indeed, the open sodium channels allow in sodium which leads to the action potential. The new action potential attracts nearby ions and produces a new action potential further along the axon.

It is now apparent that the nerve impulse is an electro-chemical event. The distribution and movement of ions across the cell membrane addresses the electrical part of the nerve impulse, and the chemical messengers released into synapse address the chemical aspects.

The Synapse
The electrical action potential travels from the soma to the end of the axon, but can not continue to the next cell in its electrical form due to a gap between the cells called the synapse. Synapses are fluid-filled spaces between the axon endings of one neuron and the somatic or dendritic membranes of another (see Figure below). A synapse, while varying in size, averages to about 200 angstroms wide. An *Angstrom unit* is one ten-millionth of a millimeter, so the synaptic gap is quite small indeed.

Because a message only travels one direction, the membranes on the two sides of the synapse are named accordingly: the transmitting neuron is called the presynaptic membrane, and that of the receiving neuron is the postsynaptic membrane. The postsynaptic membrane contains specialized protein molecules that act as "receptors" which can detect the presence of neurotransmitters in the synapse. When the released neurotransmitters diffuse across the synapse and bind at these postsynaptic receptors, the receiving neuron can initiate changes along its own membrane that will either excite or inhibit the rate of depolarization of the neuron's axon.

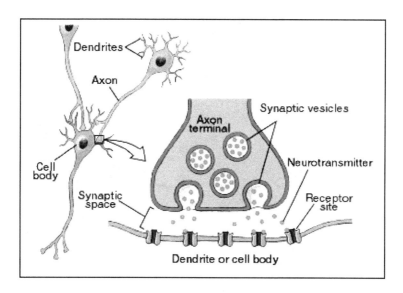

In order for electrical pulses generated by the action potential to cross a synapse, a neurotransmitter is released from one axon ending to travel across the synapse and stimulate receptors of the postsynaptic nerve.

The production of most neurotransmitters takes place in the axon endings of the neuron. The chemical reactions that produce these substances are called *enzymes* and are themselves made in the cell body. Neurotransmitter substances are stored in tiny sacs, called synaptic vesicles, after they have been produced in the axon endings.

When a neuron "fires" (producing an action potential), a number of synaptic vesicles filled with a neurotransmitter migrate to the presynaptic membrane, fasten to it, and then burst forth spilling their contents into the synapse. The whole process of synaptic transmission begins with the nerve impulse, traveling down the axon, reaching the axon endings, and triggering the vesicles' release of the neurotransmitter into the synapse. This release process occurs rather indirectly; the nerve impulse causes calcium (Ca+) ions to enter into the axon endings, and it is actually the Ca+ that triggers the release. When Ca+ enters the axon endings and facilitates the releasing process, it "primes" the vesicle to rupture and disperse the neurotransmitters into the synapse. The importance of Ca+ to synaptic transmission cannot be emphasized enough, because without it the synapse is rendered inoperative.

As a released neurotransmitter diffuses across the synapse and meets with the postsynaptic membrane, it attaches to the membrane. The postsynaptic membrane contains structural "slots" that relate to the molecular shape of the neurotransmitter (see Figure below).

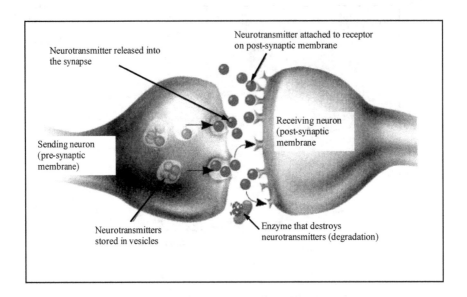

Neurotransmitter released into the synapse

Neurotransmitter attached to receptor on post-synaptic membrane

Sending neuron (pre-synaptic membrane)

Receiving neuron (post-synaptic membrane

Neurotransmitters stored in vesicles

Enzyme that destroys neurotransmitters (degradation)

These slots, called receptor sites, are specialized protein molecules embedded in the postsynaptic membrane. The process of the neurotransmitter attaching to a receptor is called *binding*. Once it binds, the postsynaptic receptor opens a neurotransmitter-dependent ion channel which then allows particular ions to pass through the membrane, changing the local membrane potential. Stating it another way, the neurotransmitter will bind at a receptor site and produce a change in the postsynaptic membrane's permeability to a certain type of ion, that either excites or inhibits a nerve impulse.

Unlike the membrane along the neuron's axon that is controlled by the electrical charge across its membrane, the postsynaptic nerve is controlled by chemical neurotransmitters that interact with the membrane. When neurotransmitters bind to receptors, they literally change the shape of the protein-molecule receptor site, opening ion channels and inhibiting the receiving neuron.

Neurotransmitters open ion channels in two ways. The primary way is where the neurotransmitter (known as the *first messenger)* binds directly at the receptor site producing changes. Some receptors can not open ion channels directly from the neurotransmitter but instead produce the so called *second messenger,* composed of cyclic nucleotides. Attached to the receptors of the postsynaptic membrane at some synapses are molecules of an enzyme called *adenylate cyclase.*

When this receptor binds with a certain type of neurotransmitter, *adenylate cylcase* activate causing *adenosine triphosphate* (ATP) to be converted into *cyclic AMP* (cyclic adenosine monophosphate). After the cyclic AMP triggers the opening of ion channels, it is destroyed by the enzyme *phosphodiesterase.* Most drugs of abuse act on second messenger systems and thus impair the nerve impulse.

The two types of binding produce different changes in neuron membrane permeability that apparently mediates different types of behavior. The direct first messenger system initiates a rapid, brief change in the membrane causing rapid behaviors such as muscle contractions and quick response movements. Second messenger systems produce slow and relatively long-lasting changes in the membrane (from minutes to hours) causing long-term alterations in behavior such as learning and memory.

Synaptic Defenses (Keys to Drug Mechanism of Action)
Whether an interaction in synapse is direct or indirect, the duration of that action and the impact it has on the postsynaptic membrane is very brief. Soon after the process initiates, the neurotransmitter is eliminated from the synaptic environment. Apparently, the human brain is extremely conservative in its chemical interactions within the synapse. That is, almost as soon as the neurotransmitter is released into synapse, it is removed or eliminated.

Behavioral homeostasis, the person's maximum capacity defined by his or her genetics and environment, is maintained by four neurological dynamics or "defenses" that take place in the synapse: *binding, reuptake, enzymatic degradation* and *autoreceptor function.*

The biological objective, an innate biological imperative which seeks to maintain behavioral homeostasis, is to keep the synapse chemically stabilized. Therefore, postsynaptic membrane activation can not be too long or too short in intensity and duration. The four synaptic defenses work in concert with each other to accommodate the biological objective for behavioral homeostasis. When the synaptic environment becomes hyperactive (too active) or hypoactive (under active), because of too much or too little neurotransmitter release, behavioral homeostasis becomes compromised.

Binding serves two primary functions. As mentioned, binding is where the neurotransmitter diffuses across the synapse and occupies a receptor site on the postsynaptic membrane where it will excite or inhibit an action potential. The second function of binding involves its role as a synaptic defense. Binding can be viewed as a process by which the neurotransmitter is removed from the synaptic environment. When a neurotransmitter binds at a receptor site, it is cleared from synapse. Thus, binding also maintains chemical stability within the synapse to further assist in maintaining homeostasis.

The postsynaptic changes induced by neurotransmitters at receptor sites are kept brief primarily through the process called *reuptake.* This is the rapid removal of the neurotransmitter from the synapse by the axon endings. When an action potential arrives, the axon endings release a small amount of neurotransmitter substance into the synapse and then take it back, giving the postsynaptic membranes only a brief exposure of the substance. Thus, reuptake essentially removes the neurotransmitter from synapse and thereby helps to maintain chemical stability.

Enzymatic Degradation is the synaptic defense where an enzyme destroys the neurotransmitter molecule. Enzymatic degradation can take place in the fluid inside of the cell (called cytoplasm or intracellular fluid) and outside of the cell within the synapse area (called extracellular fluid). Enzymatic degradation changes the structure of a neurotransmitter rendering it useless, where it eventually gets "washed out" of the synapse.

For example, neurotransmission at synapses on muscle fibers and at some points between neurons is mediated by the neurotransmitter called acetylcholine (ACh). ACh is destroyed by an enzyme called *acetylcholine esterase* (AChE) where it cleaves the ACh into its constituents of choline and acetate. Because neither of these constituents is capable of binding at receptors along the postsynaptic membrane, they are removed from the synapse. Many types of neurotransmitters have specific enzymes responsible for their degradation as well, although the type of degradation process will vary. However the manner of enzymatic degradation, the process itself is yet another way of removing neurotransmitters from synapse and thus serves to help maintain the chemical stability to insure homeostasis.

The amount of neurotransmitter released by a neuron seems to be controlled by a kind of biochemical "feedback" mechanism. Generally, after a neurotransmitter is released, it not only diffuses across the synapse and acts on postsynaptic membranes, but it also chemically "informs" the presynaptic neuron about the relative level of its own presence. In other words, presynaptic neurons have specialized receptors called *autoreceptors,* that keep the presynaptic neuron informed about the level of its own neurotransmitter in the synapse. The presynaptic receptors essentially respond to the transmitter substance that they release.

Autoreceptors can be found on the membrane of any part of the cell including the axon ending, soma or dendrite. Autoreceptors regulate internal processes of the neuron. So if there is too little or too much, the production of neurotransmitters is adjusted accordingly. When neurotransmitters are removed from the synapse by autoreceptors, the synaptic environment is helped to maintain chemical stability. Thus, in addition to the feedback function, autoreceptors are also a synaptic defense.

It is important to understand events at synapse because most psychoactive drugs act there to produce their effects. That is, drugs alter various events taking place in the synapse. Actually, *psychoactive drugs produce their effects on the nervous system by interrupting one or more of the synaptic defenses.*
The action of psychoactive drugs depends on what synaptic defense they alter;

antipsychotic drugs prevent binding by blocking receptors, methamphetamines increase production of newly synthesized neurotransmitter and blocks reuptake as well as enzymatic degradation. Some of the new antidepressants (such as mitrazepine) also affect autoreceptor function. Drugs affect one or more synaptic defenses, causing their mechanism of action as either an agonist or antagonist and also the drug's side effects.

Pharmacology of synapses

In behavioral pharmacology, scientists have discovered many drugs that affect the production, storage, release, deactivation, or re-uptake of neurotransmitters or that stimulate or block postsynaptic receptor sites. Many of these drugs are developed to study the functions of the nervous system and others are used to treat mental illness.

A drug's *mechanism of action* is its ability to produce effects. Drugs have a very general mechanism of action as either a direct-acting or indirect-acting agonist or antagonist or a combination of the two, known as a partial agonist-antagonist. As you recall from previous sections, an agonist is a drug that facilitates the effects of a particular neurotransmitter on the postsynaptic neuron, meaning that it will stimulate a receptor. An antagonist drug counteracts or inhibits the effects of a particular neurotransmitter on the postsynaptic neuron.

There are a variety of ways that drugs can act as agonists and/or antagonists. First, a neurotransmitter substance must be synthesized from its precursor (usually an amino acid). It has been noted in some cases, that the rate of neurotransmitter production and release can be affected when a precursor is administered. In these cases, the precursor itself acts as an agonist (i.e. the substance, *L-DOPA)*.

The process of converting an amino acid precursor into a neurotransmitter is controlled by enzymes. Thus, if a drug deactivates one of these enzymes, it prevents the neurotransmitter from being manufactured. The drug, *a-methyl-p-tyrosine* (AMPT) blocks the enzyme tyrosine hydroxylase and therefore prevents the synthesis of the catecholamine neurotransmitters (norepinephrine and dopamine). AMPT would thus be considered an antagonist

Neurotransmitters, when synthesized are placed in synaptic vesicles and stored until they are needed in synapse. A drug called *reserpine* deteriorates the membrane of those vesicles containing the monoamine neurotransmitters (norepinephrine, dopamine and serotonin). When the vesicle is "eaten away" by the drug, the neurotransmitters spill out of the vesicle into the cytoplasm of the presynaptic membrane where they are destroyed by enzymes. As this occurs, the neurotransmitter is eliminated before it gets placed into synapse. Resperpine, then, is considered a monoamine antagonist drug.

Other drugs act as antagonists by preventing the release of neurotransmitters from the axon endings. *Botulinum* toxin, produced by bacteria that grow in improperly canned food, prevents the release of a neurotransmitter called acetylcholine (ACh). Other drugs can act as agonists by stimulating the release of a neurotransmitter. Venom from the black widow spider, for example, causes massive ACh release.

Once the neurotransmitter is released into synapse, it must bind at receptor sites to produce an action. Some drugs act as agonists by binding with receptor sites and the activating them directly, mimicking neurotransmitters. Nicotine, for example, activates one of the acetylcholine receptor subtypes. Other drugs bind at receptor sites but do not activate them and thus prevent the neurotransmitter from any action. These drugs, called *receptor blockers*, and act as antagonists such as the anti-psychotic drugs.

Presynaptic membranes of some neurons have autoreceptors which help to regulate the amount of neurotransmitter that is released. Stimulation of these autoreceptors reduces the release of the neurotransmitter. There are drugs that selectively activate autoreceptors but do not activate the postsynaptic receptor sites and thus function as antagonists. One of the mechanisms of action of *LSD*, for example, is that it stimulates serotonin autoreceptors and thus, inhibits serotonin release.

As you know, enzymatic degradation essentially removes neurotransmitters from the synapse. Drugs that deactivate these enzymes will allow excess of neurotransmitters to remain in the synapse for a longer duration where they will continue to bind and stimulate receptor sites. For example, a drug called *phenelzine* blocks the enzyme that degrades the monoamine neurotransmitters and therefore is a monoamine agonist. Since enzyme degradation will reduce neurotransmitter activity, blocking the enzyme results in an increase in neurotransmitter activity and therefore the action would be considered an agonist.

The illustration below (see Figure below) show how agonist and antagonist dynamics can occur. Whether induced artificially by drugs or not, neurotransmitter impact is also controlled by the sensitivity of the synapse as a whole. That is, there are some compensatory actions of the postsynaptic membrane receptor sites that take place in response to a particular level of neurotransmitter activity. The postsynaptic membrane has the capacity to either increase or decrease the number of receptor sites stimulated by the neurotransmitter, depending on the level and intensity of the neurotransmitter released. In other words, the postsynaptic neuron can alter its sensitivity as a response to different levels of neurotransmitter release. It is as if the system as a whole, determined by it genetic DNA coding, inherently "knows" the optimal level of stimulation, so that when this level is not achieved, receptor sites attempt to compensate for the level of neurotransmitter release.

When the postsynaptic neuron decreases the number of receptors, usually in response to over-active stimulation of neurotransmitters, the change is called postsynaptic subsensitivity or down regulation. Basically, this is the process in which postsynaptic neurons reduce their functioning by desensitizing receptor sites. This is actually what takes place during *cellular tolerance.* Since the number of receptor sites has been reduced, there are fewer "entry points" for substances to bind and stimulate. Therefore, more of the drug may be required to initiate an effect. The postsynaptic neuron also has the ability to increase the number of its receptors, usually in response to an underactive stimulation of neurotransmitters. When this occurs it is called postsynaptic supersensitivity, or up regulation.

How drugs might produce agonist or antagonist actions

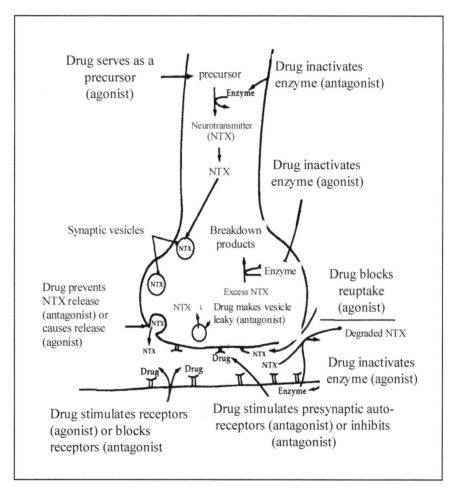

We have covered several ways the synapse can regulate its level of activity — from the synaptic defenses to changes in postsynaptic receptors. This flexibility and resilience helps maintain synaptic activity at optimal levels (homeostasis). Balance in the nervous system largely determines how well a person will respond and overcome distress produced by drugs, neural damage or even defective genes. There is a limit, however, to what the synapse might take to achieve optimal balance.

When the synapses are pushed beyond these limits, the behavioral results can be devastating, ranging from emotional difficulties to motor impairment.

Fun Facts about Neurons! Did you know . . .

- The whole of the nervous system is made up of cells called neurons and there are about 100,000,000,000 (1011) neurons in the brain. This number is too large to comprehend but it would take roughly 30,000 years to count each neuron taking one second for each cell counted.
- All neurons have the same general function; extending from the cell body are dendrites which receive impulses; and an axon which transmits impulses.
- The neuron provides the basis for all activities in the nervous system. It is the single unit of communication that underlies behavior.
- Neurons are different from other cells in two ways; 1) they can conduct electro-chemical information over long distances and 2) they relate to other neurons and tissue areas in a highly specialized manner.
- The neuron consists of a cell body (or soma), an axon which carries information away from the cell body, and dendrites which carry information toward the cell body. Some axons are surrounded by a layer of fatty tissue called a myelin sheath which serves as a protective coating and to direct the flow of the nerve impulse.
- A neuron transmits information along its fibers in the form of electric signals and transmits information to other neurons by using chemical signals.
- The ability of the neuron to transmit information from one site to another is a function of its electrochemical capability and its capacity to synthesize, store, and release transmitter substances from its axon endings.
- Each neuron is in contact with about 1,000 other neurons in the brain.
- The synapse is the microscopic area in which messages are transmitted from one neuron to another. When an electrical signal reaches the synapse, it causes the neuron to release a chemical substance which diffuses across the synaptic gap to the next neuron, which converts the chemical message back into electricity.
- There are at least 100,000,000,000,000 (1014) possible synapses in the brain. This number exceeds the number of particles in the known universe. The number of possible synapses in the human brain (1014) is also greater than the number of stars in our galaxy. However, the number of possible synaptic connections in the human brain is virtually without limit.

CHAPTER 3: SELF-STUDY QUESTIONS

TRUE/FALSE

1. *The brain is composed of two classes of cells: the nerve cell (neuron) and the glial cell.*

2. *Within the soma (cell body) is the nucleus, a structure where neurotransmitters are made from amino acids.*

3. *Neurons communicate with each other and dendrites serve as important recipients of these neurochemical messages.*

4. *The neuron, like an electrical wire, is a conductor of electricity.*

5. *A drug's mechanism of action is its ability to produce lasting and permanent neural changes in the person ingesting various substances.*

6. *Down regulation refers to the concept of cellular tolerance.*

7. *Up regulation is also referred to as postsynaptic supersensitivity.*

8. *There are five synaptic defenses: binding, reuptake, enzymatic degradation, autoreceptors and metabolism.*

9. *Neurotransmitters, when synthesized and produced, are placed in synaptic vesicles and stored until they are needed in synapse.*

10. *Receptor blockers act as antagonists and include such compounds as the antipsychotic drugs.*

* Answers to Self Study Tests are located on page 351

Chapter 3 Selected Reading

Bart, G. *et al. Neuropsychopharmacology* **30**, 417–422 (2005).

Gerrits, M.A., Petromilli, P., Westenberg, H.G., Di Chiara, G. & van Ree, J.M. *Brain Res.* **924**, 141–150 (2002).

Hamilton, L. W. & Timmons, C. R. *Principles of behavioral pharmacology: a biopsychological perspective.* Englewood Cliffs, NJ: Prentice-Hall. (1990).

Hester, R. & Garavan, H. *J. Neurosci.* **24**, 11017–11022 (2004).

Hitner, H, and Nagle, BT. *Pharmacology: An Introduction.* Career Education. (2004).

Kamienski, M, and Keogh, J. *Pharmacology Demystified.* McGraw-Hill Professional. (2005).

Katzung, BG. *Basic and Clinical Pharmacology.* McGraw-Hill Medical. 2006.
Golan, DE, et al. *Principles of Pharmacology: The Pathophysiologic Basis of Drug Therapy.* Lippincott Williams & Wilkins. (2007).

Kish, S.J. *et al. Neuropsychopharmacology* **24**, 561–567 (2001).

O'Malley, S.S., Krishnan-Sarin, S., Farren, C., Sinha, R. & Kreek, M.J. *Psychopharmacology (Berl.)* **160**, 19–29 (2002).

Oslin, D.W. *et al. Neuropsychopharmacology* **28**, 1546–1552 (2003).

Rammes, G. *et al. Neuropharmacology* **40**, 749–760 (2001).

Woodrow, R, and George, D. *Essentials of Pharmacology for Health Occupations.* Thomson Delmar Learning. (2006).

CHAPTER 4: VOCABULARY LIST

Acetylcholine (ACh) is a white crystalline derivative of choline that is released at the ends of nerve fibers in the somatic and parasympathetic nervous systems and is involved in the transmission of nerve impulses in the body. ACh associated with the biochemistry of memory and movement.

Dopamine (DA) is a monoamine neurotransmitter formed in the brain by the decarboxylation of dopa and essential to the normal functioning of the central nervous system specific to the behaviors of mood, movement, motivation and pleasure.

Gamma amino butyric acid (GABA) is the primary inhibitory neurotransmitter in the central nervous system. It plays an important role in regulating neuronal excitability. GABA is also directly responsible for the regulation of muscle tone.

Glutamate (Glu) is an amino acid, the salt (glutamate) of which functions as a neurotransmitter. Glu is secreted in many areas of the brain and by some neurons in the spinal cord where its effects are generally excitatory.

Histamine A biologically active amine that is formed by the decarboxylation of the amino acid histadine. It is widely distributed in nature and is found in tissues as well as in venoms. In humans, histamine is a mediator of inflammatory reactions, and it functions as a stimulant of hydrochloric acid secretion in the stomach.

Large molecule Neuroactive peptides weighing above 1000M, neurotransmitters including the endorphins.

Leu-enkephalin Leucine -enkephalin, critical to pain sensation and suppression (analgesia).

Met-enkephalin Methionine-enkephalin, critical to pain sensation and suppression (analgesia).

Monoamines The group of 3 neurotransmitters, norepinephrine, dopamine, and serotonin, made from a single amino precursor.

Monoamine oxidase (MAO) is the enzyme that degrades any of the monoamine neurotransmitters.

Norepinephrine   *(NE) is both a hormone and neurotransmitter, secreted by the adrenal medulla and the nerve endings of the sympathetic nervous system to cause vasoconstriction and increases in heart rate, blood pressure, and the sugar level of the blood. Also called noradrenaline. Centrally, NE needed for* mood, sleep, memory, attention and sensation.

Small molecule   *Most common neurotransmitters weighing below 1000M*
neurotransmitters   *and not proteinacious.*

Serotonin   *Also known as 5-hydroxytryptamine (5-HT), is a neurotransmitter derived from an indole-containing amino acid, tryptophan. 5-HT important in the behaviors of mood, sleep, appetite, and pain sensation.*

CHAPTER 4: THE CHEMISTRY OF BEHAVIOR

Chemical messengers that communicate neurological information from neuron to neuron are called *neurotransmitters*. While there may be over 100 different types of neurotransmitters in the brain and body, only a few have beep extensively studied with respect to their relationship in behavioral disorders.

It is not the objective of this work to describe all of the known neurotransmitters, but to provide the reader with an overview of those principal chemical messengers that are most often associated with substance abuse and mental health disorders.

Neurotransmitters produce two general effects on the postsynaptic membrane — either excitation (depolarization) or inhibition (hyperpolarization). Since there are only two general effects, one might imagine that there only needs to be two types of neurotransmitters. However, the type of behavior that a neurotransmitter produces is not simply a matter of whether it excites or inhibits.

In fact, behavior is determined by the *locus of activity* (location in the nervous system where an event takes place) and the neurotransmitter involved. Thus, the same neurotransmitter in a different part of the nervous system might create different effects, and different neurotransmitters in the same area of the nervous system will produce different behaviors. For example, the neurotransmitter dopamine in the midbrain substantia nigras coordinates movement, whereas dopamine in the medial forebrain bundle has more to do with emotions and pleasure.

Further complicating the neurobiology of behavior is the fact that no single neuron releases all neurotransmitters. Each neuron stores and releases only one or two neurotransmitters, and neurons that release a particular neurotransmitter are clustered together to form neural pathways (i.e. the "dopamine pathway"). Postsynaptic neurons, on the other hand, receive a number of different neurotransmitters at various synapses.

Finally, there are an abundance of *receptor subtypes* that produce a variance of different behavioral responses when activated. Some postsynaptic neurons have a large number of receptor subtypes, like the serotonin system which has at least eighteen identified receptor subtypes. Since these subtypes possess slightly different protein structures, drugs selective for a given subtype can be developed. Drugs with greater selectivity to target specific receptor subtypes can have significantly reduced unwanted side effects.

Many of the newer psychiatric medications, for example, have a much greater selectivity to specific receptor subtypes where the therapeutic effect is obtained with fewer side effects. Clozapine, for example, is the prototypical antipsychotic and has more selective actions at certain receptor sites.

A drug's action relates to the neurotransmitters it affects. Behavioral pharmacology seeks to understand a particular drug's mechanism of action by identifying which neurotransmitter systems the drug targets, whether it is an agonist or antagonist, and what are the observed behavioral changes, some of which may be toxic.

To qualify as a neurotransmitter, a chemical must meet four criteria as outlined in the box below.

NEUROTRANSMITTER CRITERIA

1. It is synthesized within the neuron and present within the axon endings.

2. It is released in sufficient amounts that produce a defined action on the postsynaptic neuron (or effector organ).

3. When administered from the outside (exogenously), such as a drug, it mimics the action of endogenously (from within) released neurotransmitters by activating the same ion channels or second-messenger systems in the postsynaptic neuron.

4. Specific mechanisms exist for the removal of the substance from its site of action (the synapse).

Small and Large-Molecule Neurotransmitters

Neurotransmitters are classified into two general groups, based on their molecular weights and chemical composition: small-molecule and large-molecule neurotransmitters. The *small-molecule neurotransmitters* are those chemicals normally associated with the term "neurotransmitter". These neurotransmitters have molecular weights below 1000M and are not proteinaceous. There are nine small-molecule neurotransmitters, eight amines plus the non-amine ATP, and of these eight amines, seven are amino acids or their derivatives.

The primary small-molecule neurotransmitters are dopamine, norepinephrine, serotonin, acetylcholine, glutamate, GABA (y-aminobutyric acid), and histamine (H). *Large-molecule neurotransmitters* (also called neuroactive peptides) are proteins that have molecular weights above 1000M, including endorphins, enkephalins, methionine, cholecystokinin, ACTH (adrenocortocotropic hormone), vasopressin and Substance P. The general effects on behavior of both the small and large-molecule neurotransmitters are shown in the charts below.

Principal Small-Molecule Neurotransmitters		
Type	Receptor Sites	General Functions
Dopamine (DA)	D1 through D5 in two families designated *D1* and *D2*	Mood, movement reward, pleasure, olfaction, concentration, attention
Norepinephrine (NE)	Alpha 1, Alpha 1a, Beta 1, Beta 2, and Beta 3	Mood, sleep, learning, memory, attention, concentration, mental alertness, anxiety and sensory processing
Serotonin (5-HT)	18 identified receptors designated into 8 families 5-HT1 through 5-HT 8	Mood, sleep, pain processing, appetite, sex, and aggression.
Acetylcholine(A Ch)	Muscarinic (M1 through M5) and Nicotinic (NN and NM)	Movement, motor coordination, memory, and sensory processing
Gamma-amino butyric acid (GABA)	GABA A and GABA B	Major inhibitory function within CNS
Glutamate (Glu)	NMDA, Quisqualate and Kainate	Memory, major excitatory function within the nervous system
Histamine (H)	H1 and H2	Sleep, sedation, temperature regulation

Principal Large-Molecule Neurotransmitters (neuropeptides)	
Type	General Functions
Endorphins	Suppression of pain, learning, memory and pleasure
Enkephalins Leucine	Suppression of pain, learning, memory and pleasure
Cholecystokinin	Regulation of food intake
Adrenocorticotropic hormone (ACTH)	Energy production, water intake, learning and memory
Vasopressin	Learning and memory, vasocontrcition, raises blood pressure, and reduces excretion of urine.
Substance P	Perception of pain. Transmission of pain impulses from peripheral receptors to the central nervous system.

The following provides an overview of the small-molecule neurotransmitters and their general functions within the nervous system. Included also is an overview of the receptor sub-types for each of the neurotransmitters discussed.

Dopamine

Dopamine is made from the amino acid *tyrosine*. In the CNS, DA originates in two brain areas: the substantia nigras and the ventral tegmental area (VTA). It is then extended by three major pathways into other areas of the brain including the hypothalamus, the frontal lobes and the medial forebrain bundle (MFB). DA in the midbrain substantia nigras, the nigrostriatal pathway, is involved in the control of fine skeletal muscle movement (basal ganglia).

DA activity in the hypothalamus would suggest that it plays a role in autonomic functions. Degeneration of dopamine within the substantia nigras has been linked with Parkinson's disease, a movement disorder characterized by symptoms of tremors, muscle rigidity, compromised balance and difficulty in initiating movements. In the frontal lobes, DA is important in regulating thought and, via the nucleus accumbens within the MFB, is a principal substance that provides the chemical basis for the reward circuitry. DA has also been of great interest in its association with the thought disorder of schizophrenia.

Research studies from the 1960s discovered that antipsychotic drugs were effective in alleviating the symptoms of schizophrenia. There was evidence that antipsychotics were interfering with transmission of DA synapses. Studies have shown that the primary mechanism of action of antipsychotic drugs is binding and blocking a DA receptor sub-type called D2.

Interestingly, in contrast to the blocking actions of the antipsychotic drugs, DA agonist drugs such as cocaine or amphetamine, that mimic the actions of DA, can induce psychotic features. While it is tempting indeed to believe that schizophrenia is the result of a hyperactive DA system, studies have shown that DA, by itself, is not the single cause of the disorder. Nonetheless, DA is strongly associated with the condition of schizophrenia, although the disorder includes other systems and neurotransmitters.

It is generally agreed upon that the brain's reward circuitry is the main area where DA reinforces drug abuse, the DA-rich circuit that involves the mesolimbic pathway, the nucleus accumbens and the ventral tegmental area. Studies have demonstrated that drugs which have the potential for abuse demonstrate their agonist actions within the mesolimbic pathway involving the reward circuitry. DA's role in governing the brain's pleasure center is well documented, and the section on the neurobiology of reward will provide a detailed account of that information.

Most DA, when released into synapse, is eliminated through reuptake. However, there are two enzymes that are active in degrading excess DA. The first is called *monoamine oxidase* (MAO), found in both presynaptic and postsynaptic membranes. The second enzyme is called *catechol-O-methyltransferase* (COMT) located in the synaptic gap.

There are five DA receptor sub-types that have been identified to dart, labeled D1 through D5. D1 and D5 receptors will stimulate the synthesis of cAMP second messenger systems whereas D2 will inhibit cAMP activity. The action of receptors D3 and D4 have not yet been fully determined. Interestingly however, the some antipsychotic drugs like Clozaril and Olanzapine possess a mechanism of action that includes blocking the D4 receptor site. Yet, the function of this particular receptor site in behavioral health is not fully known.

The Dopamine Pathways in the Brain
Dopamine is transmitted via three major pathways. The first extends from the substantia nigra to the caudate nucleus-putamen (striatum) and is concerned with sensory stimuli and movement. The second pathway projects from the ventral tegmentum to the mesolimbic forebrain and is associated with cognitive, reward and emotional behavior. The third pathway is concerned with neuronal control of the hypothalmic-pituatory endocrine system.

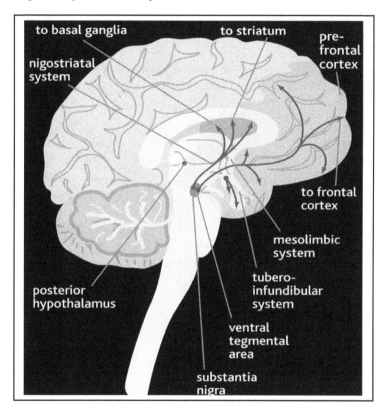

Norepinephrine
Norepinephrine (NE) is found in both the peripheral and central nervous systems, and is synthesized from the amino acid *tyrosine,* as is dopamine. In fact, DA can be considered a precursor to norepinephrine because it is the second step of a three-step process in converting tyrosine to NE. In the PNS, NE is the main neurotransmitter within the sympathetic nervous system, and is the primary substance where nerves innervate at target organs (involved in the fight-or-flight response). In the CNS, NE is involved in mood control, cortical arousal, pleasure, and cognitive behaviors of attenuation, concentration and focusing.

The Noradrenaline Pathways in the Brain

Many regions of the brain are supplied by the noradrenergic systems. The principal centers for noradrenergic neurons are the locus coeruleus and the caudal raphe nuclei. The ascending nerves of the locus coeruleus project to the frontal cortex, thalamus, hypothalamus and limbic system. Noradrenaline is also transmitted from the locus coeruleus to the cerebellum. Nerves projecting from the caudal raphe nuclei ascend to the amygdala and descend to the midbrain.

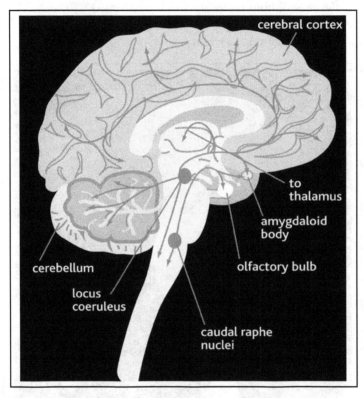

Synapses that use NE are called *adrenergic* or *noradrenergic* synapses. With depolarization and Ca+ intake, the NE is released and acts on postsynaptic receptors, called -*alpha*-adrenergic receptors (αl). This primarily affects Ca+ channels mediated through second messengers. In addition, the released NE acts on presynaptic axon endings at receptors called α2-adrenergic receptors. It is known that α2-adrenergic receptors will control the activity at synapse. In norepinephrine systems, there is a second type of adrenergic receptor called the *beta* (β) receptor. This receptor differs from the alpha receptor mainly by being primarily postsynaptic and connected to the c-AMP second messenger system.

Stimulant drugs act as agonists within the NE system, but with a variety of different mechanisms. Cocaine will increase NE synaptic activity by increasing biosynthesis and release of newly formed NE molecules then blocking reuptake. Methamphetamine will do the same, but will also inhibit enzyme degradation.

Contrasting this, noradrenergic antagonists, such as some antipsychotic drugs, will reduce NE activity, thus significantly reducing excitement and hypomania.

The alpha receptors, located in the PNS (peripheral nervous system) affect sympathetic responses including blood vessel constriction. As such, antagonist drugs specific to these receptors are useful in treating high blood pressure. Other adrenergic receptors within the PNS govern additional sympathetic responses. β receptors located on the heart muscle can be antagonized by "beta-blockers" to treat cardiac arrhythmia (irregular heart beat). NE activity is terminated by two mechanisms: reuptake (the primary method of terminating the NE), and enzymatic degradation by both MAO and COMT (the same enzymes that terminate DA).

Currently there are five NE receptor sub-types which are grouped into two categories: the *alpha-adrenergic* and *beta-adrenergic* receptors. Within the a-adrenergic system are the receptors Alpha 1 and Alpha 1a. Within the β-adrenergic systems are the receptors Beta 1, Beta 2, and Beta 3.

Serotonin
Approximately 98% of serotonin (5-HT, for *5- hydroxytryptamine)* is located outside of the CNS and in the gastrointestinal tracts and platelets. 5-HT is synthesized from the amino acid *tryptophan.* The storage, release and termination of serotonin is essentially the same as for DA and NE, with the exception that 5-HT is only metabolized by MAO enzymes. The reuptake process for 5-HT is also identical to the termination of DA and NE.

The interest in the behavioral actions of 5-HT began in the 1950s with the realization that its molecular structure resembled *d-lysergic acid diethylamide* (LSD), and the discovery that LSD antagonized intestinal smooth muscles. 5-HT has been the focus of research in the 1980s and 1990s, with many new discoveries about its extensive role in behavior. The 5-HT system has the largest number of receptor subtypes, numbering eighteen to date, which are divided into eight families or categories.

The Serotonin Pathways in the Brain
The principal center for serotonergic neurons is the raphe nuclei. From the raphe nuclei axons ascend to the cerebral cortex, limbic regions and specifically to the basal ganglia. Serotonergic nuclei in the brain stem give rise to descending axons, some of which terminate in the medulla, while others descend the spinal cord.

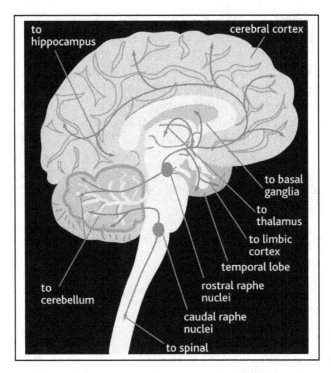

The following briefly summarizes the current understanding of the most widely studied serotonin (5-HT) receptors. Note that some 5-HT receptors affect other neurotransmitter systems. For example, when a particular 5-HT receptor site is stimulated, it may act as an antagonist to other neurotransmitter systems (i.e 5-HT3 receptors will cause a decrease in acetylcholine). Still other 5-HT receptor sites, when stimulated, will influence the release of neurotransmitters from different systems (i.e., 5-HT1B receptors will indirectly cause an increase in dopamine release).

5-HT1 Receptors
These receptors appear to be involved in the processes of smooth muscle relaxation, contraction of some cardiac and vascular smooth muscle, rejunctional inhibition of neurotransmitter release, and effects in the CNS. Five subtypes have been proposed, four of which appear to play a major role in humans.

5-HT1A
This represents perhaps the most widely studied 5-HT receptor subtype. These receptors are located primarily in the CNS. Agonists facilitate male sexual behavior in rats, increase food intake, produce hypothermia and hypotension, and reduce anxiety. This receptor has also been widely implicated in depression. When multiple 5-HT agonist drugs are used concurrently, such as the antidepressants Prozac, Zoloft and Paxil, the overactivity can result in the serotonin syndrome, marked by symptoms of confusion, hyperreflexia, ataxia and hypertension. Over activation of

the 5-HT1A receptors is most likely the cause of this syndrome. In the hippocampus, postsynaptic 5- HT1A receptors play an important role in preventing the adverse physiologic effects of chronic stress.

5-HT1B

These may serve as autoreceptors; thus, their activation causes inhibition of neurotransmitter release. Agonists inhibit aggressive behavior and food intake in rodents. 5-HT1B receptors, which have been identified only in rodents and are apparently absent in humans, are therefore only of theoretical interest at present. These receptors may be the counterpart of the 5-HT1D receptor found in other species

5-HT1c

These receptors belong to the same receptor subfamily as the 5-HT2 receptor and have been recently renamed as 5-HT2c receptors. They are located in high density in the choroid plexus and may regulate cerebrospinal fluid production and cerebral circulation. This subtype is speculated to be involved in the regulation of analgesia, sleep and cardiovascular function.

5-HT1D

Located primarily in the CNS, this subtype may play a role as a presynaptic heteroreceptor or as a terminal autoreceptor, inhibiting neurotransmitter release by mediating a negative feedback effect. This subtype is the most abundant 5-HT1 receptor in the CNS but is also found in vascular smooth muscle mediating contraction. While the role of activation of this receptor subtype is not fully understood, agonists at this site are effective in treating acute migraine headaches. The development of selective antagonists of this receptor should clarify the functional role of 5- HT1D receptors in the CNS.

5-HT2 Receptors

Located primarily in vascular smooth muscles, platelets, lungs, CNS, and the GI tract, these appear to be involved in gastrointestinal and vascular smooth muscle contraction, blood platelet aggregation, hypertension, migraine, and neuronal depolarization. Antagonists have potential use as antipsychotic agents. Because these receptors belong to the same receptor subfamily as the former 5-HT1c receptors, they have been recently renamed as 5-HT2A receptors. The activation of the 5-HT2A receptors seems to increase the release of the neurotransmitters dopamine, acetylcholine, GABA and glutamate.

5-HT2A receptors are implicated in behavioral problems of hallucinations and depression, and may play a role in sleep as well. 5-HT2B receptors are located in the cortex, hypothalamus, and parts of the limbic system, and also found on postsynaptic membranes in these areas. These receptors are involved in anxiety states. The 5-HT2c receptors may play a role in depression, hallucinations, appetite, anxiety, memory and migraines.

They also seem to be important in producing cerebrospinal fluid. The 5-HT2A and 5-HT2c receptors (where most hallucinogens are partial agonists), become downregulated with prolonged use of antidepressants. Serotonin itself has a greater affinity for 5-HT2c receptors than for 5-HT2A receptors. Some of the newer antipsychotic drugs, such as *risperidone*, are antagonists at both 5-HT2A and 5-HT2c receptors.

5-HT3 Receptors
Located primarily in peripheral and central neurons, these receptors appear to be involved in the activation of peripheral neurons, pain, and the emesis (vomiting) reflex. The 5-HT3 receptors are excitatory and may be involved in anxiety. Agents acting at this site have potential use for curing migraines, anxiety or cognitive and psychotic disorders. Discovered in the 1950's, the 5-HT3 receptors were originally called M receptors because morphine was an antagonist on them. They are also involved in euphoria as the activation of 5-HT3 receptors decreases acetylcholine release which, in turn, augments dopamine release.

Drugs such as ondansetron and zacopride are antagonists of the 5-HT3 receptors and have been used as anti-emetics, and in other cases, for memory augmentation in Alzheimer's patients. Their use is being explored for possible anti-craving treatments for alcoholism and cocaine addiction.

5-HT4 Receptors
These receptors are found in the CNS, the heart, and the GI tract. Their activation produces an increase in cyclic adenosine monophosphate (cAMP), and appears to involve activation of neurotransmitter release. The neurotransmitters norepinephrine, dopamine and serotonin are sometimes categorically referred to as the monoamines, of which there are two sub-categories: the catecholamines, including norepinephrine and dopamine (since they are built from a catechol nuclear structure), and the indolamines, which include serotonin. One may often come across the words *catecholaminergic* or *indolaminergic,* which indicate the type of monoamines a drug is acting on. For example, Paxil is an indolaminergic antidepressant drug in that it is selective in its effects on serotonin systems. Methamphetamine may be considered catecholaminergic, for example.

Acetylcholine
Acetylcholine (ACh) is perhaps the most widely distributed neurotransmitter in the nervous system. In the 1930's, scientists determined that the nerve impulse could not be an entirely electrical event, contrary to popular belief at that time. Scientists confirmed this notion with the discovery of the neurotransmitter acetylcholine (then identified as *vagus stuffe* since it was obtained from the vagus nerve). ACh is synthesized from *acetyl co-enzyme A (acetyl-CoA)* and choline, and is stored in vesicles much like other neurotransmitters. When released into synapse, ACh chemically binds at receptor sites and is terminated by the enzyme *acetylcholinesterase.*

The degradation of acetylcholine results in the liberation of choline, which is then taken back into the presynaptic axon ending and is re-synthesized into newly formed ACh. There are seven acetylcholinergic (also called *cholinergic)* receptor sub-types. These are divided into two families based on whether they are blocked by nicotine or muscarine. The two families are therefore called *muscarinic,* with receptors M1 through M5, and *nicotinic,* containing the receptors NN and NM. The nicotinic cholinergic receptors in the autonomic nervous system are significant in the coordination of movement, where ACh has an excitatory role in the control of skeletal muscles.

Direct binding of ACh at the nicotinic cholinergic receptors in the autonomic nervous system, along with the rapid degradation of the substance at synapse, facilitate quick action as needed for control of the skeletal muscles. In contrast to the nicotinic receptors, muscarinic receptors are typically found where the synapse actions are slower such as in the synapses of motor nerves onto the autonomic ganglia, glands, cardiac and smooth muscle.

Remember that the key substance which chemically drives the autonomic nervous system is acetylcholine. In the CNS, ACh is found in several areas including the brain stem, midbrain regions, hypothalamus, cortical areas and the spinal cord. In the hindbrain, ACh is located within the reticular formation where it is involved in the control of the level of arousal. In the hypothalamus, ACh is involved in the release of *antidiuretic hormone* (ADH) and *adrenocorticotropic hormone* (ACTH) and plays a role in the regulation of body temperature.

The behavioral effects of ACh have been determined by using certain drugs, such as atropine, an antagonist to muscarinic receptors. Muscarinic receptors are largely found in the CNS. Atropine is a drug used medically by ophthamologists who administer it in eye drops to dilate the pupils. Large doses of atropine, however, where excessive muscarinic cholinergic receptor sites have been blocked, will produce an *atropine psychosis* characterized by symptoms of memory impairment, confusion, hallucinations, slurred speech and drowsiness.

Two other cholinergic drugs produce interesting behavioral effects: *curare, a* cholingeric antagonist, and *"nerve gas"* (di-isopropyl fluorophosphate, or *DFP),* a cholinergic agonist. Curare *(d-tubocurarine)* is the substance used by the Jivaro Indians of South America, where they place it on the tips of arrows to paralyze prey. The mechanism of action of curare is an antagonist at the nicotinic cholinergic receptor sites. Nicotinic receptors are largely found in the PNS, as mentioned previously. Curare occupies nicotinic receptors in skeletal muscles and therefore prohibits ACh from binding (an antagonist function). Therefore, the animal struck by a curare-soaked arrow is paralyzed from muscular inhibition since ACh cannot bind and stimulate the nicotinic receptors.

The other drug, Diisopropyl fluorophosphate (DFP), is a nerve gas used in

World War II as a chemical weapon. This cholinergic agonist acts in a unique way in that it inhibits the synaptic defense of enzymatic degradation in cholinergic systems. As you recall, when ACh is released into the synapse it is rapidly removed by the enzyme acetylcholinesterase (AChE). DFP essentially disables AchE, resulting in a hyperactivity of ACh stimulation of postsynaptic neurons. The constant stimulation of receptors produces a flurry of action potentials in the nerves of skeletal muscles which become unable to relax. Constriction of muscles in this way leads to paralysis and eventually asphyxiation.

Some psychiatric medications can inadvertently decrease ACh activity and produce side effects called the anticholinergic syndrome. This syndrome is characterized by urinary retention, dry mouth, photosensitivity, delirium, motor incoordination and tachycardia (rapid heart beat). Drugs such as the typical antipsychotics (i.e. the phenothiazines) and some anti-depressant drugs have greater liability for producing the anticholinergic syndrome. Marijuana produces anticholinergic *symptoms,* but not the syndrome as defined above.

Gamma Aminobutyric Acid

GABA (gamma aminobutyric acid) is considered the most important inhibitory neurotransmitter in the CNS. When binding at the postsynaptic receptor site, it hyperpolarizes the neuron by facilitating chloride (Cl-) ions through the channels which prevents the neuron from depolarization. GABA is terminated at synapse through reuptake into the presynaptic neuron and also in the glial cells. Because GABA is a powerful neural inhibitor, GABA agonists have been developed as sedatives, tranquilizers, antiseizure drugs and anesthetics.

Two categories of GABA receptors have been identified: GABAA and GABAB. Many subunits were found within GABAA receptors, categorized into three different groups *a (alpha), fi (beta)* and *y (gamma).* Each group contains several different subunits, but the exact composition of most GABAA receptors is not known.

In addition, different subunits within each group also differ in pharmacological properties (sensitivity). As a result, the specific subunit composition of a GABAA receptor determines its overall characteristics. GABAA receptors in different parts of the brain also differ in their pharmacological properties. GABAA receptors are found in abundance throughout the brain. This wide distribution may be related to the spectrum of behaviors (i.e., sedation, relaxation or staggering gait) produced by various drugs that are GABAA agonists such as alcohol, benzodiazepines, the barbiturates.

Alcohol significantly alters GABA neurotransmission, and provides some evidence that the GABAA receptors may play a critical role in the tolerance and dependence on alcohol while contributing to the predisposition to alcoholism. GABAB is the other receptor type of which not much is known.

GABA Pathways in the Normal Brain

GABA is the main inhibitory neurotransmitter in the central nervous system (CNS). GABAergic inhibition is seen at all levels of the CNS including the hypothalamus, hippocampus, cerebral cortex and cerebellar cortex. As well as the large well-established GABA pathways, GABA interneurons are abundant in the brain, with 50% of the inhibitory synapses in the brain being GABA mediated.

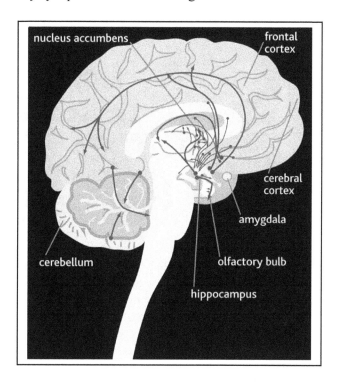

Glutamate

Glutamate (Glu) is a potent neural excitatory substance. It has been known for some time that glutamic acid (Glu) is highly concentrated throughout the brain. Glu is synthesized from glutamine, stored in vesicles, and released depending on the presence of Ca+. Glu acts on postsynaptic receptors that are linked directly to those channels that depolarize the neuron's membrane and create action potentials. Glu is terminated from synapse by reuptake into both the presynaptic neuron and by glial cells as well.

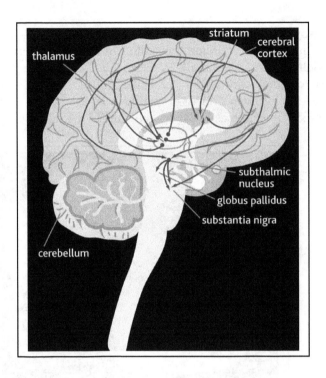

Glu has three receptor subtypes: NMDA (N-methyl-d-aspartate), AMPA (alpha-amino-3- hydroxy-5-methyl-4-isoxazole proprionic acid) and kainate. Of these receptors, NMDA plays a particularly important role in controlling the brain's ability to adapt to environmental and genetic influences.

Glu and its receptor subtype NMDA have been recently studied extensively for their role in addiction. Alcohol, for example, is a potent inhibitor of the function of NMDA receptor. Following chronic exposure of animals to alcohol, there is evidence for an up-regulation of NMDA receptors and a change in the NMDA receptor subunit composition. The time elapsed for this up-regulation parallels the cycle of alcohol withdrawal seizures, which can be attenuated by NMDA receptor antagonists.

Another recent study has provided evidence that the drug *dextromethorphan* – an uncompetitive NMDA antagonist, may facilitate detoxification from heroin and inhibit cravings. Also, after repeated exposure to amphetamine, dopamine neurons within the ventral tegmental area (VTA) are supersensitive to the excitatory effects of Glu and AMPA. Increases in excitatory drive may also reflect effects of amphetamine within the VTA, since studies demonstrate a delayed response in Glu eflux after local amphetamine.

The drug, *acamprosate (Campral) (calcium acetylhomotaurinate)* is being used as an anti-craving medicine in the treatment of alcoholism. Acamprosate,

90

a synthetic compound similar in structure to GABA, is thought to act via several mechanisms affecting multiple neurotransmitter systems including the inhibition of neural excitability by antagonism of NMDA activity and the reduction of Ca+ ion fluxes.

Histamine (H)

Histamine (H) is found in high concentration in both the hypothalamus and reticular formation. Within these areas, H is made from *histadine* and increases cAMP levels by stimulation of adenyl cyclase. The effects of histamine at these sites is primarily inhibitory. There are currently two identified H receptor subtypes: Hi and H2. In the periphery, H is released as part of the body's reaction to allergens (producing common allergy symptoms including coughing and sneezing).

Nitric Oxide: A Novel Neurotransmitter

Nitric oxide (NO), an endogenous substance, relaxes blood vessels, the lungs, the gut, and the genitourinary tract. It is also involved with immunologic defense, and appears to play a role in the function of neurotransmission, insulin secretion, and memory formation.

Only a few years ago, nitric oxide was considered a primarily toxic contributor to smog, acid rain and ozone problems. One reason it may have taken researchers so long to discover its importance is that NO is a very small compound, not stored in vesicles but rather diffuses from its formation directly to its site of action (since it is both water and lipid soluble, it diffuses freely within tissues). As discussed, neurotransmitters are large molecules stored in vesicles and released by specific properties, after which they move to a site of action and bind at a postsynaptic receptor.

In the CNS, NO is a neuronal mediator that may be involved in neurotransmitter release and even memory formation. NO formation in the CNS can be triggered by stimulation of the glutamate receptor. Glutamate, as you recall, is an excitatory neurotransmitter implicated in brain damage after *cerebral ischemia* and stroke. It now appears that stimulation of the glutamate receptor during ischemia causes a prolonged release of NO, with subsequent tissue damage.

Thus, NO can be considered both beneficial (by protecting, enhancing, and mediating neural activity) as well as toxic, where under certain conditions, it indiscriminately destroys neurons.

In the peripheral nervous system, NO seems to function as a transmitter substance of sorts. It is located in nerves of the gastrointestinal (GI) and urogenital systems (so-called nitrogenic neurons) where it is involved in GI peristalsis and penile erection. NO may also cause insulin release, and excess NO may destroy 13 cells during the development of diabetes. More information on this rather unique and new transmitter substance is being discovered as the research continues.

Neuropeptides (Large-Molecule Neurotransmitters)

A peptide is a protein consisting of amino acid chains (many amino acids linked together in a specific sequence). Neuropeptides simply mean those peptides that are neuroactive (i.e. act in the nervous system). A variety of neuropeptides have been discovered and characterized as you noticed in the illustration of large-molecule neurotransmitters.

Enkephalin, the endogenous morphine-like substance, is the best known neuropeptide. There are two types of enkephalins: methionineenkephalin (met-enkephalins) and leucineenkephalin (leu-enkephalins). These substances play a critical role in pain sensation and pain suppression (analgesia). The enkephalins are released throughout the neural pain circuitry, where morphine mimics its action and thus reduces pain. Enkephalins are also found in the limbic system, where their role in pain suppression may be related to how they reduce the emotional response to pain sensation.

Substance P (Sub P), is released by the primary pain fibers in the periphery where sensory neurons signal transmission of pain sensations from the spinal cord to the brain. Substance P is also found throughout the CNS and most notably within the substantia nigras of the midbrain region.

Where enkephalin is an analgesic that suppresses pain, Sub P is the substance that promotes the actual pain sensation. Part of the analgesic mechanism of action of the enkephalins is to block the effect of Sub P.

Cholecystokinin (CCK), the gut peptide known for contracting the gall bladder, is found within the CNS. Many of the neuropeptides (especially cholecystokinin) are "co-localized" with the small-molecule neurotransmitters and function together in a unique way.

For example, dopamine neurons within the substantia nigras and the ventral tegmental area (VTA) increase their rate of depolarization when CCK is applied. Interestingly, there are no current CNS drugs that selectively influence the action of any neuropeptide other than enkephalin and Sub P. This is because the neuropeptides are proteins of large-molecular weight that do not easily enter the brain, and their actions in the CNS cannot be effectively studied following systematic administration. This is disappointing, since many neuropeptides are know to influence very specific regions of the brain.

What neurotransmitter systems best describe drug addiction?

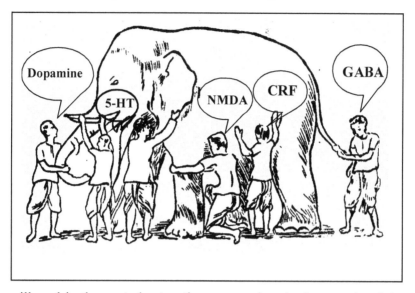

As you will read in the next chapter, there are various brain areas involving several neurotransmitter systems when discussing the neurobiological aspects of drug addiction.

CHAPTER 4: SELF-STUDY QUESTIONS

TRUE/FALSE

1. *Chemical messengers that communicate neurological information from neuron to neuron are called neurotransmitters.*

2. *A drug's mechanism of action is related to the neurotransmitter(s) it affects.*

3. *Neurotransmitters are classified into three general groups based on their molecular weights and chemical composition; small-molecule neurotransmitters, medium-sized neurotransmitters and large-molecule neurotransmitters.*

4. *Large-molecule neurotransmitters are sometimes called neuroactive peptides and include the endorphins.*

5. *There are five dopamine receptor sub-types that have been identified to date, labeled D1 through D5.*

6. *Approximately 98% of the serotonin neurotransmitter systems are located outside of the central nervous system.*

7. *Acetylcholine is perhaps the most widely distributed neurotransmitter in the nervous system.*

8. *GABA is considered the most important excitatory neurotransmitter in the central nervous system.*

9. *Glutamate is a potent neural excitatory substance in the brain with three major receptor sub-types; NMDA, AMPA and kainate.*

10. *Nitric oxide formation in the central nervous system can be triggered by stimulation of the glutamate receptor.*

* Answers to Self Study Tests are located on page 351

Chapter 4 Selected Reading

Agahjanian, G.K., Sprouse, J.S. and Rasmussen, K., "Physiology of the Midbrain Serotonin System," H.Y. Meltzer (editor), *Psychopharmacology: The Third Generation,* Raven Press, New York, 1987.

Alberts, B., A. Johnson, J. Lewis, M. Raff, K. Roberts, and P. Walter. *Molecular Biology of the Cell.* New York: Garland Publishers, 2002.

Ashton, H., *Brain Function and Psychotropic Drugs,* Oxford Press, New York, 1992.

Balster, R.L, L.B. Wingard, Jr., T.M. Brody, J. Lamer, et al (editors), *Human Pharmacology,* Mosby Yearbook, St. Louis, MO, 1991.

Boulton, A,. Baker, GB, and Juorio, AV. *Drugs as Tools in Neurotransmitter Research.* Humana Press. 1989.

Bellen, HJ. *Neurotransmitter Release.* Oxford University Press. 1999.

Carvey, P.M., *Drug Action in the Central Nervous System,* Oxford University Press, New York, 1998

King, M. W., Indiana State University. *Biochemistry of Neurotransmitters.* http://www.indstate.edu/theme/mwking/nerves.html (2004).

Südhof, TC and Starke, K. Pharmacology of Neurotransmitter Release. Springer. 2008.

Von Bohlen, O, and Dermietzel, R. *Neurotransmitters and Neuromodulars-Handbook of Receptors and Biological Effects.* Wiley-VCH. 2006.

Washington State University. "Neurotransmitters and Neuroactive Peptides." *Neuroscience for Kids.* http://faculty.washington.edu/chudler.chnt1.html (2004).

Webster, R. Neurotransmitters, *Drugs and Brain Function.* Wiley. 2001.

SECTION II: BEHAVIORAL PHARMACOLOGY OF SUBSTANCE ABUSE

SECTION INTRODUCTION

At one time, drug addiction was viewed as a failure of willpower or a flaw of moral character. It was not recognized as a disease of the brain, in the same way that mental illnesses previously were not viewed as such. Medical authorities have now accepted drug addiction as a chronic, relapsing condition that alters normal brain function, just as any other neurological or psychiatric illness. Its development and expression are influenced by genetic, biological, psychosocial, and environmental factors. Outwardly, drug addiction is often characterized by impaired control over continued drug use, compulsive use despite harmful consequences, and/or intolerable drug craving.

To understand drug addiction in the 21st century, you need to have the largest possible picture of the associated science, the facts which shape your perceptions, and the existing and emerging approaches to understand and appreciate the new directions of treatment. Investigators have found that drugs like methamphetamine, heroin and alcohol increase the brain's production of dopamine, the neurotransmitter that regulates pleasure, among other things. This helps account for the euphoric high drug users feel. But these drugs deplete the dopamine pathway, disrupting the individual's ability to function.

At the Brookhaven National Laboratory on Long Island, for instance, Dr. Nora D. Volkow has found that even 100 days after a cocaine addict's last dose, there is significant disruption in the brain's frontal cortical area, which governs such attributes as impulse, motivation and drive. Dr. Volkow says that "the disruption of the dopamine pathways leads to a decrease in the reinforcing value of normal things, and this pushes the individual to take drugs to compensate." Other researchers have found a physiological basis for the craving so many addicts experience, but it is not yet clear how long such physiological changes remain.

Dr. Herbert D. Kleber, the medical director of the National Center on Addiction and Substance Abuse in New York, says that the brain-disease concept fits with his experience with thousands of addicts over the years. "No one wants to be an addict," he says. "All anyone wants to be able to do is knock back a few drinks with the guys on Friday or have a cigarette with coffee or take a toke on a crack pipe. But very few addicts can do this. When someone goes from being able to control their habit to mugging their grandmother to get money for their next fix, that convinces me that something has changed in their brain."

From the evidence of the new science of addiction, it seems that drug addiction is a brain disease expressed as compulsive behavior; both its development and the recovery from it depend on the individual's behavior.

Alcohol and drug use begins with an individual's conscious choice, but addiction is not simply using alcohol and drugs in excess. Recent scientific research provides overwhelming evidence that not only do alcohol and other drugs interfere with normal brain functioning by creating powerful feelings of pleasure, but they also have long-term effects on brain metabolism and activity. At some point, changes occur in the brain that produce conditioned urges to repeat drug use, while simultaneously reducing awareness, caution and judgment. It is clear that these are predictable, physiological consequences of substance use, and they explain why those addicted to alcohol and other drugs suffer from a compulsive craving for, and use of, these substances and cannot quit by themselves. Treatment is necessary to end this compulsive behavior.

The word "treatment" may be a misnomer as applied to addiction because it implies a one-time strategy to eliminate the adverse effects of a physiological condition. Like other chronic illnesses such as heart disease or diabetes, treatment of addiction actually refers to an extended process of diagnosis, treatment of acute symptoms, identification and management of circumstances that initially may have promoted the alcohol and/or drug use, and development of life-long strategies to minimize the likelihood of ongoing use and its attendant consequences.

In this context, treatment is best viewed as a continuum of different types and intensities of services over a long period of time. A phrase more and more commonly used in the new treatment paradigm is "sustained recovery management," referring to the structured process of accessing and completing a range of services on the road to health and self-sufficiency.

That addiction is a chronic, relapsing disease of the brain is a completely new concept for much of the general public, for many policymakers, and, sadly, for many health care professionals. The consequence of this enormous informational disconnect is a significant delay in the progress of developing improved standards of treatment.

There is gaining momentum in the addictions treatment arena shifting from long-standing pathology and intervention paradigms to a solution-focused recovery paradigm. The shift toward a recovery paradigm is evident in a number of quarters: the international growth of addiction recovery mutual aid societies, a new recovery advocacy movement, and calls to shift the design of addiction treatment from a model of acute biopsychosocial stabilization to a model of sustained recovery management.

CHAPTER 5: VOCABULARY LIST

Abuse liability   *A measure of the likelihood that a drug's use will result in continued repeated use despite adverse consequences.*

Cued reactivity   *A learned conditioned response where both internal and external triggers are associated with the anticipation of drug reward. Explains the dynamics of relapse.*

Drug discrimination   *The perception of the specific effects of a drug, usually in relation to a placebo.*

Genetic component   *Multiple genes that control biological drug creating predisposition to use drugs.*

MCLP   *The brain's pleasure or reward circuitry called the mesocorticolimbic pathway or MCLP.*

Pharmacological equivalence   *When a particular drug class cause similar effects that constitute their profile.*

Physical dependence   *Through repeated drug use, the development of tolerance to the drug's effects and a withdrawal syndrome upon abrupt cessation. Physical dependence is not drug addiction.*

Rate-limited   *Drug adaptation that gradually dissipates as the brain readapts to drug absence*

Residual neuroadaptation   *Cellular adaptations to drugs with symptoms that last for months or years in abstinence.*

Sensitization   *When the drug effects increase after repeated use; the opposite of tolerance.*

Tolerance   *The body's adaptive process to repeated exposure of drugs and alcohol. As a result, there are reduced effects that require progressively larger doses to achieve desired effect.*

Withdrawal syndrome   *The body's de-adaptive process drug use is discontinued or reduced. Anxiety, insomnia, nausea, perspiration, body aches, and tremors are a few of the symptoms of the withdrawal syndrome.*

CHAPTER 5: NEUROBIOLOGICAL ASPECTS OF SUBSTANCE ABUSE

Studies on the pharmacological results from drugs of abuse indicate that their reinforcing properties may be due to actions on a common neural circuit. While the mechanisms for all drugs of abuse are not completely described, many activate the mesocorticolimbic pathway (MCLP). Such drugs include cocaine, amphetamines, opiates, sedatives, and nicotine. For other drugs of abuse, the precise relationship, if any, to the brain reward system is unclear.

Repeated administration of all drugs of abuse is associated with neuro-adaptive responses. In general, tolerance develops to at least some of their effects, although the details of the biological mechanisms underlying these changes are not completely understood. A prominent aspect of substance abuse is tolerance to the reinforcing properties of drugs, where higher doses are needed to achieve the same result.

Withdrawal is associated with most drugs of abuse, though the severity varies. Barbiturates, alcohol, stimulants, opiates and benzodiazepines produce pronounced and sometimes severe withdrawal symptoms, while those for nicotine and caffeine are less intense. A withdrawal syndrome has also been associated with cannabis use, while there is no evidence of a withdrawal syndrome related to LSD. Certain aspects of withdrawal, such as changes in mood and motivation induced by the chronic drug state, are key factors to relapse and drug-seeking behavior.

Psychoactive drugs alter the brain's normal balance and level of biochemical activity by altering one or more of the brain's synaptic defenses. As you recall, synaptic defenses are specific neurobiological mechanisms that work in concert to keep the chemistry stabilized at synapse in order to maintain behavioral homeostasis. Drugs of abuse interrupt this delicate process and compromise homeostasis.

Drugs alter the neuropharmacological activity in the brain and body through many different mechanisms. They effect the production, release or reuptake of the neurotransmitters, they can mimic or block the neurotransmitters at a receptor, or they can interfere with other cellular activity. Prolonged drug use potentially alters these processes, and the ultimate effect either excites or inhibits activity in different brain regions. Both the immediate and long-term effects of drug abuse will change normal brain behavior, and ultimately have very strong reinforcing effects that increase their use

Reinforcement is defined as the increased likelihood that the consequences of taking the drug will increase the behavior directed toward that drug. More simply stated, individuals who use drugs experience some effect, such as pleasure, detachment or relief from distress that initially establishes and then maintains drug use. Thus, taking the drug enhances the prospect that it will be relied upon for some real or perceived effect which creates a need state, hence engendering compulsive self-administration.

What separates drugs of abuse from other psychoactive drugs is that these drugs act, at least in part, on those areas of the brain that mediate feelings of pleasure and reward. By stimulating the brain reward system, drugs of abuse create positive reinforcement that provoke and supports their continued use and abuse.

Beyond their immediate rewarding effects, drugs used on a chronic, long-term basis can cause either permanent changes in the brain or alterations that may take hours, days, months, even years, to reverse after the drug use has stopped. These changes are adaptive responses that occur in the brain to counter the immediate effects of a drug. When drug taking is stopped, these changes often appear opposite to the initial pleasurable drug response. The continued administration of drugs to avoid aversive effects of drug cessation creates negative reinforcement which also contributes to an individual's addiction to a drug.

In addition to their reinforcing effects, drugs of abuse can have a variety of pharmacological actions in other areas of the brain and the body. The ultimate effect of a drug will also be shaped by other factors including the dose of the drug, the route of administration, the physiological status of the user, and the environmental context in which the drug is taken. The subjective experience of the drug user and his overt behavior is the result of a combination of these factors and the drug's pharmacologic mechanism of action.

The Brain Reward System
Eating, drinking, sexual and maternal behaviors are essential for the survival of the individual and the species. To ensure these behaviors occur, natural selection has ensured their powerful rewarding properties. Bioanthropologists also suggest that the brain reward system apparently evolved to process these natural reinforcers.

Recent studies have shown that direct stimulation of certain areas of the brain produces extreme pleasure. Such stimulation activates neural pathways that carry natural rewarding stimuli. The fact that lab animals will forego food and drink or willingly experience pain to receive the reward attests to the power of these reinforcing characteristics. In the case of addiction, administration of most drugs of abuse reduces the amount of electrical stimulation needed to produce self-stimulation responding.

The reward system is made up of various brain structures. The central component is a neural pathway that interconnects structures in the middle part of the brain (hypothalamus and ventral tegmental area [VTA]) to structures in the front part of the brain (frontal cortex and limbic system). A key part of this drug reward pathway appears to be the mesocorticolimbic pathway (MCLP).

The MCLP is made up of the axons of neuronal cell bodies in the ventral tegmental area projecting to the nucleus accumbens, a nucleus in the limbic system. The limbic system is a network of brain structures that controls emotion, behavior and specifically perception, motivation, gratification, and memory. MCLP also connects the ventral tegmental area with parts of the frontal cortex (medial prefrontal cortex). The VTA consists of dopaminergic neurons which respond to glutamate. These cells respond when stimuli indicative of a reward are present. The VTA supports learning and sensitization development and releases dopamine into the forebrain. These neurons also project and release dopamine into the nucleus accubems through the mesoliombic pathway. Ventral tegmental neurons release dopamine to regulate activity of cells in the nucleus accumbens and the prefrontal cortex. Virtually all drugs causing drug addiction increase the dopamine release in the mesolimbic pathway, in addition to their specific effects.

The nucleus accumbens (NAcc), consisting of mainly of GABA neurons, is associated with acquiring and eliciting conditioned behaviors and involved in the increased sensitivity to drugs as addiction progresses. The prefrontal cortex, more specifically the anterior cingulate and orbitalfrontal cortices, is important for the integration of information which contributes to whether a behavior will be elicited. It appears to be the area in which motivation originates and the salience of stimuli are determined. The basolateral amygdala projects into the NAcc and is important for motivation as well. More evidence is pointing towards the role of the hippocampus in drug addiction because of its importance in learning and memory. Much of this evidence stems from investigations manipulating cells in the hippocampus alters dopamine levels in NAcc and firing rates of VTA dopaminergic cells.

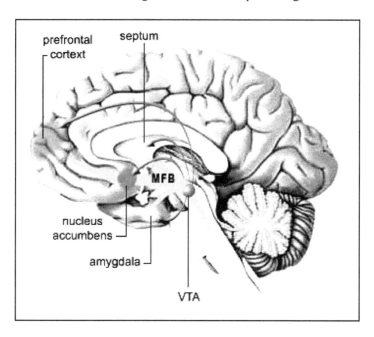

Key Common Brain Areas in Addiction
- *Nucleus Accumbens Central Nucleus of the Amygdala* – Forebrain

structures involved in the rewarding effects of drugs of abuse and drive the binge intoxication stage of addiction. Contains key reward neurotransmitters: dopamine and opioid peptides.

- *Extended Amygdala* – Composed of central nucleus of the amygdala, bed nucleus of the stria terminalis, and a transition zone on the medial part of the nucleus accumbens. Contains "brain stress" neurotransmitter, corticotropin-releasing-factor (CRF) that controls hormonal, sympathetic, and behavioral responses to stressors, and is involved in the anti-reward effects of drug addiction.
- *Medial Prefrontal Cortex* – neurobiological substrate for "executive function" that is compromised in drug addiction and plays a key role in facilitating relapse. Contains major glutamatergic projection to nucleus accumbens and the amygdala.

These structures play a significant role in reinforcing drug use, although some precise mechanisms involved lack thorough description. The MCLP is critical in reinforcing stimulant drugs as well, like cocaine and amphetamines. Also, both the ventral tegmental area and the nucleus accumbens appear to be important for opiate reward, while these same structures and their connections to other limbic areas, like the amygdala may play a role in the rewarding aspects of barbiturates and alcohol. PCP is also a strong reinforcer but its relationship, if any, to activity in MCLP has not been well established.

Other drugs are either weak reinforcers or have not been shown to support self-administration in animal experiments at all. Nicotine activates dopamine neurons in the MCLP system; however, when compared with cocaine or amphetamine, this effect is modest. Likewise, caffeine is a weak reinforcer, but the precise mechanisms of its reinforcement still remain unclear. Finally, while cannabis and lysergic acid diethylamide (LSD) produce positive effects that clearly support their use, there is currently little empirical evidence that they act as reinforcers in controlled experiments. Interestingly, a new study has shown that while dopaminergic pathways of the brain's reward circuitry do indeed play a major role in the reinforcing effects of many drugs, they are not the only mechanisms involved.

Corticotropin-Releasing Factor
In addition to the reward circuit, it is hypothesized that stress mechanisms also play a role in addiction. Researchers have hypothesized that during drug use corticotropin-releasing factor (CRF) activates the hypothalamic-pituitary-adrenal axis (HPA) and other stress systems in the extended amygdala. This activation influences the dysregulated emotional state associated with drug addiction. They have found that as drug use escalates, so does the presence of CRF in human cerebrospinal fluid (CSF). In animal models, the separate use of CRF antagonists and CRF receptor antagonists both decreased self-administration of the drug of study. Other studies in this review showed a dysregulation in other hormones associated with the HPA axis, including

enkephalin which is an endogenous opioid peptides that regulates pain. It also appears that the mu opioid receptor system, which enkephalin acts on, is influential in the reward system and can regulate the expression of stress hormones.

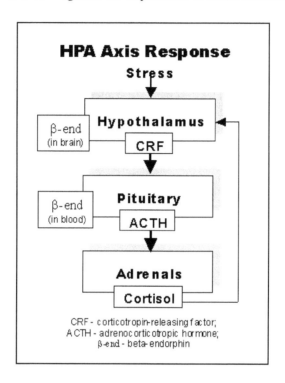

Cycle of Addiction

As addiction develops, neuroplastic brain reward systems eventually become transformed. This is what some refer to as the "dark side" of drug addiction. That is, the decline in normal reward-related neural mechanisms and persistent recruitment of the brain's anti-reward systems that accompany drug use. Progressive worsening of the brain reward system perpetuates compulsive use of the drug.

Drug addiction has elements of both an impulse control disorder and a compulsive disorder that are mediated by separate but overlapping neural circuits. The individual with an impulse control disorder experiences an increasing sense of tension or arousal before committing the impulsive act such as drug-taking; pleasure, gratification or relief during the act; and in some cases, regret, self-reproach or guilt following the act. The individual with a compulsive disorder feels anxiety and stress before the compulsive, repetitive act, and relief from stress by performing the act. In the progression from an impulsive disorder to a compulsive disorder, the motivation for the behavior shifts from positive reinforcement to negative reinforcement, when removal of the aversive state increases the probability of the behavior. Drug addiction follows this pattern in a collapsed cycle of addiction involving 3 stages:

1. Binge/intoxication;
2. Withdrawal/negative affect; and
3. Preoccupation/anticipation (craving).

Addiction involves a long-term persistent plasticity of the neural circuits that control two different reward systems: declining function of brain reward systems driven by natural rewards and stimulation of anti-reward systems that bring on aversive states. Studies of the acute reinforcing effects of drugs of abuse in the binge/intoxication stage have identified the neurobiological substrates involved in the reward response. Drugs with the potential for abuse and dependence, such as the opioid analgesics, initially produce positive reinforcing effects from actions at the ventral tegmental area in the midbrain and the nucleus accumbens and amygdala of the basal forebrain. Activation of the mesocorticolimbic dopamine pathway is the primary route of positive reinforcement in addiction for psychostimulant drugs, but the opioid peptides (endorphins), serotonin, and gamma-aminobutyric acid (GABA) have key roles for nonpsychostimulant drugs. These so-called "reward neurotransmitters" induce hedonic effects of euphoria and a feeling of well-being.

Reward Neurotransmitters Implicated in the Motivational Effects of Drugs Abuse	
Positive Pleasurable Effects	Negative Unpleasant Effects of Withdrawal
Increased dopamine	Decreased dopamine (dysphoria)
Increased opioid peptides	Decreased opioid peptides (pain)
Increased serotonin	Decreased serotonin (dysphoria)
Increased GABA	Decreased GABA (anxiety, panic attacks)

The Brain Anti-Reward System

Withdrawal from a drug induces symptoms of negative affect such as dysphoria, depression, irritability, and anxiety. Dysregulation of brain reward systems involves some of the same neurochemical pathways implicated in the drug's acute reinforcing effects, but in this case, they represent an opponent process. During acute abstinence, increases in brain reward thresholds (a higher set point for drug reward) are a consequence of altered reward neurotransmitters. This in turn may contribute to the negative motivational state of withdrawal and vulnerability to relapse. Neurochemical changes during opioid withdrawal include decreases in dopaminergic and serotonergic transmission and increased sensitivity of opioid receptor transduction mechanisms. Escalating doses of opioids, like those seen in the human pattern of morphine or heroin use, are associated with profound alterations in the function of mu-opioid receptors. A decrease in baseline reward mechanisms leads to an increase in drug intake to compensate for the shift in reward baseline.

Stress response systems of the body contribute to the negative emotional state associated with abstinence and can exacerbate drug taking throughout the addiction cycle. In response to taking the drug, the neuroendocrine system kicks in trying to restore the brain to normal function. Chronic drug use adversely affects the hypothalamic-pituitary-adrenal axis, disrupting regulation of hypothalamic corticotropin releasing factor (CRF). Particularly important is activation of CRF in the extended amygdala. CRF, as you have read, controls hormonal, sympathetic, and behavioral responses to stress. During acute withdrawal of the drug, production of adrenocorticotropic hormone, corticosterone, amygdala CRF, norepinephrine, dynorphin, and inhibition of neuropeptide Y (NPY) induce brain arousal, stress-like responses, and a dysphoric, aversive state. The activation and recruitment of brain and hormonal stress responses contribute to a deviation in brain reward set point. These are the sources of negative reinforcement that lead to compulsive drug-seeking behavior and addiction.

Anti-Reward Transmitters Implicated in the Motivational Effects of Drugs of Abuse
• Increased dynorphin (dysphoria)
• Increased CRF (sress)
• Increased norepinephrine (stress)
• Decreased neuropeptide Y (NPY) (anti-stress)

Craving and Relapse
The preoccupation/anticipation stage of the addiction cycle is mediated via afferent projections to the extended amygdala and nucleus accumbens. There are different stimuli for craving a drug of abuse, leading to relapse. It can be drug-induced, cue-induced, or stress-induced. Chronic relapse is a significant problem in drug addiction, with about half of all addicts relapsing into drug taking. Addicts can return to compulsive drug taking long after acute withdrawal exhibiting behavior that corresponds to the preoccupation/anticipation stage of addiction. Drug-related cues and stressors are a powerful inducement to return to drug use. Areas of the brain associated with drug and cue-induced reinstatement are the prefrontal cortex (orbitofrontal, medical prefrontal, prelimbic/cingulate), and the basolateral amygdala. The neurotransmitters involved in relapse are dopamine, opioid peptides, glutamate, and GABA. Relapse can also be precipitated by stress and the release of CRF, glucocorticoids and norepinephrine. Many different stressors can provoke drug craving and drug-seeking behavior

Neurobiological Actions
One thing is certain – changes will occur in the brain when it is exposed to drugs. Beyond the immediate reward, chronic and long-term drug abuse can cause alterations in brain function that can take years to reverse or improve, if at all. These changes are adaptive responses to the pharmacological action of drugs in order to counter their disruptive effects. Remember, the biological system is genetically coded to always find and maintain healthy balance. Therefore, the adaptive responses to repeat drug exposure are biological expressions of the system attempting to regain its homeostasis.

As you recall, one such adaptive response is tolerance, where the intensity of the drug's effects are reduced. Tolerance can contribute to drug-taking behavior by requiring that an individual take progressively larger doses of a drug to achieve a desired effect. While it is unclear from available data whether or not tolerance develops to cocaine's rewarding effects, the notion is supported by experiments and anecdotal reports that the drug's euphoric actions diminish with repeated use. This decrease of effects may be related to decreasing levels of available dopamine to work on. *Dependence* is when cells adapt to prolonged use of a drug so that use is required to maintain comfortable body functioning. Upon abrupt cessation of the drug, neurons may behave abnormally, causing a *withdrawal syndrome.* Generally, the withdrawal syndrome is characterized by signs and symptoms that are *opposite* to those of the acute effects of the drug. The figure below provides an example.

Substance	Global acute Effects	Global Withdrawal Effects
Stimulants (amphetamines, cocaine)	Euphoria, increased energy, insomnia, decreased appetite	dysphoria, depression, fatigue, increased appetite
Sedatives (alcohol, benzodiazepines)	Sedation, sleep inducing, anti-seizure, anti- anxiety	irritability, insomnia, anxiety, agitation, seizure
Opiates (morphine, heroin)	Euphoria, analgesia, constipation	dysphoria, depression, hypersensitivity to pain, diarrhea

Understanding the basic acute symptoms of drugs will lend to understanding withdrawal symptoms because they are generally the opposite in nature. Withdrawal also creates a craving state where there is a strong desire for the drug. Drug craving behaviors play a strong role in patterns of relapse, and also in maintaining drug seeking behavior to forestall the withdrawal syndrome.

Sensitization occurs when the effects of a given dose of a drug will increase after repeated administration; sensitization is the opposite of tolerance. Sensitization to a drug's behavioral effects seem also to play a significant role in supporting drug-taking behavior. For example, while tolerance to some of the effects of cocaine and amphetamines develops, sensitization to other effects can also occur.

The *abuse liability* of a drug is a measure of the likelihood that its use will result in addiction. Many factors ultimately play a role in a person's drug usage. Nevertheless, abuse potential of a drug is due to its intrinsic rewarding properties and neuroadaptive responses that result from its prolonged use. Drugs can be screened for their abuse liability using animals as models. The criteria to classify a drug as addictive include: pharmacological equivalence to known drugs of abuse, demonstration of reinforcing effects, tolerance, and physical dependence. The reinforcing capacity is essential in determining abuse potential, whereas tolerance and physical dependence might occur, but are not absolutely required to make this determination.

The main feature of all drugs with abuse potential is that they are *self-administered.* In fact, self-administration to the point where behavior becomes obsessive and detrimental is the principal criterion that classifies a drug as having significant potential for addiction. Another contributing factor to abuse liability is the notion of craving and the tendency of individuals to relapse to drug use during withdrawal. Although craving is a difficult term to quantify, once a drug is voluntarily or involuntarily withdrawn, the desire to take the drug can create relapse to substance abuse.

Another measure in the assessment of abuse liability is *drug discrimination,* the perception of the specific effects of a drug. Specifically, animal or human subjects that can discriminate a drug from a *placebo* show a remarkable ability to distinguish that drug from other drugs with different properties. These procedures also permit the subject to consider the drug to be the equivalent of another drug. *Pharmacological equivalence* is when drugs of a particular class, such as stimulants or depressants, cause a series of similar effects on the body that collectively constitute their pharmacological profile.

Residual Tolerance
In general, expression of tolerance and dependence has been considered to be *rate-limited* in that adaptation to drugs gradually dissipates with time as the brain readapts to the disappearance of the drug; withdrawal peaks within hours or days after discontinued use but then disappears. However, there is a significant amount of evidence indicating that there may be persistent or *residual neuroadaptation* that lasts for months or years. For example, craving and drug-seeking behavior have been reported to last for years with nicotine, alcohol and cocaine, suggesting some residual effect of drug use that may not dissipate with time. Moreover, there is a phenomenon that characterizes specific drug-dependent individuals.

Specifically, with repeated cycles of abstinence and reinitiation of drug use, the time required to elicit drug dependence grows shorter and shorter. Furthermore, there is evidence that naloxone, a drug that blocks the actions of opiates, may elicit a withdrawal syndrome in individuals who have abstained from opiate use for an extensive time. These findings indicate that some residual neuroadaptive changes induced by drugs can persist for as yet undefined periods of time. Little information is available about the mechanisms involved in this effect, but it is clear that long-term residual changes do persist for some former drug users, which may account for the striking relapses that occur after long-term abstinence.

Testing new pharmaceuticals for their abuse potential is an important precaution in new drug development. The emphasis of many major pharmaceutical firms today is to develop new and safer drugs to treat chronic pain and mental disorders. In particular, scientific advances in understanding the brain, neurological disease, psychiatric disturbances and aging are fueling research into treatment of brain disorders. As such psychoactive compounds become available, they must be screened for abuse potential. The *abuse liability assessment* of new products is not simply a choice for the manufacturer. Various federal laws mandate testing and regulatory agencies are charged with seeing that testing is carried out.

Animal models are generally used to screen for the abuse potential of new drugs either in earlier stages of development or drugs that cannot be readily studied in humans. Laboratory methods for abuse potential evaluation in humans are also well developed, since this is an area of active research. However, factors such as the heterogeneity of drug-using populations, the use of multiple drugs, and the other biological, social, and environmental factors involved in human drug use make human studies complex.

At first glance, it seems impossible to mimic the highly complex syndrome of drug abuse in humans using lab animals. Paradoxically, the apparent limitations of animal models are actually their strengths. Specifically, the simplicity of an animal model obviates the problems inherent in the complexity of humans; the experimenter has strict control over environmental factors, drug use patterns, and individual differences that permit study of the pharmacological and biological mechanisms associated with addiction potential. Thus, the use of animal models permits the highly complex syndrome of human drug addiction to be dissected into separate components without the intrusion of a series of confounding variables found in humans.

Are animal models valid as a means of studying human drug addiction? An excellent correlation exists between animals and humans to predict the abuse liability of specific classes of drugs.

However, it must be recognized that animal models are not perfect. In fact, there are examples of drugs that proved to have significant abuse potential in humans, whereas the preclinical testing in animals revealed relatively minimal abuse potential. Thus, the ultimate answer to the question about abuse potential is long-term experience with the drug once it has become available, either legally or illegally. Nevertheless, animal models serve as the only practical means of initially screening for abuse liability, and have proven to be the most effective means of detecting any likely problems in humans.

Conditioned Biobehavioral Responses
Another significant factor in drug abuse is the *learning* that can occur during an individual's drug-taking activity. In addition to producing pleasant feelings, drugs of abuse produce changes in numerous organ systems such as the

cardiovascular, digestive, and endocrine systems. The effects of a drug occur in the context of an individual's drug-seeking and drug-using environment. As a result, there are environmental cues present before and during a person's drug use that are consistently associated with behavioral and physiological effects. With repetition, these cues become *conditioned stimuli* that automatically change organ systems and cause severe craving even after long-term absence of the drug.

This is analogous to Pavlov's classical conditioning experiments in which dogs salivate on the cue of a bell, following repeated association of food with a ringing bell. Evidence for this effect is seen in numerous studies showing that animals seek out places associated with reinforcing drugs, and that the physiological effects of drugs can be classically conditioned in both animals and humans. Thus, exposure to environmental cues associated with drug use in the past can act as a stimulus for voluntary drug-seeking behavior. If the individual succeeds in finding and taking the drug, the chain of behaviors is further reinforced by the drug-induced reward and the effects of the drug on other organ systems. Drug conditioning can explain why many drug abusers often return to environments associated with drug use, even after being counseled not to. The effects of environmental stimuli are similar to the priming effects of a dose of the drug.

Also, it has long been known that conditioning may stimulate withdrawal effects of drugs. It was observed that opiate addicts who were drug free for months and thus should not have had any signs of opiate withdrawal developed withdrawal symptoms (e.g., yawning, sniffling, tearing of the eyes, etc.) when talking about drugs in group therapy sessions. This phenomenon, termed *conditioned withdrawal,* results from environmental ability to elicit signs and symptoms of pharmacological withdrawal.

Conditioned withdrawal can also play a role in relapse to drug use in abstinent individuals. The emergence of withdrawal symptoms resulting from conditioned exposure can motivate a person to seek out and use drugs. Relapse prevention protocols address this conditioning process to re-condition cellular response.

Studies have also demonstrated that conditioned associations are difficult to reverse. In theory, repeated presentation of the environmental cues, without the drug, should extinguish the conditioned association. Animal studies indicate that extinction is difficult to achieve and does not erase the original learning. As a result, once established, the extinction is easily reversed. Research has found that various aspects of extinguished responses can either be reinstated with a single pairing of the drug and environmental cue, a single dose of drug in the absence of the environmental cue, or can spontaneously recover.

The biological mechanisms underlying conditioned drug effects are just beginning to be understood. Recent evidence links the mesocorticolimbic pathway (MCLP) to these effects. Studies have found increased release of dopamine in the nucleus accumbens associated with anticipated voluntary alcohol consumption. Other studies have presented evidence that destruction of the MCLP blocks the conditioned reinforcing effects of opiates.

Studies using the technique of genetic linkage analysis have attempted to identify genes that might be associated with alcoholism in humans. However, the findings of these studies are inconclusive. While some studies have reported a link between alcoholism and a gene that regulates the number of a type of dopamine receptor in the brain (i.e. allele D2 studies) others have not. The reason for this discrepancy is unclear, but one study has found relationship between the presence of the gene not only in alcoholism, but also in other disorders such as autism, attention deficit hyperactivity disorder, and Tourette's syndrome. Thus, the presence of the gene may cause an alteration in the dopamine system that somehow exacerbates or contributes to alcohol abuse, but is not uniquely specific for alcoholism.

Another study indicates that inherited differences of neural mechanisms in the MCLP contribute to a genetic predilection to drug addiction. In a comparison of rats with high and low rates of self-administering drugs of abuse, the higher self-administering strain exhibited impaired control over activity in the neurons of the ventral tegmental area and nucleus accumbens. Further examination of causal relationships between inherited neurochemical alterations and behavioral traits would produce valuable information about genetic factors of substance abuse.

Additional studies exploring the role of genes in drug response are needed to more fully understand the range of biological factors that underlie drug abuse. The recent development of new and more sensitive techniques to analyze brain activity and processes should facilitate these studies.

CHAPTER 5: SELF-STUDY QUESTIONS

TRUE/FALSE

1. *Psychoactive drugs alter the brain's normal balance and level of biochemical activity by altering one or more of the brain's synaptic defenses.*

2. *A key part of the brain's reward circuitry, and where drugs of abuse exert their reinforcing action, is the mesocorticolimbic pathway (MCLP).*

3. *Dependence occurs when neurons in the brain adapt to prolonged use of a drug, such that the drug's presence is required to maintain normal function.*

4. *Generally, the withdrawal syndrome is characterized by symptoms that are the same as those of the acute effects of the drug.*

5. *Sensitization occurs when the effects of a given dose of a drug increase after repeated administration.*

6. *The abuse liability of a drug is a measure of how little it may cause drug craving behaviors.*

7. *The predominant feature of all drugs with significant abuse potential is that they are self-administered.*

8. *The behavioral pharmacological effects of a drug will often occur in the context of an individual's drug-seeking and drug-using environment.*

9. *Conditioned withdrawal can play a role in relapse to drug use in abstinent individuals.*

10. *While it seems likely that inherited differences exist, a genetic component alone is insufficient to produce substance abuse and addiction.*

* Answers to Self Study Tests are located on page 351

Chapter 5 Selected Reading

Brick J. and Erickso C.K., *Drugs, The Brain, and Behavior: The Pharmacology of Abuse and Dependence* . Haworth Press. 1999.

Brick J., (ed)., *Handbook of the Medical Consequences of Alcohol and Drug Abuse*, The Haworth Press. 2004.

Cami, J. and Farre, M., Drug addiction. *New Engl. J. Med.* 349: 975-86. 2003.

Erickson, C.K., *The Science of Addiction: From Neurobiology to Treatment* . W.W. Norton & Co. 2007.

Gardner, EL. Brain-Reward Mechanisms. Lowinson, JH, Ruiz, P, Millman, RB, and Langrod, JG (editors), *Substance Abuse A Comprehensive Sourcebook*. Fourth Edition. Lippincott Williams & Wilkins. 2005.

Gass JT, Olive MF. Glutamatergic substrates of drug addiction and alcoholism. *Biochem. Pharmacol.* **75** (1): 218–65. 2008.

Goldstein, A. *Addiction: From Biology to Drug Policy*. Oxford University Press. 2001.

Kalivas PW, Volkow ND. The neural basis of addiction: a pathology of motivation and choice. Am J Psychiatry **162** (8): 1403–13. 2005.

Kandel, E.R., Schwart, J.H. and Jessell, T.M., *Essentials of Neural Science and Behavior,* Appleton and Lange. 1995.

Koob G, Kreek MJ . Stress, dysregulation of drug reward pathways, and the transition to drug dependence. *Am J Psychiatry* **164** (8): 1149–59. 2007.

Koob, GF, and Le Moal, M. *Neurobiology of Addiction*. Academic Press. 2005.

Koob, G.F. Drugs of Abuse: Anatomy, Pharmacology and Function of Reward Pathways. *Trends in Pharmacological Science,* Volume 13: 177-183, 1992.

Koob GF, Le Moal M. Drug addiction, dysregulation of reward, and allostasis. *Neuropsychopharmacology*. 2001;24:97-129.

Koob, G.F., Ahmed, S.H., Boutrel, B., Chen, S.A., Kenny, P.J., Markou, A., O'Dell, L.E., Parsons, L.H., Sanna, P.P., Neurobiological mechanisms in the transition from drug use to drug dependence. Neurosci. Biobeh. Rev. 27: 739-749, 2004.

Leshner, A.I. Addiction is a brain disease and it matters. *Science 278:45-47. 1997.*

Liebman, J.M. and Cooper, S.J. (editors), *The Neuropharmacological Basis of Reward,* Claredon Press. 1989.

McLellan, A.T., Lewis, D.C., O'Brien, C.P., and Kleber, H.D., Drug dependence, a chronic medical illness. <u>J. Am. Med. Assoc.</u> 284: 1689-1695 (2000).

Nestler, E.J., Molecular Neurobiology of Drug Addiction, *Neuropsychopharmacology,* Volume 11:77-87, 1994.

O'Brien, C.P., Childress, A.R. and McLellan, A.T., et al. Classical Conditioning in Drug-Dependent Humans. P.W. Kalivas and H.H. Samson (editors), *The Neurobiology of Drug and Alcohol Addiciton, Annals of the American Academy of Sciences,* Volume 654: 400-415, 1992.

Robinson, TE, and Berridge, RC. The Neural Basis of Drug Craving: An Incentive-Sensitization Theory of Addiction. *Brain Research,* Volume 18: 247-291, 1993.

Robinson, TE and Berridge, RC. The psychology and neurobiology of addiction: an incentive-sensitization view. *Addiction* 95 (Suppl. 2): S91-S117, 2000.

Volkow, N.D. and Li, T.-K., Drug addiction: The neurobiology of behaviour gone awry. *Nature. Rev./Neurosci.* 5: 963-970, 2004.

Wise, R.A. The Role of Reward Pathways in the Development of Drug Dependence. *Pharmacological Therapeutics,* Volume 35, 227-263, 1987.

CHAPTER 6: VOCABULARY LIST

Acetaldehyde
Metabolite that alcohol oxidizes into, with the help of a zinc-containing enzyme.

Aldehyde dehydrogenase
Enzyme that metabolizes acetaldehyde into acetic acid, where it can be excreted.

Antabuse
(disulfiram) A drug that inhibits alcohol's full metabolism resulting in extreme discomfort.

Antidiuretic Hormone
(ADH) Posterior pituitary hormone when decreased can cause profound diuresis.

Anxiolytics
The benzodiazepine class of drugs introduced in the 1960s as anti-anxiety agents.

Cardiac arrhythmias
(Irregular Heart Beat) One of the direct effects of alcohol on the heart muscle.

Cardiomyopathy
(Heart Swelling) One of the direct effects of alcohol on the heart muscle.

Delirium Tremens
(DTs) Severe, potentially fatal symptom of delirium of the alcohol withdrawal syndrome.

Hepatitis
(Fatty Liver) Liver damage caused by decrease in hepatic (liver) vitamin A levels.

Idiopathic
Loss of iron metabolism caused by chronic drinking, hemochromatosis contributes to iron overload.

MEOS
(Mixed Enzyme Oxidizing System) Liver enzymes that converts alcohol into acetaldehyde.

NAD
(Nicotinamide Adenine Dinucleotide) Alcohol co-enzyme depleted in alcoholics.

Peripheral neuropathy
Thiamine deficiency in alcoholics, caused by demyelination of peripheral nerve fibers.

Protracted abstinence syndrome
Syndrome that follows withdrawal, marked by depression and sleep disturbances.

CHAPTER 6: ALCOHOL AND ANTI-ANXIETY DRUGS

Alcohol, barbiturates, and benzodiazepines are drugs that inhibit CNS activity similar to many abuse inhalants which also produce sedative depressant effects. Although all these drugs have different specific mechanisms of action in the brain, they all share the ability to enhance the activity of the inhibitory amino acid neurotransmitter gamma amino butyric acid (GABA). In some cases, GABA activation in turn alters other inhibitory pathways. Thus, the final outcome of inhibiting an inhibitory pathway is the net activation of a brain region. This mechanism of interfering with other inhibitory pathways is thought to play a role in the abuse of these drugs.

ALCOHOL

In the United States, two out of three men and women are drinkers at some point in their lives, even higher numbers of people have consumed caffeinated beverages; at least among individuals in their 20s and 30s, 70% or more have had experience with marijuana; 20% - 40% of members of subgroups have used amphetamines or cocaine on occasion, and perhaps 10% - 20% have had experience with any variety of other drugs including hallucinogens, brain depressants other than alcohol, and solvents.

The lifetime risk for alcohol abuse or dependence is 15% to 20% for men, with lower but still substantial figures for women. Repetitive use of alcohol and other drugs can:
1. cause a wide range of psychiatric symptoms;
2. contribute to problems in the workplace;
3. contribute as a factor in many fatal accidents;
4. exacerbate almost all major medical problems.

Alcohol (ethyl alcohol or ethanol) differs from most other drugs of abuse in that it has no known target receptor system in the brain. Ethanol affects a number of neurotransmitter systems through its action on membranes of neurons and the ion channels inside, particularly calcium (CA+) and chloride (CL-). In general, ethanol inhibits receptors for excitatory neurotransmitters and augments activity at inhibitory neurotransmitters.

For example, ethanol enhances the activity of GABA by slowing ion channels associated with GABAA receptor subtype and the excitatory amino acid neurotransmitter glutamate, through inhibition of the NMDA receptor. The net effect of ethanol is to depress activity in the brain, producing paradoxical sedative and intoxicating effects. A similar spectrum of effects is seen with benzodiazepines and barbiturates.

Alcohol and Neurotransmitters: A Review of the Research

A general working hypothesis is that alcoholics who are sensitive to the low-dose rewarding properties of alcohol are less sensitive to the high-dose actions of ethanol, and develop tolerance to the aversive toxic effects of alcohol.

Studies were conducted under experimental conditions where the animal was allowed to receive alcohol as a reward for performing a task. The fact that lab animals can be selectively bred to have such alcohol drinking characteristics supports a genetic link to these traits.

Animals that have been bred for specific characteristics are a valuable tool in drug use and abuse research. For example, certain strains of rodents differ in their response to the analgesic effects of morphine, the motor activating effects of stimulant drugs, and the convulsive properties of benzodiazepines. Since the essential characteristic of addiction is persistent drug-seeking behavior, the most salient models are those of genetic preferences for drug self-administration and related symptoms and tolerance. While there are some genetic models of preference for harder drugs (like opiates or cocaine), more information is available about the hereditary mechanisms that underlie the self-administration of alcohol than any other drugs.

Dopamine and Ethanol

Studies have found up to 30 percent lower levels of dopamine in the nucleus accumbens and the olfactory tubercle in alcohol-preferring rats. No other differences in dopamine content have been observed in other brain areas. This data suggest an abnormality in the dopamine system projecting from the ventral tegmental area to limbic regions (nucleus accumbens) of rats bred to prefer alcohol.

Since this system is thought to mediate various drugs of abuse, and ethanol is thought to increase dopamine levels in the system, it may indicate that abnormal functioning of mesocorticolimbic dopamine system might promote alcoholic behavior. That is, alcohol preference may be due to the ability of ethanol to compensate for abnormalities in the mesocorticolimbic pathway. The nature of this abnormality is unknown, but may be due to one or more of the following factors: decreased dopamine synthesis, a lower number of dopamine neurofibers or reduced functional activity of dopamine neurons.

Some evidence exists that the MCLP may respond to systemic ethanol administration to a greater degree in the alcohol-preferring than in the nonpreferring animals. Studies have found that levels of dopamine metabolites were higher in areas of this system after ingestion of ethanol in alcohol-preferring rats.

One study reported that oral self-administration of alcohol increased the synaptic levels of dopamine significantly more in the nucleus accumbens of these alcohol-preferring rats than in nonpreferring rats. It was also established that the alcohol-preferring strain receives alcohol directly into the ventral tegmental area. These studies suggest that the mesocorticolimbic dopamine system is involved in regulating alcohol drinking behavior and that ethanol may be a strong positive reinforcer.

Differences in dopamine receptor populations have also been reported. Two genetically determined alcoholic lines of rats had fewer of one type of dopamine receptor (the D2 receptor) in their limbic system compared with the nonalcoholic rats. 20 percent fewer D2 receptors were also observed in the nucleus accumbens of these rats. These studies, along with genetic linkage studies, provide a foundation for relating the D2 receptor to alcohol preference.

Serotonin and Ethanol
Evidence suggests that the serotonin system is involved in regulating the activity of the dopamine system. Further examination has indicated a relationship between high alcohol preference and a deficiency in CNS serotonin. A number of studies have reported 10 to 30 percent lower levels of serotonin and its metabolites in the brains of alcohol-preferring rats. Only one study, using a strain of rats not used in any other tests, did not find lower brain serotonin levels. Areas of the brain found to have low serotonin include the cerebral cortex, frontal cortex, nucleus accumbens, anterior and corpus striatum, septal nuclei, hippocampus, olfactory tubercle, thalamus and hypothalamus.

Since several of these CNS regions may be mediate the rewards of drugs of abuse, these findings suggest a relationship between lower brain serotonin and high alcohol preference. Also, some of the areas found to have less serotonin (the hypothalamus and hippocampus) may be involved in mediating the aversive effects of ethanol. Since tolerance is a possible characteristic of alcoholic abuse, a deficiency in serotonin in these areas may be an innate factor promoting tolerance to the aversive effects of ethanol in alcohol-preferring lines of rodents.

Further study of one of the rat strains showed that low serotonin in the alcoholic line was due to fewer serotonin containing axons. This study found fewer serotonin presynaptic fibers forming synapses in the nucleus accumbens, frontal cortex, cingulate cortex and hippocampus of alcohol-preferring rats. These results suggest that low serotonin is caused by structural differences in the CNS serotonin system rather than lower production of serotonin.

Examination of this same strain of rats found increased numbers of one type of post-synaptic serotonin receptor in areas of the frontal cortex and hippocampus. This increase in the number of serotonin receptors may represent a compensation for lower presynaptic serotonin fibers. No such increase in receptors was found in the strain of rats with normal levels of brain serotonin activity discussed earlier.

Overall, the animal data shows an inverse relationship between the functioning of the CNS serotonin system and alcohol behavior. Thus, innate low functioning of the serotonin system may be associated with high alcohol preference. In support of this concept, some studies found lower serotonin metabolite concentrations in cerebrospinal fluid of alcoholics than in various control populations.

GABA and Ethanol

Research indicates that alcohol can exert some of its anti-anxiety and intoxicating effects by potentiating the actions of the neurotransmitter gamma amino butyric acid (GABA) receptor.

GABA receptors seem to be involved in mediating alcohol drinking behavior of alcohol-preferring rats. However, little has been published to associate innate abnormality in GABA system with alcohol preference.

A recent study examined the density of GABA fibers in the nucleus accumbens and other brain areas of both alcoholic and non-preferring rats. The results of this study indicated a higher density of GABA fibers in the nucleus accumbens of the alcohol-preferring rats. There was no difference between the respective lines in the other regions. These results suggest alcohol preference may involve an innate, abnormal GABA system within the nucleus accumbens.

The experimental drug *RO 15-4513* binds to the GABAA BDZ-chloride channel receptor complex and is known to block the actions of alcohol at this receptor (the BDZ-chloride channel refers to a benzodiazepine-like receptor site in the GABA system). The administration of RO 15-4513 reduced alcohol but not water intake in a study using alcohol-preferring rats. The effect of RO 15-4513 on alcohol intake could itself be blocked by administration of a drug that blocks the benzodiazepine receptor. These results indicate that the GABAA BDZ -chloride channel receptor complex may reinforce the actions of ethanol that promote alcoholism in these rats. Furthermore, treatment with drugs that activate the GABAA receptor was shown to markedly increase the acquisition of voluntary ethanol consumption in laboratory rats. Also, in animals sensitive to alcohol intoxication, GABAA receptor function is enhanced by alcohol, but alcohol has little effect on GABAA receptors of animals with resistance to alcohol intoxication. These results support findings that GABAA receptors regulate alcohol consumption.

Alcohol Withdrawal Severity

Animal models have helped differentiate genetic susceptibility to alcohol withdrawal. For example, mice prone to seizures display a higher incidence of convulsions than do seizure-resistant mice when exposed to identical alcohol concentrations. Other studies suggest that this withdrawal reaction is mediated by an increased sensitivity of channels for calcium ions, coupled to receptors for excitatory amino acids. Several important results have emerged in studies of these mice to understanding drug abuse.

For example, studies indicate that independent genetic factors control alcohol sensitivity, tolerance, and dependence, suggesting that these features of drug abuse are maintained by different neurobiological mechanisms. In addition, the withdrawal seizure-prone mice have more severe withdrawal to other depressant drugs (like diazepam and phenobarbitol) suggesting that a group of genes acts to influence drug withdrawal severity not only to alcohol but also to a number of other depressant drugs.

Symptoms of Alcohol Withdrawal Syndrome

Symptom	Time Appearance After Cessation of Alcohol Use
Insomnia, tremulousness, mild anxiety, gastrointestinal upset, headache, diaphoresis, palpitations, anorexia	6 to 12 hours
Alcoholic hallucinosis: visual, auditory, or tactile hallucinations	12 to 24 hours
Withdrawal seizures: generalized tonic-clonic seizures	24 to 48 hours
Alcohol withdrawal delirium (delirium tremens): hallucinations (predominately visual), disorientation, tachycardia, hypertension, low-grade fever, agitation, diaphoresis	48 to 72 hours

Alcohol Abuse
Alcohol is a CNS depressant and as with all depressants, induces a dose-response relationship leading to disinhibition, ataxia, impaired judgment, sedation, slurred speech, and eventually coma, respiratory depression and death. Once absorbed, alcohol is distributed rather uniformly through all tissues and fluids. Measuring the levels of alcohol in the body is accomplished by evaluating the amount of alcohol in the blood. Blood-levels of alcohol are measured in grams of alcohol present in 100 milliliters (mls) of blood.

That is, .08 g percent is 80 mg of alcohol in 100 mls of blood. The dose-response relationship effects of alcohol are related to the blood alcohol level (BAL) which is the concentration of alcohol in the blood. The illustration below shows that effects of alcohol with the corresponding blood alcohol levels (BALs).

The Behavioral Effects of Blood-Alcohol Levels	
Levels of Alcohol in the Blood	Behavioral Effects
0.05%	Feels good; less alert
0.10%	Slower to react; less cautious
0.15%	Reaction time much slower
0.20%	Sensory-motor abilities suppressed
0.25%	Staggering gait (motor abilities severely impaired; inability to walk heal-to-toe in straight line); perception is limited
0.30%	Semistupor
0.35%	Level of anesthesia; death is possible
0.40%	Death is likely via respiratory failure)

Note: Approximate dose-response ranges are for a 150-pound person. Levels may be lower for certain individuals.)

Absorption

After ingestion, alcohol is absorbed from the stomach and small intestine, and is then distributed uniformly throughout the body. Absorption of alcohol from the stomach will increase as gastric alcohol increases. As alcohol concentrations rise, the rate of absorption decreases as the astringent actions of alcohol will restrict the blood supply to the stomach. Carbohydrates may actually enhance alcohol absorption by the small intestines. The complete absorption of alcohol takes from 2 to 6 hours.

Metabolism

Most alcohol is metabolized in the liver. Alcohol is oxidized into acetaldehyde with the assistance of a zinc-containing enzyme called alcohol dehydrogenase. When alcohol is present in large concentrations, another liver-enzyme system, called the microsomal ethanol oxidizing system (MEOS), is induced to convert alcohol into the metabolite of acetaldehyde. Aldehyde dehydrogenase is the enzyme that assists in the further metabolization of acetaldehyde into acetic acid where it then becomes excreted.

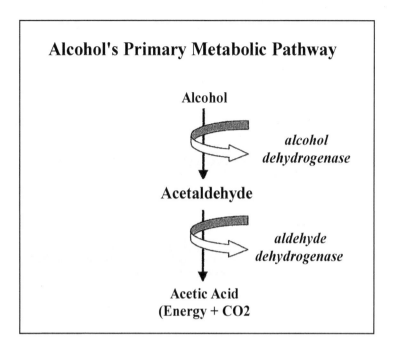

Alcohol's Primary Metabolic Pathway

Alcohol

alcohol dehydrogenase

Acetaldehyde

aldehyde dehydrogenase

**Acetic Acid
(Energy + CO2**

Alcohol Effects on the Brain

Alcohol has two major actions on the brain: increasing neuronal inhibition mediated through the inhibitory gamma-aminobutyric acid (GABA), glycine, and adenosine—prolonged alcohol use down-regulates these receptors and decreases inhibitory neurotransmission; and inhibiting excitatory neurotransmission by inhibiting both N-methyl-d-aspartate (NMDA) and non-NMDA (kainite and α-amino-3-hydroxy-5-methisoxizole-4-propionic acid [AMPA]) receptors. Up-regulation of these glutamate receptors compensates for alcohol's antagonistic effect after prolonged exposure and results in increased neuroexcitation. Cessation or reduction of alcohol use initiates an imbalance between the decreased neuroinhibition and increased neuroexcitation. This causes the clinical manifestations of the alcohol withdrawal syndrome.

Alcohol Withdrawal Syndrome

Alcohol withdrawal is a classic example of *neuroadaptation,* often characterized by CNS hyperexcitability, resulting in anxiety, anorexia, insomnia, tremors and disorientation. In severe withdrawal a syndrome called delirium tremens may develop as well, marked by hallucinations, disorientation, and outbursts of irrational behavior. The syndrome peaks 24 to 48 hours after the drug is cleared. Potentially fatal convulsions and cardiovascular collapse can also occur after a week. Protracted abstinence syndrome generally follows and is often marked by depression and sleep disturbances.

The CNS hyperexcitability associated with alcohol withdrawal is thought to be related to alcohol-induced alterations in the sensitivity of GABA and glutamate receptors. Experimental evidence indicates that prolonged alcohol exposure decreases the sensitivity of GABA receptors and increases the sensitivity of glutamate receptors. With the cessation of alcohol intake, these changes are manifested throughout the brain as a decrease in the inhibitory neurotransmitter GABA and an increase in the excitatory amino acid neurotransmitter glutamate.

Alcohol-Induced Biomedical Conditions

In humans, acute consumption of alcohol produces a sense of well being and mild euphoria. As the previous studies have shown, animals will also self-administer alcohol. This research has also provided evidence implicating dopamine, serotonin, GABA and opioid peptides in alcohol reinforcement.

Alcohol is also thought to enhance GABA activity in specific parts of the brain. GABA enhancement mirrors the reinforcing effects of alcohol, since drugs that block GABA activity also decrease alcohol intake, while drugs that increase GABA activity increase alcohol preference forestalling withdrawal. Part of alcohol's reinforcement is possibly due to increased GABA inhibition on other inhibitory neurons that decrease the activity of the dopamine neurons in the ventral tegmental area. This chain of action would have the ultimate effect of increasing the activity of the dopamine neurons. However, the experimental evidence supporting this idea is equivocal. While it is clear that both GABA and dopamine are involved in the reinforcing affects of alcohol, the relationship between these systems in this action is yet to be fully defined. The following medical conditions have been associated with chronic alcohol abuse.

Liver and organ effects are caused by enzyme depletion. Alcohol metabolism requires a coenzyme called *nicotinamide adenine dinucleotide (NAD)* which can get depleted in alcoholics. NAD depletion can result in the build-up of glutamate, maleate, and lactate which contribute to liver impairment and damage. This can lead to fatty liver (hyperlipemia), hepatitis and cirrhosis. Depletion of NAD can also lead to alcoholic hypoglycemia which contributes to alcohol's mental effects since the brain is an insulin-dependent organ. Alcohol also disrupts the gastrointestinal function by reducing the water-soluble vitamins, and increasing secretion of hydrochloric acid (HCL) and digestive juices that contribute to gastritis and pancreatitis.

Vitamin and mineral deficiencies can result from alcohol's "empty calories", which are of no nutritional value. The ingestion of large amounts of alcohol also results in limited or sporadic food consumption, resulting in vitamin deficiencies.

Secondary deficiencies may develop, due to impaired absorption and storage of vitamins. These alcohol-related defects involve the liver, which is the primary organ that stores and converts precursor forms of vitamins to their active metabolites. B vitamin deficiencies are common in chronic alcoholics. Vitamin B deficiency is associated with cardiovascular symptoms, alcohol neuritis, Korsakoff s psychosis and Wernicke's syndrome. *Peripheral neuropathy,* a thiamine deficiency, is actually demyelination of peripheral nerve fibers, also common in many alcoholics. This condition is associated with less sensory acuity, *paresthesias* and reduced conductance velocity.

Deficiencies in vitamins D, K and A are also common in chronic alcoholics. Alcoholics with liver damage such as hepatitis (fatty liver) have an 80% decrease in hepatic (liver) vitamin A levels. The combination of impaired vitamin D metabolism, chronic intake of antacids containing aluminum, and high corticosteroid levels may also result in osteoporosis in both alcoholic women and men. The metabolism of iron is impaired by alcohol, even when the person is well nourished and has no anemia. The loss of iron metabolism caused by chronic drinking is important in contributing to idiopathic hemochromatosis (iron overload).

High blood pressure and *cardiac irregularities* are observed in both acute and chronic alcohol ingestion due to the combined effects of more norepinephrine, depression of cardioregulatory centers *in* the brainstem, and the reflex response to peripheral vasodilation. The direct effects of alcohol on the heart muscle itself may eventually lead to *cardiomyopathy* (heart swelling) with associated *arrhythmias* (irregular beat). Peripheral neuropathies that accompany chronic use also contribute to cardiovascular impairment.

Alcohol-induced CNS depression produces a marked decrease in *antidiuretic hormone (ADH)* from the posterior pituitary. The sudden decrease in ADH, coupled with the increase in liquid volume consumption, can lead to a profound and dramatic diuresis.

Contrary to what many believe, alcohol actually lowers body temperature. Even though the vasodilation from acute alcohol ingestion produces a warm sensation (due to increased vascular flow to the cutaneous vessels), the restricted blood flow to the periphery causes heat loss. Also, alcohol at high doses produces hypothalamic depression and will compromise the temperature-regulating systems of the body. These combined factors can be potentially fatal to the homeless alcoholic living on the street, because their systems can not respond to changes in weather. There are also dangers when alcohol is used in combination with certain antipsychotic medications that further impair response to temperature changes. The dually diagnosed patient, for example, who is taking an anti-psychotic medication and is at risk for alcohol relapse would require careful case management in this regard.

Prenatal exposure to alcohol can produce a variety of problems for children. Fetal alcohol syndrome includes mental retardation, congenital heart defects, and abnormal morphological conditions including microencephaly, under-development and facial abnormalities.

High Risk Populations and Alcoholism
Genetic influences on normal and pathological consumption of alcohol are shown in family studies, twin studies and adoption studies, as well as animal research. Animal studies have established that alcohol preference and the reinforcing actions of alcohol are influenced by genetic factors. While there have been fewer studies examining the genetic component of drug abuse, evidence from animal studies also supports a genetic influence on the use and abuse of drugs other than alcohol.

The study of nonalcoholic drug abuse in humans is more difficult because of substantially smaller populations that use these drugs and marked changes in exposure to these agents. Investigation in this area is further hampered by the complexity of subjects' drug use, since most drug abusers have used multiple agents. This has led researchers either to concentrate on one class of drug or to treat all illicit drug use as equivalent. The tendency to lump all illicit drugs into one category makes results difficult to interpret or compare. In the case of alcohol, studies indicate that low doses of alcohol are stimulating and produce a strong positive reward in animals susceptible to the alcohol addiction.

Another component of excessive alcohol consumption might be that alcoholics have a high threshold to the aversive effects of ethanol. This could be a result of an innate low sensitivity to medium and high doses of alcohol or acute tolerance to its aversive effects. Results from animal studies suggest an association between high alcohol preference and acute tolerance to high-dose effects of ethanol.

Neurobiological evidence points to common pathways mediating the positive reinforcing actions of alcohol and other drugs of abuse. Most evidence shows the involvement of the mesocorticolimbic pathway dopamine system in drug reinforcement. Other neural pathways that regulate MCLP activity may also increase the rewarding effects of ethanol and other drugs of abuse. In the case of serotonin, innate genetic factors appear to reduce CNS activity of serotonin, and induce heavy drinking.

Animal and human studies additionally suggest an inherited difference in dopamine response to alcohol consumption and possibly an anomaly in the D2 receptor for dopamine associated with alcohol abuse. Continued studies with animals and humans are needed to clarify these differences and to explore the relationship of other neurobiological mechanisms related to the inherited components of other drugs of abuse.

Twin Studies
Evidence from twin studies suggests genetic influences on drinking patterns and alcohol problems. Results from twin studies demonstrate genetic determination of alcohol consumption such as abstention, average alcohol intake or heavy alcohol use. Twin studies also indicate an inherited risk for smoking.

When evaluating how alcoholism develops, twin studies generally show mutual development of a disorder. One study found a higher concordance rate for alcohol abuse between identical twins (54 percent) versus fraternal twins (28 percent), while two subsequent studies found no such relationship. A 1991 study examined 50 male and 31 female identical twin pairs and 64 male and 24 female fraternal twin pairs, with 1 member of the pair meeting alcohol abuse or dependence criteria. The study found that identical male twins differed from fraternal male twins in the frequencies of both alcohol abuse and dependence as well as other substance abuse and dependence. On the other hand, female identical and fraternal twins were equally likely to abuse alcohol and/or become dependent on other substances, but identical female twins were more likely to become alcohol dependent.

Another study of 356 twin pairs also found higher identical than fraternal rates of concordance for problems related to alcohol and drug use as well as conduct disorder. The same study also noted that among men, heritability was greater for early rather than late onset of alcohol problems, whereas no such effect was seen for women. Finally, a study of 1,030 female twin pairs found evidence for substantial heritability of liability to alcoholism, ranging from 50 to 60 percent.

Thus, twin studies provide general agreement that genetic factors influence certain aspects of drinking. Most twin studies also show genetic influence over pathological drinking, including the diagnosis of alcoholism, which appears (like many psychiatric disorders) to be moderately heritable. Whether genetic factors operate comparably in men and women, and whether severity of alcoholism influences twin concordance is less clear. How psychiatric comorbidity may affect heritability of alcoholism also remains to be studied.

Adoption Studies
Adoption studies have also supported the role of heritable factors in risk for alcoholism. The results from a series of studies conducted in Denmark during the 1970s are typical. Of 5,483 adoption cases from Copenhagen between 1924 and 1947, the researchers compared 20 adoptees with 30 nonadopted brothers. They also studied 49 female adoptees, comparing them with 81 non-adopted daughters of alcoholics. Comparisons also were made with matched control adoptees.

The Copenhagen study revealed that adopted sons of alcoholic parents were *four times* as likely as sons of nonalcoholics to have developed alcoholism. Evidence also suggested that the alcoholism in these cases was more severe. The groups differed little on other variables, including prevalence of other psychiatric illness or heavy drinking. Being raised by an alcoholic biological parent did not further increase the likelihood of developing alcoholism. That is, rates of alcoholism did not differ between the adopted children and their nonadopted brothers.

In contrast, daughters of alcoholics were not at elevated risk of alcoholism. Among adoptees, 2 percent had alcoholism (another 2 percent had drinking problems), compared with 4 percent of alcoholism among the adopted controls and 3 percent among nonadopted daughters.

Another analysis examined factors promoting drug abuse as well. In this study, all classes of illicit drugs were collapsed into a single category of "drug abuse." Most of the 40 adopted drug abusers had coexisting anti-social personality disorder; the presence of ASPD correlated highly with drug abuse. For those without ASPD, family history of alcoholism accompanied drug abuse. Also, turmoil in the adoptive family (divorce or psychiatric disturbance) was also associated with increased drug abuse.

Finally, results from other adoption studies suggest two possible forms of alcohol abuse. The two forms have been classified as "milieu- limited" or *Type I alcohol abuse* in contrast to "male-limited" or *Type 2 alcohol abuse.* Type 1 alcohol abuse is generally mild, characterized by mild alcohol problems and minimal criminal behavior in the parents, but it can be occasionally severe, depending on a provocative environment. Type 2 is associated with severe alcohol abuse and criminality in biological fathers. In the adoptees, it was associated with recurrent problems and appeared to be unaffected by postnatal environment.

In summary, adoption studies of alcoholism clearly indicate the role of biological, presumably genetic, factors in the genesis of alcoholism. They do not exclude, however, a possible role for environmental factors as well. Moreover, evidence suggests several biological backgrounds are conducive to alcoholism. In particular, one pattern of inheritance suggests a relationship between parental antisocial behavior and alcoholism in the next generation. Thus, adoption studies, like other designs, suggest that even at the genetic level, alcoholism is not a homogeneous construct.

Electro-Physiological Activity
Attempts to correlate distinctive patterns of spontaneous electrical activity of the brain with alcoholism and substance abuse have been conclusive. A few studies have found distinctive *electroencephalograph (EEG)* patterns in individuals at risk for alcoholism, but others have not. Similarly, the use of alcohol challenge (i.e., giving the subject alcohol and then recording EEG) on subjects at high risk for alcoholism has likewise yielded inconclusive results. The rationale for challenge studies rests on the observation that alcohol has been shown to affect resting EEG, and thus might have a differential effect on those at low and high risk for alcoholism. Again, some studies have seen distinctive responses, while others have not.

A logical extension of studying resting EEG activity is examining event-related potentials (ERPs). ERPs are patterns of brain electrical activity produced in response to a particular stimulus (e.g., auditory, visual); they can reflect a variety of sensory and cognitive processes. Since ERPs may reflect heritable differences in cognitive function or capability that may in turn contribute to liability to alcoholism, some have suggested that ERP changes may allow discrimination between those at low and high genetic risk for alcoholism. The results of these studies have also been equivocal. Some have found characteristic responses among individuals at risk for alcoholism while others have not. The specificity for alcoholism of such findings is unclear. In particular, it is not yet known whether similar findings might be identified in subjects at risk for illicit drug abuse.

Currently, both EEG and ERP findings seem best viewed as possible markers. Further studies are needed to confirm the positive results that have been observed. In addition, while ERP findings in particular might relate to aspects of cognitive functioning that may differ among those at risk for alcoholism how such differences contribute to risk for alcoholism and perhaps substance abuse is not well understood.

BIOCHEMICAL ASSAYS

Serotonin

Results over the last two decades from both human and animal studies have supported a relationship between low levels of serotonin in the central nervous system (CNS) and impulsive violent behavior. Since problematic drug use has long been associated with a wide range of violent behavior, scientists have examined the relationship between alcoholism and serotonergic abnormalities. While a consistent relationship is lacking between alcoholism and low CNS levels of serotonin and its metabolites, mounting evidence supports low serotonin in a subgroup of alcoholics with early-onset problems and a history of violence.

Because measures of serotonin activity are difficult to obtain, researchers have used pharmacological probes of serotonin function, such as hormonal response to drugs that affect serotonin. These indirect measures have also indicated a relationship between impulsivity, substance abuse, and abnormal serotonin function.

Given that early-onset alcoholism and ASPD overlap substantially, the specificity of the serotonin findings is unclear, especially as similar results have been found in substance abusers with ASPD. However, at least one report has indicated that, even after controlling for the presence of ASPD and illicit drug abuse, other neurochemical findings remained significantly associated with alcoholism. While research might delineate the relationship between decreased CNS serotonin levels and specific psychiatric syndromes, current evidence suggests relatively specific biological differences may exist between early- and late-onset alcoholics, raising the possibility of defining biologically homogeneous subgroups.

Aldehyde and Alcohol Dehydrogenase

Many Asians rapidly develop a prominent facial flush following ingestion of a small amount of alcohol. Continued drinking leads to nausea, dizziness, palpitations and faintness. This reaction is due to inactivity in the individuals' aldehyde dehydrogenase, an enzyme, as you will recall, that helps metabolize alcohol in the body. Ineffective enzyme activity results in a buildup of acetaldehyde in the blood following alcohol consumption which can be toxic. Interestingly, a mutant form of alcohol dehydrogenase also produces a transient increase in the acetaldehyde concentration after alcohol ingestion. This form of the enzyme also has been reported in Asian populations.

The two enzymes, aldehyde and alcohol dehydrogenase, interact in some individuals to amplify the adverse reaction to alcohol consumption. Since this reaction discourages heavy drinking and occurs in populations where alcoholism is relatively rare, this suggests that alcohol and aldehyde dehydrogenase mutations might be a major determinant of alcohol consumption, abuse, and dependence. This holds true in Taiwan and Japan where the reaction occurs in 30 to 50 percent of individuals.

The genetics of aldehyde and alcohol dehydrogenase are well described. Different forms of these enzymes are by variations of their normal genes. The presence of these gene variations in an individual accounts for variations in the metabolism of alcohol. Thus, these genes can also effect alcohol consumption. For example, the gene variation that code for the ineffective form of aldehyde dehydrogenase is not only rare in alcoholics, but is also rare in Japanese patients with alcoholic liver disease. Despite identification of such genes, the relationship between their inheritance and family transmission of alcoholism remains unstudied.

Alcohol Challenge

A number of studies have been conducted investigating the effect of administering alcohol to young adult sons of alcoholics. These studies indicate that, despite similarity of blood alcohol levels, sons of alcoholics demonstrate less intense subjective responses to alcohol, as well as less intense upper body sway. Since these individuals have less of a reaction to alcohol, they might find it more difficult to self-regulate alcohol consumption, thus increasing the risk of developing alcoholism. In conjunction with these findings, other studies have found that sons of alcoholics demonstrate slightly lower levels of certain hormones (prolactin, cortisol or ACTH) after ingesting alcohol. The relationship, if any, of these decreased hormonal levels to alcohol consumption is provocative yet unclear.

Cognitive Differences

Study of high-risk populations (e.g., sons of alcoholics) has revealed temperamental as well as biological differences between high-risk and control subjects, suggesting that vulnerability to alcoholism can be conceptualized from a behavior-genetic perspective. In other words, heritable constitutional differences might affect temperament and increase risk for alcoholism and addiction. In particular these differences might influence cognitive styles, learning ability, and capability to control one's own behavior.

In general, it appears that sons of alcoholics tend to have greater impairment on tests of cognitive development, academic achievement, and neuropsychological function. However, the magnitude of these differences may depend greatly on how the population is categorized. To date, little is known of what specific psychological, temperamental, or cognitive factors ascertain high risk subjects who actually go on to develop alcoholism.

Alcoholism and drug abuse are complex conditions that result from multiple causal factors. Alcoholism and other forms of addiction have a genetic component but require specific environmental influences. Thus, consideration of genetic factors must also take into account general social conditions such as availability and cost of substances, acceptability of use, influences on initiation of use, maintenance or cessation of use, and development of use-related problems. A major goal of clinical addiction research is to determine who is vulnerable under what conditions. Understanding this interaction might lead to better prediction of relapse as well as improved matching of patients and treatments.

Barbiturates

Barbiturates are a class of drugs that depress CNS activity. First introduced in the early 1900s, barbiturates were widely prescribed as antianxiety agents and sleep aids, and treatment for other psychiatric conditions. However, their lethal overdose potential and high abuse potential, coupled with the advent of the safer benzodiazepine compounds, curtailed their use starting in the 1960s.

The sedative effects of barbiturates result from their ability to increase GABA activity. Their mechanism of action is an augmentation of the activity of the GABAA receptor. This receptor is linked to a chloride ion channel. Stimulation of the receptor by GABA opens the channel and increases the flow of chloride into the neuron, which inhibits the cell's activity. Barbiturates increase the time the chloride channel stays open, thus increasing the inhibitory effects of GABA.

Acute Administration

The reinforcing properties of barbiturates have been clearly demonstrated in both animal and human studies. Animals readily self-administer barbiturates in a variety of different experimental paradigms. Human studies have demonstrated that drug-experienced subjects, blind to the identity of the drug, consistently give barbiturates high rankings when asked to rate a series of drugs. Human subjects will work to receive barbiturates and will do more work to receive the drug if the available dosage is increased.

The mechanism of barbiturate reward is still unclear. Since one of the major effects is to enhance GABA activity, barbiturates, like alcohol, may increase GABA inhibition of other inhibitory neurons, thus increasing the net activity of the dopamine neurons in the ventral tegmental area. Further studies are necessary to confirm this possibility.

Chronic Administration
With continued use, some tolerance develops to most effects of barbiturates. However, little tolerance develops to prevent a lethal dose. Unlike most other drugs of abuse, both metabolic and pharmacodynamic tolerance are important in the development of barbiturate tolerance. Barbiturate withdrawal is marked by a severe and sometimes life-threatening condition similar to alcohol withdrawal. Both anxiety and depression are common, and with prolonged use, the development of severe grand mal tonic epileptic seizures can occur.

The neurochemical changes responsible for the pharmacodynamic tolerance and withdrawal syndrome have yet to be clearly established, but may be related to rebounding NE systems. Some evidence suggests that tolerance is the result of the GABAA receptors becoming less sensitive to the effects of barbiturates. After cessation, the barbiturate stimulation of GABA activity ceases, and the desensitized receptors create an overall decrease in GABA activity causing withdrawal symptoms. The hyperexcitability that results is very similar to what occurs in the alcohol withdrawal. In fact, barbiturates are sometimes referred to as "solid alcohols" because of the similarity in mechanism of action.

Benzodiazepines (Anxiolytics)
Benzodiazepines, also known as the *anxiolytics* (reducing anxiousness), are a class of drugs introduced in the 1960s as anti-anxiety agents. They rapidly replaced barbiturates, which have significant abuse potential, to treat psychiatric conditions. Like barbiturates, they generally inhibit brain activity by enhancing GABA. However, unlike barbiturates, which create a nonspecific effect on chloride ion channels, benzodiazepines act by binding to a specific receptor (BDZ receptor) within the GABA system. The presence of a BDZ receptor suggests a natural endogenous chemical that normally interacts with it.

The benzodiazepine receptor is coupled with the GABAA receptor. Stimulation of the BDZ receptor increases the frequency of chloride ion channel opening in response to GABA binding to the GABAA receptor. Also, benzodiazepines enhance GABA binding to its receptor, and the presence of GABA enhances benzodiazepine binding. The net effect of benzodiazepines augments activity at the GABAA receptor and enhances GABA action, creating sedative results.

Acute Administration

Most benzodiazepines support only modest levels of self-administration, much below the levels observed with barbiturates, when given intravenously in animal studies. When given orally, benzodiazepines do not induce self-administration in animal studies. Human studies, similar to those used for barbiturates, have demonstrated that benzodiazepines yield modest rankings of liking and that given a choice, subjects consistently prefer barbiturates over benzodiazepines. Since benzodiazepines act selectively on GABA activity, their mild reinforcing properties might be due to activating GABA mechanisms similar to those for alcohol. However, combining benzodiazepines with alcohol or other sedatives produces an additive effect that can be extremely toxic.

Chronic Administration

Prolonged exposure to benzodiazepines results in tolerance to their therapeutic effects. This may be due to a reduction in the functional activity of GABA as a result of a desensitization of the benzodiazepine receptor caused by prolonged exposure to the drug. As with alcohol and the barbiturates, a withdrawal syndrome can occur following benzodiazepine cessation. In general, the characteristics of benzodiazepine withdrawal are similar to barbiturate withdrawal but at therapeutic doses, the magnitude of the symptoms are less severe than with barbiturates. Nonetheless, since benzodiazepines are widely prescribed, their abuse potential physicians to use careful administration.

Medications in the Treatment of Alcoholism

Disulfiram (Antabuse)

Disulfiram (Antabuse) was the first medicine approved for the treatment of alcohol abuse and alcohol dependence by the U.S. Food and Drug Administration. Antabuse is prescribed to help people who want to quit drinking by causing a negative reaction if the person drinks while they are taking Antabuse.

As you have read, alcohol is metabolized by the liver into acetaldehyde, a very toxic substance that causes many hangover symptoms heavy drinker's experience. Usually, the body continues to oxidize acetaldehyde into acetic acid, which is harmless. Antabuse interferes with this metabolic process, stops the process with the production of acetaldehyde and prevents the oxidation of acetaldehyde into acetic acid. Because of this, Antabuse will cause a build up of acetaldehyde five or ten times greater than normally occurs when someone drinks alcohol.

The high concentration of acetaldehyde that occurs when someone drinks while taking Antabuse can cause reactions that range in severity. Some of the principal symptoms that can occur with acetaldehyde buildup include flushing, nausea, vomiting, sweating, throbbing headache, breathing difficulty, chest pains, heart palpitations, tachycardia, hypotension, and blurred vision.

Antabuse serves merely as an aversive treatment for someone trying to stop drinking. It does not reduce the person's craving for alcohol, nor does it treat any of the alcohol withdrawal syndrome. Remember, some things seem to work more or less for some people some of the time. All treatment has a role in certain situations. And, like all other forms for behavioral healthcare, medications alone is not a best practice. Rather, medications combined with counseling is a standard of care.

Vivitrol (naltrexone)
The FDA has approved naltrexone extended-release injectable suspension (*Vivitrol*) for the treatment of alcohol dependence in patients who are able to abstain from drinking in an outpatient setting and who are not actively drinking on therapy initiation. It must be administered by a healthcare professional and used in combination with psychosocial support, such as counseling or group therapy.

Naltrexone is a medication that blocks the effects of drugs known as opioids. It competes with these drugs for opioid receptors in the brain. Originally used to treat dependence on opioid drugs, nalrexone is also approved by the FDA as treatment for alcoholism (Vivitrol). In clinical trials evaluating the effectiveness of naltrexone, patients who received naltrexone were twice as successful in remaining abstinent and in avoiding relapse as patients who received placebo-an inactive pill. Vivitrol must be administered by a healthcare professional. It is administered once a month or every 4 weeks as a gluteal IM injection. Vivitrol is contraindicated in patients receiving or dependent on opioids, in acute opioid withdrawal, and in those who have failed the naloxone challenge test or have a positive urine screen for opioids; and in those with previous hypersensitivity to naltrexone, PLG or any other components of the diluent.

Acamprosate (Campral)
Acamprosate has in vitro affinity for GABA type A and GABA type B receptors, so it's been assumed that the therapeutic effects of acamprosate are due to actions on GABA receptors. However, acamprosate does not share most of the other effects of GABA receptor modifying drugs, such as antianxiety, hypnotic, or muscle relaxant activity. It's therefore possible, perhaps likely, that the effects are mediated some other way. Acamprosate is structurally related to l-glutamic acid (l-gutamate), which is an excitatory neurotransmitter. It's been proposed that acamprosate decreases the effects of the naturally-occurring excitatory neurotransmitter glutamate in the body.

Since chronic alcohol consumption disrupts this system, and the changes last many months after alcohol ingestion is stopped, it's possible that acamprosate somehow restores the glutamate system towards normal. It's thought, no matter how it acts, that Campral decreases the pleasant "high" associated with alcohol consumption, and thus decrease the frequency of relapse during abstinence.

Treatment with acamprosate calcium typically starts between 2 and 7 days after ceasing alcohol consumption. The medication is taken orally, in a 333mg pill, taken three times daily, and treatment traditionally lasts around six months. Acamprosate produces best results when combined with counseling treatment and recovery support services.

Vitamins

a. Common nutritional deficiencies of alcoholic patients: e.g., magnesium, zinc, various vitamins.

b. Administration of supplemental thiamine to all patients with a history of chronic alcoholism and in the treatment of Wernicke's encephalopathy, alcoholic amblyopia (a decrease of vision).

c. Multiple mega-B therapy recommended for amblyopia.

(NOTE: Thiamine, 100 mg daily and a multivitamin supplement, provided patient shows no significant neurologic or hematologic problems secondary to chronic excessive alcohol intake is a rather standard vitamin regime for this population.)

Intesting Research!

No Prototypic "Alcoholic"

Americans with alcohol addiction tend to fit into one of five personality types, putting to rest theories that there is a "typical alcoholic." A study described in *Drug and Alcohol Dependence* analyzed the clinical features of 1,484 persons found to be alcohol-dependent through the 2001-2002 National Epidemiological Survey on Alcohol and Related Conditions and then grouped those persons according to their clinical features. The study found that there is no such thing as a "typical alcoholic," rather that alcohol-dependent subjects tend to fall into five subtypes.

The findings should help dispel the notion of the 'typical alcoholic. Young adults comprise the largest group of alcoholics and nearly 20 percent of alcoholics are highly functional and well educated with good incomes. More than half of the alcoholics in the United States have no multigenerational family history of the disease, suggesting that their form of alcoholism was unlikely to have genetic causes.

Clinicians have long recognized diverse manifestations of alcoholism and researchers have tried to understand why some alcoholics improve with specific medications and therapies while others do not.

In the study, the researchers identified 5 unique subtypes of alcoholism based on respondents' family history of alcoholism, age of onset of regular drinking and alcohol problems, symptom patterns of alcohol dependence and abuse, and the presence of additional substance abuse and mental disorders.

- **Young adult subtype.** This is the most common alcohol-dependent subtype, constituting **32 %** of alcohol-dependent Americans. They are typically young, male adult drinkers with relatively low rates of co-occurring substance abuse and other mental disorders. They have a 22% rate of familial alcoholism and rarely seek help for their drinking.

- **Young antisocial subtype.** This is the second most common category of alcohol-dependent individuals, constituting **21%** of alcohol-dependent Americans. They are apt to be in their mid-20s and to have started drinking early. About half come from families with alcoholism, and about half have a diagnosis of antisocial personality disorder. Three-fourths of these individuals smoke cigarettes; two-thirds meet criteria for marijuana abuse or dependence. About a fourth use cocaine, and about a fifth abuse opioids. About one-third seek treatment for their drinking problem.

- **Intermediate familial subtype. 19%** of alcohol-dependent Americans fall into this category. They tend to be middle-aged, with about half coming from families in which a member has alcoholism. Almost half have experienced a major depression, and almost a quarter have been diagnosed with bipolar disorder. About one-fifth abuse marijuana or cocaine. One quarter of these people seek treatment for their drinking problem.

- **Functional subtype. 19.5%** of alcohol-dependent Americans fall into this category. They are, on average, older than other subtype members and tend to drink in an excessive, although less severe, manner than other subtypes. They have the highest family income, are college-educated, and are most likely to be married. They also include the highest proportion of retired individuals. From a psychosocial perspective, they represent the highest functioning subtype of alcohol-dependent persons. Seventeen percent seek treatment for their drinking problem.

- **Chronic severe subtype.** This is the smallest category of alcohol-dependent Americans, constituting **9%** of them. The subtype is composed mostly of middle-aged persons who had early onset of drinking. Over three-fourths come from families afflicted with alcoholism. This subtype has the highest probability of all the subtypes of having both first- and second-degree family members with alcohol dependence. Almost half have antisocial personality disorder. Of all the subtypes, they have the highest rate of major depression, social phobia, and bipolar, anxiety, and panic disorders. Over three-fourths smoke cigarettes. They often abuse substances in addition to alcohol. Two-thirds seek help for their drinking and are the largest subgroup who seek treatment.

The study results suggest that certain therapies might work better with certain subtypes than with others.

For example and these ideas have not yet been tested, the young adult subtype may be addressed with screening and brief intervention techniques rather than much more expensive approaches to therapeutic intervention. It may also be that certain types of pharmacotherapies now available could be better targeted to this subgroup. For example, this subgroup might benefit from pharmacotherapy that reduces the reinforcing effect of alcohol. Since the antisocial group has the worst prognosis of any of the subtypes, the focus has to be on complete abstinence and elimination of other forms of substance abuse.

The functional subtype represents individuals who essentially have fewer psychosocial consequences from their alcohol addiction. So the focus of the therapy might be on the recognition of the impairment that their alcohol dependence is producing in their life and focusing on either abstinence or a return to a much less hazardous level of drinking.

As for individuals with chronic severe alcohol dependence, it is assumed that they need substantial treatment. They might benefit from therapies that are directed toward relapse prevention. Furthermore, this subtype is going to have greater psychiatric comorbidity.

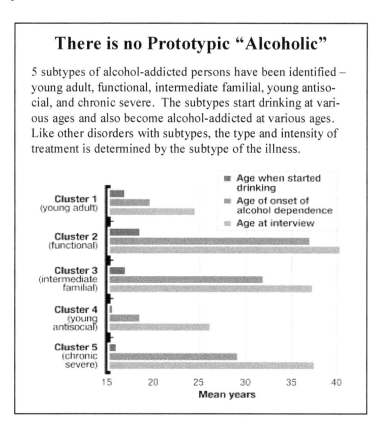

There is no Prototypic "Alcoholic"

5 subtypes of alcohol-addicted persons have been identified – young adult, functional, intermediate familial, young antisocial, and chronic severe. The subtypes start drinking at various ages and also become alcohol-addicted at various ages. Like other disorders with subtypes, the type and intensity of treatment is determined by the subtype of the illness.

CHAPTER 6: SELF-STUDY QUESTIONS

TRUE/FALSE

1. *Alcohol differs from most other drugs of abuse in that it has no known receptor system in the brain.*

2. *Once absorbed, alcohol is distributed rather uniformly through all tissues and fluids.*

3. *The dose-response relationship effects of alcohol are related to the blood alcohol level (BAL) which is the concentration of alcohol in the blood.*

4. *After ingestion, alcohol is absorbed from the esophagus into the large intestine where it gets metabolized by the liver.*

5. *Most alcohol is metabolized by specialized enzymes within the kidneys.*

6. *Antabuse (disulfiram) is a drug that was developed as a conditioning reward response treatment approach to alcoholism.*

7. *The ingestion of large amounts of alcohol often results in limited or sporadic food consumption, resulting in vitamin deficiencies.*

8. *Alcoholics with liver damage such as fatty liver or hepatitis have an 80% to 90% decrease in liver vitamin A levels.*

9. *Vitamin B1 deficiency, common in chronic alcoholics, is associated with Korsakoff's psychosis.*

10. *Alcohol actually lowers body temperature.*

* Answers to Self Study Tests are located on page 351

Chapter 6 Selected Reading

Abbott PJ, Quinn D, Knox L. Ambulatory medical detoxification for alcohol. Am J Drug Alcohol Abuse 1995;21:549-63.

Begleiter, H., Projesz, B. and Bihari, B., "Auditory Brainstem Potentials in Sons of Alcoholic Fathers," *Alcohol and Clinical Experimental Research,* Volume 11 (Number 5): 477-480, 1987.

Boehm, SL, Valenzuela, CF, and Harris, RA. Alcohol: Neurobiology. Lowinson, JH, Ruiz, P, Millman, RB, and Langrod, JG (editors), *Substance Abuse A Comprehensive Sourcebook.* Fourth Edition. Lippincott Williams & Wilkins. 2005.

Bouza C, Angeles M, Magro A, Muñoz A, Amate JM. Efficacy and safety of naltrexone and acamprosate in the treatment of alcohol dependence: a systematic review. *Addiction* 99 (7): 811–28. 2004.

Chang PH, Steinberg MB. Alcohol withdrawal. Med Clin North Am 2001;85:1191-212 Johnson BA, Ait-Dowd N. Neuropharmacological treatments for alcoholism: scientific basis and clinical findings. *Psychopharmacology*. 2000;149:327-344.

Gianoulakis, C. and Dai, X., Levels and circadian rhythmicity of plasma ACTH, cortisol, and beta-endorphin as a function of family history of alcoholism. *Psychopharm._* 181: 437-444. 2005.

Grant, K.A., Valverius, P. and Hudspith, M., "Ethanol Withdrawal Seizures and NMDAReceptor Complex," *European Journal of Pharmacology,* Volume 176: 289-296, 1990.

Johnson, B.A., Swift, R.M., Ait-Doud, N., DiClemente, C.C., Javors, M.A., Malcom, R.J., Development of novel pharmacotherapies for the treatment of alcohol dependence: Focus on antiepileptics. *Alc. Clin. Exp. Res._* 28: 295-301 (2004).

Kenna GA, Wood MD. Alcohol use, dysfunction and abuse in healthcare professionals. *Alcohol Clin Exp Res*. 2003;27:32A.

Kranzler, H.R., Koob, G., Gastfriend, D.R., Swift, R.M., & Willenbring, M.L. Advances in the pharmacotherapy of alcoholism: Challenging misconceptions. *Alc. Clin. Exp. Res., 30,* 272-281, 2006.

Longo LP, Bohn MJ. Alcoholism pharmacotherapy: new approaches to an old disease. *Hospital Physician*. 2001;6:33-43.

Malcolm R, Herron JE, Anton RF, Roberts J, Moore J. Recurrent detoxification may elevate alcohol craving as measured by the Obsessive Compulsive Drinking scale.

Alcohol 2000;20:181-5.

Moss, HB, Chen, CM, and Yi, Hsiao-ye. Subtypes of alcohol dependence in a nationally representative sample. *Drug and Alcohol Dependence, Volume 91, Issues 2-3, 1.* 2007.

Myrick H, Anton RF. Clinical management of alcohol withdrawal. CNS Spectr 2000;5:22-32.

O'Malley, S.S., Rounsaville, B.J., Farren, C., Namkoong, K., Wu, R., Robinson, J., O'Connor, P.G., Initial and maintenance naltrexone treatment for alcohol dependence using primary care vs. specialty care. *Arch. Intern. Med.* 163: 1695-1704 (2003).

Pettinati HM, Rabinowitz AR. Choosing the right medication for the treatment of alcoholism. *Curr Psychiatry Rep* **8** (5): 383–8. 2006.

Rounsaville, BJ, O'Malley, S, and O'Connor, P. Guidelines for the Use of Naltrexone in the Treatment of Alcoholism - *The APT Foundation*, 904 Howard Avenue, New Haven, CT 06519.

Sanchis-Segura, C., Borchardt, T., Vengeliene, V., Zghoul, T., Bachteler, D., Gass, P., Sprengel, R., and Spanagel, R., Involvement of the AMPA receptor GluR-C subunit in alcohol-seeking behavior and relapse. *J. Neurosci.* 26: 1231-1238, 2006.

Soyka M, Roesner S. New pharmacological approaches for the treatment of alcoholism. *Expert Opin Pharmacother* 7 (17): 2341–53. 2006.

Sullivan JT, Sykora K, Schneiderman J, Naranjo CA, Sellers EM. Assessment of alcohol withdrawal: the revised Clinical Institute Withdrawal Assessment for Alcohol scale (CIWA-Ar). Br J Addict 1989;84:1353-7.

Swift RM. Drug therapy in alcohol dependence. *N Engl J Med.* 1999;340:1482-1490.

Swift RM. Medications and alcohol craving. *Alcohol Res World.* 1999; 23 (3): p. 209.

Williams SH. Medications for treating alcohol dependence. *Am Fam Physician* **72** (9): 1775–80. 2005.

CHAPTER 7: VOCABULARY LIST

Ephedrine
Naturally occurring chemical from the ephedra plant that forms the foundation for amphetamines.

Erythroxylon Coca
A large shrub indigenous to South America; cocaine is extracted from its leaves.

MDMA
(methylenedioxymethamphetamine) an analog of methamphetamine that is chemically related to mescaline and amphetamine and is used illicitly for its euphoric and hallucinogenic effects.

Methylxanthines
A class o f CNS stimulant compounds, to which caffeine belongs.

Monoamine oxidase
(MAO) The enzyme that degrades the monoamine neurotransmitters but is inhibited by amphetamines, so that NE, DA and 5-HT activity is more pronounced.

Nicotinic receptor
The acetylcholine receptor subtype which is most commonly activated by nicotine.

Sympathomimetic
A group of drugs that stimulate the sympathetic nervous system, increasing mental alertness, and increasing blood flow to muscles. Adverse effects of high doses include raised blood pressure, increased heart rate, and increased anxiety.

Tweaking
Slang for someone exhibiting OCD-like, compulsive or repetitive behaviors, often making insignificant tiny adjustments to things or behaviors, while in a slightly agitated or confused state.

CHAPTER 7: PSYCHOSTIMULANTS

As the name implies, stimulant drugs have an energizing effect that promotes an increase in psychological and/or motor activity. Stimulants such as cocaine and the amphetamines have their most pronounced effect on the monoamine neurotransmitters like norepinephrine (NE), epinephrine (E), dopamine (DA) and serotonin (5-HT). This results from their combined actions as reuptake inhibitors, neurotransmitter releasers and monoamine oxidase inhibitors (MAOIs). The arousing and euphoric effects associated with these drugs are caused by these various actions. Stimulants also affect mechanisms triggered in stress situations (the fight-or-flight response) via activation of the sympathetic nervous system (sympathomimetic effects), including increases in heart rate (tachycardia), blood pressure (hypertension) and the release of various hormones.

AMPHETAMINES

Amphetamine is a generic term that applies to a group of synthetic compounds derived from naturally occurring ephedrine found in the ephedra plant indigenous to Eastern Africa. Amphetamines are all classified as indirect-acting agonists at NE, DA and 5-HT synapses. Amphetamine users describe the euphoric effects of the drug in the same terms used by cocaine users, and in the laboratory, subjects cannot distinguish between the effects of cocaine and amphetamines. This is not to suggest that cocaine and amphetamines have similar mechanisms of action. In fact under proper conditions, differences between their effects can be demonstrated. For example, cocaine effects are relatively brief after intravenous injection, whereas those of methamphetamine may last for hours. Oral ingestion is a common route of amphetamine administration, but like cocaine, intravenous injection, smoking, and snorting are also common.

Methamphetamines
First synthesized in 1887 Germany, amphetamine was for a long time, a drug in search of a disease. Nothing was done with the drug, from its discovery (synthesis) until the late 1920's, when it was investigated as a cure or treatment against nearly everything from depression to decongestion. In the 1930's, amphetamine was marketed as Benzedrine, an over-the-counter inhaler to treat nasal congestion (for asthmatics, hay fever sufferers, and people with colds). By 1937 amphetamine was available by prescription in tablet form.

Methamphetamine, more potent and easy to make, was discovered in Japan in 1919. The crystalline powder was soluble in water, making it a perfect candidate for injection. It is still legally produced in the U.S., sold under the trade name Desoxyn. During World War II, amphetamines were widely used to keep the fighting men going (Note -during the Vietnam War, American soldiers used more amphetamines than the rest of the world did during WWII). In Japan, intravenous methamphetamine abuse reached epidemic proportions immediately after World War II, when supplies stored for military use became available to the public.

In the United States in the 1950s, legally manufactured tablets of both dextroamphetamine (Dexedrine) and methamphetamine (Methedrine) became readily available and were used non medically by college students, truck drivers, and athletes, As use of amphetamines spread, so did their abuse. Amphetamines became a cure-all for such things as weight control and treating mild depression. This pattern changed drastically in the 1960s with the increased availability of injectable methamphetamine. The 1970 Controlled Substances Act severely restricted the legal production of injectable methamphetamine, causing its use to decrease greatly.

Methamphetamine trafficking and abuse in the United States have been on the rise over the past few years, as indicated by investigative, seizure, price, purity, and abuse data . As a result, this drug is having a devastating impact in many communities across the nation. Although more common in western areas of the country, this impact increasingly is being felt in areas not previously familiar with the harmful effects of this powerful stimulant.

Clandestine production accounts for almost all of the methamphetamine trafficked and abused in the United States. The illicit manufacture of methamphetamine can be accomplished in a variety of ways, but is produced most commonly using the ephedrine/pseudoephedrine reduction method.

Domestically, large-scale production of methamphetamine is centered in California. In addition, methamphetamine increasingly is produced in Mexico or in labs within the United State that are sponsored by Mexican mafia. Not only are methamphetamine laboratories used to manufacture illegal, often deadly drugs, but the clandestine nature of the manufacturing process and the presence of ignitable, corrosive, reactive, and toxic chemicals at the sites have resulted in explosions, fires, toxic fumes, and irreparable damage to human health and to the environment.

Traditionally, the suppliers of methamphetamine throughout the United States have been outlaw motorcycle gangs and numerous other independent trafficking groups. Although these groups continue to produce and distribute methamphetamine, organized crime drug groups operating from Mexico currently dominate wholesale methamphetamine trafficking in the United States for several reasons: these organizations established access to wholesale ephedrine sources of supply on the international market; these organizations are producing unprecedented quantities of high-purity methamphetamine on a regular basis; and, they already control well-established cocaine, heroin, and marijuana distribution networks throughout the western United States, enabling them to supply methamphetamine to a large retail-level market. Their expansion into the methamphetamine trade has added a new dimension to their role in the U.S. drug market and has redefined the methamphetamine problem in the United States.

Patterns of Abuse

Methamphetamine is a drug that strongly activates certain systems in the brain. Methamphetamine is closely related chemically to amphetamine, but the central nervous system effects of methamphetamine are greater. Both drugs have some medical uses, primarily in the treatment of obesity and attention deficit disorder (ADD) but their therapeutic use is limited. Methamphetamine is made in illegal laboratories and has a high potential for abuse and dependence. It has many street names, such as "speed," "meth". Clear chunks of methamphetamine hydrochloride resembling ice crystals, which can be inhaled by smoking, is referred to as "crystal", "shabu", "ice" and "glass."

Methamphetamine is taken orally or intranasally (snorting the powder), and by injection. Immediately after inhalation or injection, the methamphetamine user experiences an intense sensation, called a "rush" or "flash," that lasts only a few minutes and is described as extremely pleasurable. Oral or intranasal use produces euphoric high, but not a rush. Because methamphetamine elevates mood, people who experiment with it tend to drastically increase frequency and doses, although this was not their original intent.

Adverse Effects

Not surprisingly, the action of amphetamines is similar to cocaine. The reinforcing properties of these drugs result from their ability to enhance dopamine action in mesocorticolimbic pathway (MCLP). While amphetamines also block dopamine reuptake, their most significant action is to directly stimulate the release of dopamine from neurons (see Figure below). Thus, unlike cocaine, which blocks dopamine reuptake following normal release of the transmitter from the terminal, amphetamines increase dopamine activity independent from neuronal activity. As a result of this difference, amphetamines are more potent than cocaine in increasing the levels of dopamine in the synapse. Contributing to this as well, there is evidence that amphetamines, unlike cocaine, inhibits the enzyme monoamine oxidase, so newly released neurotransmitters remain in synapse longer where binding to and stimulating postsynaptic receptors occurs at a heightened frequency .

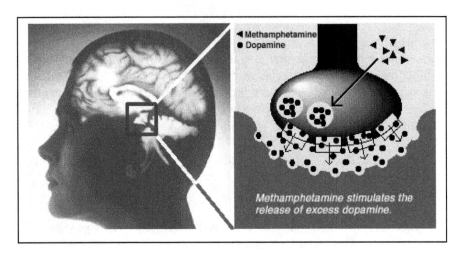

Methamphetamine stimulates the release of excess dopamine.

Amphetamines also directly stimulate the release of norepinephrine, epinephrine, and serotonin from neurons. Among the amphetamines, the balance between their actions on these different neurotransmitter systems varies. For example, methylenedioxymethamphetamine (MDMA) has a particularly potent effect on the serotonin system, which provides this drug with a psychedelic effect.

The central nervous system (CNS) actions that result from taking even small amounts of methamphetamine include increased wakefulness, increased physical activity, decreased appetite, increased respiration, hyperthermia, and euphoria. Other CNS effects include irritability, insomnia, confusion, tremors, convulsions, anxiety, paranoia, and aggressiveness. Hyperthermia and convulsions can result in death. Cardiovascular side effects, which include chest pain and hypertension, also can result in cardiovascular collapse and death. In addition, methamphetamine causes increased heart rate and blood pressure and can cause irreversible damage to blood vessels in the brain, producing strokes. Other effects of methamphetamine include respiratory problems, irregular heartbeat, and extreme anorexia.

Like cocaine, acute amphetamine administration results in mood elevation and increased energy. In addition, the user may experience feelings of markedly enhanced physical strength and mental capacity. Amphetamines also stimulate the sympathetic nervous system and produce the physiological effects associated with sympathetic activation. High doses of amphetamine produce a toxic syndrome that is characterized by visual, auditory, and sometimes tactile hallucinations. There is paranoia and disruption of normal thought processes. The toxic reaction to amphetamines can often be indistinguishable from an episode of schizophrenia.

The chart below shows the drug-induced neurotransmitter systems commonly affected by methamphetamine use and the behavioral toxic reactions as a result.

Methamphetamine-Induced Behavioral Toxicity		
Symptom	Complication	Neurotransmitter
paranoia	psychotic episode	increased DA
hypertension	cerebral hemorrhage	increased NE
tachycardia	cardiac arrhythmia	increased NE
increased physical energy	hyperexcitability	increased NE
anorexia	malnutrition	increased NE
hyperthermia	heat stroke	increased NE
insomnia	exacerbates paranoia	increased NE
euphoria	dysphoria	increased DA, then after repeated use, decreased DA
hypersexuality and increased susceptibility to STDs	hyposexuality and depression	increased DA, then after repeated use, decreased DA

Chronic Effects

As with cocaine, both sensitization and tolerance to different effects of amphetamines occur. Animal studies have shown that intermittent administration of amphetamines results in sensitization to the motor stimulating effects. This sensitization is thought to be due to an augmentation of dopamine release after intermittent, repeated drug administration.

Tolerance to the euphoric effects of amphetamine develops after prolonged, continuous use. Such tolerance is believed to be caused by depletion of stored neurotransmitters, especially dopamine, in the presynaptic terminals as a result of the continued stimulation of release from the stores by the drug. Drug craving is increased with continued amphetamine use.

Withdrawal from high doses produces prolonged sleep, dysphoria, severe depression, lassitude, increased appetite, and craving for the drug. Chronic abuse produces a psychosis resembling the primary symptoms of schizophrenia and is characterized by paranoia, and auditory and visual hallucinations. The most dangerous stage of the binge cycle is known as *tweaking*. Typically, during this stage, the abuser has not slept in three to fifteen days and is extremely irritable and paranoid. The "tweaker" has an intense craving for more methamphetamine; however, no dosage will help recreate the euphoric high. This causes frustration and can lead to unpredictability and a potential for violence.

Methamphetamine Analogs

Several dozen analogs of amphetamine and methamphetamine are hallucinogenic; many have been scheduled under the Controlled Substances Act (CSA). The methamphetamine analog most commonly used is

MDMA (3,4- methylenedioxy-methamphetamine), also know as *Ecstasy or XTC*.

MDMA is structurally similar to both methamphetamine and mescaline, and stimulates hallucinations. MDMA was first synthesized in the early 1950s as an appetite suppressant, although it was never used as such. It was first made illegally in 1972, but was not widely abused until the 1980s. Beliefs about MDMA are reminiscent of similar claims made about LSD in the 1950s and 1960s, which proved to be untrue. According to its proponents, MDMA can make people trust each other and break down barriers between therapists and patients, lovers, and family members. In fact, various claims have been made by a few psychiatrists for the use of MDMA to enhance psychotherapy. However, no evidence has been presented to document these few anecdotal reports.

Many of the problems that users encounter with MDMA are similar to those found with the use of amphetamines and cocaine. These psychological difficulties include confusion, depression, sleep problems, drug craving, severe anxiety, and paranoia which sometimes occur weeks after taking MDMA along with psychotic episodes.

Physical symptoms include muscle tension, teeth- clenching, nausea, blurred vision, rapid eye movements, faintness, and chills. Increased heart rate and blood pressure pose a special risk for people with circulatory or heart disease.

Cocaine
Cocaine is found in the leaves of the *Erythroxylon coca* plant, a large shrub indigenous to South America. The compound is extracted from the leaves and processed into either rudimentary paste, powder or free-base form. Adding hydrochloric acid to the paste makes cocaine powder (cocaine hydrochloride). The only clinical application of cocaine is as a local anesthetic (in preparation to pass a tube in the nose or throat).

Patterns of Abuse
Cocaine use ranges from occasional episodic experimentation to repeated or compulsive use, with several patterns between these extremes. The major methods of administration of cocaine are snorting, injecting, and smoking (including free-base and crack cocaine). Snorting is the process of inhaling cocaine powder through the nostrils where it is absorbed into the bloodstream via the nasal tissues. Injecting is using a needle to release the drug directly into the bloodstream. Smoking involves the inhalation of cocaine vapor or smoke into the lungs where absorption into the bloodstream is as rapid as by injection.

There is great risk no matter how cocaine is ingested. It appears that compulsive cocaine use may develop even more rapidly if the substance is smoked rather than taken intranasal. Most clinicians estimate that approximately 10 percent of people who begin to use the drug "recreationally" will go on to serious, heavy use. Smoking allows extremely high doses of cocaine to reach the brain very quickly and brings an intense and immediate high. The injecting drug user is at risk for transmitting or acquiring a variety of sexually transmitted diseases (STD's) including syphilis, gonorrhea and HIV /AIDS if needles or other injection equipment is shared.

"Crack" is the street name given to cocaine that has been processed from cocaine hydrochloride to a free base for smoking. To avoid the more volatile method of using ether to process cocaine for smoking, crack is made with ammonia or sodium bicarbonate (baking soda) and water and heated to remove the hydrochloride, thus producing a form of cocaine that can be smoked. The term "crack" is a reference to the crackling sound when the mixture is smoked, presumably from the sodium bicarbonate.

Adverse Effects
Physical effects of cocaine use include constricted peripheral blood vessels, dilated pupils, and increased body temperature, heart rate, and blood pressure. The duration of cocaine's immediate euphoric effects, which include hyperstimulation, reduced fatigue, and mental clarity, depends on the route of administration. The faster the absorption, the more intense the high. On the other hand, the faster the absorption, the shorter the duration of action. The high from snorting may last 15 to 30 minutes, while that from smoking may last 5 to 10 minutes. Increased use can reduce the period of stimulation.

Some cocaine users report feelings of restlessness, irritability and anxiety. An appreciable tolerance to the high may develop, and many addicts report that they seek but fail to achieve as much pleasure as they did from their first exposure. Scientific evidence suggests that the powerful reinforcing property of cocaine is responsible for an individual's continued use, despite harmful physical and social consequences. In rare instances, sudden death can occur on the first use of cocaine or unexpectedly thereafter. However, there is no way to determine who is prone to sudden death.

High doses of cocaine and/or prolonged use can trigger paranoia. Smoking crack cocaine can produce a particularly aggressive paranoid behavior in users. When addicted individuals stop using cocaine, they often become depressed. This also may lead to further cocaine use to alleviate the depression. Prolonged cocaine snorting can result in ulceration of the mucous membrane of the nose and can damage the nasal septum enough to cause it to collapse.

Cocaine-related deaths are often a result of cardiac arrest or seizures followed by respiratory arrest. Other toxic effects of high doses of cocaine include delirium, seizures, stupor, cardiac arrhythmias, and coma. Seizures can sometimes result in sustained convulsions where multiple seizure episodes one right after the other (called, status epilepticus).

The most prominent pharmacological effect of cocaine is blocking dopamine reuptake back into the presynaptic terminal once it has been released from a neuron terminal, resulting in increased levels of dopamine at its synapses in the brain. The specific uptake site for dopamine has been identified and cocaine's actions on the mechanism that transports dopamine back into the neuron is an active area of research. Within the brain mesocorticolimbic pathway (MCLP), levels of dopamine increase in the synapses between the terminals of the neurons projecting from the ventral tegmental area and the neurons in the nucleus accumbens and medial prefrontal cortex. In addition to blocking dopamine reuptake, cocaine also blocks the reuptake of norepinephrine and serotonin.

The acute behavioral effects of cocaine are the result of these neurochemical actions. The acute reinforcing properties of cocaine are due to its capacity to enhance the activity of dopamine in MCLP. The reinforcing properties of cocaine are mediated via dopamine activation of at least two receptor subtypes, the D1 and D2 dopamine receptor subtypes, and more recently there is evidence for an action at D3 receptors as well.

The increase in dopamine activity via D2 and DI receptors is also important in the other behavioral effects of cocaine. When combining cocaine and alcohol consumption, research shows that the human liver combines both drugs and makes a third substance, cocaethylene, that intensifies cocaine's euphoric effects, while potentially increasing the risk of sudden death.

Chronic Effects
Chronic administration of cocaine activates a number of brain neurochemical compensatory mechanisms. Both short and long-term changes in the dynamics of neurotransmission following repeated cocaine administration have been well documented. Animal studies indicate that continued administration results in a sustained increase in dopamine levels within the synapses of the nucleus accumbens. This is believed to be due to a decreased sensitivity of dopamine autoreceptors, which regulate the release of dopamine from the presynaptic terminal. In their normal state, these autoreceptors decrease the amount of dopamine released into the synapse. Changes also seem to occur in the number of postsynaptic receptors for dopamine, but the exact nature of these changes has yet to be characterized. Both increases and decreases in receptor numbers have been reported.

A number of changes occur in the intracellular mechanisms, including second messenger systems, involved in dopamine neurons in the ventral tegmental area and nucleus accumbens have been described following chronic cocaine administration. The changes are thought to be due to alterations in the expression of the genes that regulate and control the intracellular mechanisms. The net effect of these changes is to reduce the capacity of ventral tegmental neurons to transmit dopamine signals to the neurons in the nucleus accumbens. These represent a mechanism by which tolerance to the rewarding properties of cocaine would develop and could contribute to overall cocaine craving. Importantly, these changes are lacking in other dopamine pathways not involved in drug reward. Similar changes were observed following chronic morphine administration. These findings suggest a common physiological response to chronic administration of these drugs of abuse.

Finally, repeated administration of cocaine changes the levels of other neurotransmitters, most notably the neuropeptides. These changes may result from alterations in dopamine transmission that affects other areas of the brain. These secondary responses indicate that the neurochemical adaptive response to repetitive cocaine administration involves a complex interaction between multiple neuronal pathways and neurotransmitter systems. Much like the pharmacological profile, the behavioral response to repeated cocaine administration is complex. Studies suggest that how the drug is administered affects whether sensitization or tolerance occurs.

Intermittent administration of cocaine can trigger sensitization to some of its specific motor effects, such as stimulating levels of activity. Conversely, tolerance to these motor effects develops when the drug is taken continuously. Research suggests that tolerance develops to cocaine's reinforcing effects, and cocaine users report that the euphoric actions of the drug diminish with repeated use. Chronic cocaine administration also increases drug craving.

A withdrawal syndrome occurs with the abrupt cessation of cocaine after repeated use. This syndrome is marked by prolonged sleep, depression, lassitude, increased appetite, and craving for the drug. In animal studies, cocaine withdrawal results in an increase in the level of electrical stimulation necessary to induce a rat to self-stimulate the brain reward system. This indicates that during cocaine withdrawal, the brain reward system is less sensitive.

It is suspected that the pharmacological mechanism underlying cocaine withdrawal is related to the hypoactivity in dopamine functioning within the brain reward system. Changes in the expression of genes that control intracellular mechanisms represent a possible mechanism that could account for this change and could contribute to the drug craving associated with chronic cocaine use. Avoidance of the withdrawal reaction is another important determinant factor in continued cocaine use (negative reinforcement).

Caffeine
Caffeine is the most widely used psychoactive substance in the world. Surveys indicate that 92 percent of adults in North America regularly consume caffeine, mostly in coffee or tea. Caffeine belongs to a class of compounds called *methylxanthines,* CNS stimulants. Caffeine blocks both the A1 and A2 receptors for inhibitory neurotransmitter adenosine, causing neural stimulation. Adenosine inhibits the release of various neurotransmitters, in particular the excitatory amino

acid glutamate. Therefore, caffeine block of adenosine receptors results in increased glutamate activity.

Caffeine also increases the levels of norepinephrine and serotonin, which contributes to the drug's CNS stimulating effects. Caffeine's effects on dopamine are unclear in that increases, decreases, or no change in the release of dopamine have been observed following caffeine administration in various experiments.

In humans, caffeine has a general alerting affect, and it has been shown to increase locomotor activity in laboratory animals. However, evidence shows great individual variability in caffeine's effects, linked to differences in rates of caffeine absorption from the gastrointestinal system and metabolism in the body. Age also seems to affect the response to caffeine, in that older people show an increased sensitivity to caffeine's stimulating effects. This is particularly true of caffeine's disruptive effects on sleep.

Caffeine exhibits weak reinforcing effects in animal self-administration experiments. The level of responding induced by caffeine is much less than that seen with other stimulants such as amphetamine and cocaine. Caffeine's reinforcing actions are also minimal and dose-dependent. Low doses are mildly reinforcing with subjects reporting positive effects, while higher doses produce adverse effects. The results from human studies show that reinforcement occurs only under certain conditions and certain individuals.

The mechanism of caffeine's reinforcing actions is unknown. Tolerance may develop to many of the physical manifestations of caffeine's actions such as increased heart rate and higher blood pressure. There is, evidence that tolerance develops to its behavioral consequences including alertness and wakefulness. In animals, tolerance develops to some of caffeine's behavioral effects such as the stimulation of locomotor activity.

A withdrawal syndrome has clearly and repeatedly been demonstrated after the cessation of chronic caffeine consumption. Changes in mood and behavior can occur with lethargy and headache being the two most common symptoms of caffeine withdrawal. These changes may be the result of a compensation increase in adenosine receptors resulting from the chronic blockade by caffeine. However, more studies are needed to confirm this possibility.

Nicotine
It is generally accepted that while people smoke tobacco for many social or cultural reasons, the majority of people smoke in order to experience the psychoactive properties of nicotine. Furthermore, a significant proportion of habitual smokers become dependent on nicotine and tobacco smoking has all the attributes of drug use considered to be addicting. Nicotine activates one of the receptor subtypes for the neurotransmitter acetylcholine. As a result, this receptor is called the nicotine

receptor. The psychological effects of nicotine are fairly subtle and include mood changes, stress reduction, and some performance enhancement.

When tobacco is smoked, nicotine is readily absorbed by the lungs. Studies of smoking patterns have shown that habitual smokers tend to smoke more efficiently, because they inhale longer, have shorter intervals between puffs, and take a greater number of puffs per cigarette thus increasing the dose of nicotine they receive.

Smokeless tobacco involves either chewing tobacco leaves or placing tobacco between the cheek and gums. The blood nicotine level achieved using smokeless tobacco can be as high as that achieved from smoking cigarettes. Because of the route of administration, however, blood nicotine levels remain higher longer.

Evidence indicates that the diseases related to the use of tobacco may be caused by different constituents of tobacco or tobacco smoke. For example, cardiovascular effects are related to carbon monoxide in the smoke, and the effects on the heart and various cancers are probably due to carcinogens in the tobacco.

Nicotine stimulates the release of dopamine from dopamine neurons in the MCLP. Activation of nicotine receptors stimulates activity in dopamine neurons in the ventral tegmental area. However, when compared to the effects of cocaine or amphetamine, the nicotine increase in dopamine release is modest, and as a result, nicotine is a comparatively weak reinforcer in animal experiments. Nonetheless, nicotine reinforcing properties are thought to be the result of this action. Animal study results indicate that activation of nicotine receptors also stimulates the release of noradrenaline from neurons in the locus ceruleus and may reduce serotonin activity in the hippocampus. However, the exact nature of these changes and the role they may play in the behavioral effects of nicotine is unclear.

Tolerance develops to many of the effects of nicotine, and a withdrawal syndrome is marked by irritability, anxiety, restlessness, and difficulty concentrating. In addition, a craving for tobacco occurs but may subside in a few days although the mechanisms underlying these changes are unknown. Animal studies suggest that chronic administration of nicotine increases the number of nicotine receptors, yet the action that mediates this increase and its possible involvement in nicotine tolerance and withdrawal remains to be clarified.

Within 12 hours after a smoker has his last cigarette, the levels of carbon monoxide and nicotine in the system declines rapidly, and the individual's heart and lungs begin to repair the damage caused by cigarette smoke. Within a few days, the individual probably will begin to notice some remarkable physical changes. The sense of smell and taste may improve. As a person's body begins to repair itself from the damages of smoking, the individual may feel worse for awhile, before feeling better.

Immediately after quitting, many ex-smokers experience "symptoms of recovery" such as temporary weight gain caused by fluid retention, irregularity, and dry, sore gums or tongue. They may feel edgy, hungry, tired, and short-tempered, with trouble sleeping and frequent coughing. These symptoms are the result of the body clearing itself of nicotine, and most of the nicotine is eliminated in 2 to 3 days.

Medications in the Treatment of Stimulant Addiction

Vigabatrin (gamma-vinyl GABA [GVG])

Vigabatrin increases the amount of the brain chemical GABA. It is thought that epileptic seizures are the result of low levels of GABA. By increasing the amount of GABA, vigabatrin, under the name of Sabril, reduces the likelihood of an epileptic seizure. Vigabatrin has been "fast-tracked" by the Food and Drug Administration (FDA) and could one day become approved as a treatment for cocaine and methamphetamine dependence.

The drug is though to work by blocking craving and euphoria by increasing the level of gamma-amino-butyric acid (GABA). Animal testing and two small-scale human trials have shown that the drug inhibits both craving and euphoria. Sabril has already been approved by the FDA for treatment of seizures and infantile spasms.

A rapid elevation in nucleus accumbens dopamine characterizes the neurochemical response to cocaine, methamphetamine, and other drugs of abuse. Research has demonstrated that this response and associated behaviors are attenuated or even blocked by vigabatrin. The drug is not yet approved as a medication for methamphetamine and cocaine addiction.

Nicotine

Inhaled tobacco smoke delivers nicotine to the brain which causes an increase in dopamine activity. Smoking everyday essentially establishes a nicotine/dopamine maintenance level in the brain. The abrupt cessation of smoking means that the nicotine blood levels drop suddenly causing a decrease in dopamine which is the basis for the discomfort of the nicotine withdrawal syndrome. This syndrome is characterized by symptoms of irritability, insomnia and difficulty concentrating. The nicotine withdrawal syndrome can begin as early as 2 hours after the last cigarette and can last over several months with varying degrees if symptom intensity. Nicotine replacement products, including the patch, gum and lozenges, and the antidepressant bupropion (Zyban) are associated with the release low levels of dopamine in the brain. In this way, these medications decrease the craving for nicotine and reduce the signs and symptoms of nicotine withdrawal.

Nicotine Replacement Therapy

Nicotine gum and lozenges release nicotine slowly into the mouth. Nicotine patches applied to the skin and slowly release nicotine through the pores of the skin into the bloodstream. The nicotine inhaler has a holder that contains nicotine. The inhaler delivers a puff of nicotine vapor into the mouth and throat.

Nicotine replacement therapy (NRT) helps reduce nicotine withdrawal and craving by supplying the body with nicotine. It contains about one-third to one-half the amount of nicotine found in most cigarettes. Tars, carbon monoxide, and other toxic chemicals in tobacco cause harmful effects, not the nicotine. When tobacco smoke is inhaled, the nicotine in the smoke moves quickly from the lungs into the bloodstream. The nicotine in replacement products takes much longer to get into the system. This is why nicotine replacement medications are much less likely to cause dependence on nicotine than are cigarettes and other tobacco products. Nicotine by itself is not nearly as harmful as smoking.

Chantix (varenicline)
Chantix works by blocking the effect that nicotine has on the brain. As with other smoking cessation medications, Chantix also stimulates the release of low levels of dopamine in the brain to help reduce the symptoms of nicotine craving and withdrawal. In addition, Chantix blocks nicotinic receptors in the brain. The idea of blocking is that if the person relapses, the cigarette will not stimulate the brain's receptors with much intensity. Cigarettes, ideally, become markedly less pleasurable, and the desire to return to regular smoking is reduced.

Zyban (bupropion hydrochloride)
Zyban is a non-nicotine aid to smoking cessation. Zyban is chemically unrelated to nicotine or other agents currently used in the treatment of nicotine addiction. Initially developed and marketed as the antidepressant Wellbutrin. It works by increasing levels of brain dopamine and norepinephrine that is associated with the decrease in withdrawal intensity from nicotine.

New In Research: Methamphetamine-Nicotine-Cocaine Vaccine

Cocaine and many other drugs consist of particles so tiny that the human body cannot fight it by making antibodies, which are proteins used by the immune system to identify and neutralize foreign and potentially harmful particles, usually bacteria or viruses.

The only way you can get people's bodies to make antibodies is to "trick" the immune system. That is how scientists of Baylor Medical College (BCM) have engineered the cocaine vaccine to work. They used inactivated cholera toxin proteins and attached cocaine to the outside. Inactivating the cholera proteins prevents them from causing disease, but the immune system can see them when they are injected. It makes antibodies to cholera and cocaine at the same time. That means the person is vaccinated against both cholera and cocaine in the same injection.

During early studies in humans, researchers vaccinated subjects repeatedly over a period of three months. During this time, the subjects made large amounts of cocaine-specific antibodies. While the antibody levels drop within a year, they remain significantly high during the first few months. In that early period, if a vaccinated subject used cocaine, the antibodies prevented it from entering the brain and giving the person the cocaine "rush" that is attractive to addicts.

Blood vessels are distributed all over the brain, but the cocaine does not get into the brain because when it is bound to the antibodies, which are fairly large proteins, it cannot get through the blood-brain barrier. A common tenet in psychology is if there is no reward, the behavior will ultimately stop. Preliminary results from the first clinical trials in humans suggest that the vaccine holds tremendous promise.

Scientists at BCM found that twice as many people who were vaccinated were able to achieve at least a 50 percent reduction in cocaine use compared to those who received a placebo. Some who were vaccinated even stopped using drugs completely.

Aside from developing and testing a cocaine vaccine, scientists at BCM have developed a methamphetamine vaccine with which they hope to run a clinical trial in humans soon. There are also plans in the works to start a study on a nicotine vaccine in collaboration with The University of Texas M. D. Anderson Cancer Center.

CHAPTER 7: SELF-STUDY QUESTIONS

TRUE/FALSE

1. *Amphetamine is a generic term that applies to a group of synthetic compounds derived from the naturally occurring opium poppy.*

2. *Amphetamines are all classified as indirect acting agonists at NE, DA and 5-HT synapses.*

3. *Methamphetamine is closely related chemically to amphetamine but the CNS effects of methamphetamine are greater.*

4. *MDMA, also known as the designer drug "XTC", is a synthetic psychoactive drug with hallucinogenic and amphetamine-like properties.*

5. *The only clinical application of cocaine is as a local anesthetic medically used as a surgical preparation on membranes of the nose, pharynx, mouth, and throat to pass a tube through the nose or throat.*

6. *High doses of cocaine and/or prolonged use can trigger paranoia.*

7. *The most prominent pharmacological effect of cocaine is to block the liver metabolism of aldehyde dehydrogenase.*

8. *A withdrawal syndrome has clearly and repeatedly been demonstrated after cessation of chronic caffeine consumption.*

9. *Nicotine stimulates the release of dopamine from dopamine neurons in the MCLP.*

10. *Studies have shown that nicotine does not appear to produce tolerance and withdrawal syndromes in tobacco users.*

* Answers to Self Study Tests are located on page 351

Chapter 7 Selected Reading

Balfour, D.J.K., "The Neurochemical Mechanisms Underlying Nicotine Tolerance and Dependence," J. Pratt (editor), The Biological Basis of Drug Tolerance and Dependence, Academic Press, London. 1991.

Frishman WH. Smoking cessation pharmacotherapy--nicotine and non-nicotine preparations" *Prev Cardiol* **10** (2 Suppl 1): 10–22. 2007.

Hughes, J. R., Helzer, J.E., Lindberg, S.A., Prevalence of DSM/ICD-defined nicotine dependence. *Drug Alc. Depend.* 85:91-102. 2006.

King, GR, and Ellinwood, EH. Amphetamines and Other Stimulants. Lowinson, JH, Ruiz, P, Millman, RB, and Langrod, JG (editors), *Substance Abuse A Comprehensive Sourcebook.* Fourth Edition. Lippincott Williams & Wilkins. 2005.

Ling W, Rawson R, Shoptaw S. Management of methamphetamine abuse and dependence". *Curr Psychiatry Rep* **8** (5): 345–54. 2006.

London ED, Simon SL, Berman SM, et al.. Mood disturbances and regional cerebral metabolic abnormalities in recently abstinent methamphetamine abusers. *Arch Gen Psychiatry* 61:73–84, 2004.

National Institute on Drug Abuse. *Epidemiologic Trends in Drug Abuse: Advance Report, Community Epidemiology Work Group, January 2006*. NIH Pub. No. 06-5878, Bethesda, MD: NIH, DHHS, 2006.

National Institute on Drug Abuse. *Epidemiologic Trends in Drug Abuse: Vol. I., Proceedings of the Community Epidemiology Work Group, Highlights and Executive Summary, January 2006*. NIH Pub. No. 06-5879, Bethesda, MD: NIH, DHHS, 2006.

National Institute on Drug Abuse. *Epidemiologic Trends in Drug Abuse: Vol. II., Proceedings of the Community Epidemiology Work Group, January 2006*. NIH Pub. No. 06-5880, Bethesda, MD: NIH, DHHS, 2006.

Pentel, P., and Malin, D., A vaccine for nicotine dependence: Targeting the drug rather than the brain. *Respir.* 69: 193-197, 2002.

Preti A. New developments in the pharmacotherapy of cocaine abuse. *Addict Biol* **12** (2): 133–51. 2007.

SAMHSA, Office of Applied Studies. *Treatment Episode Data Set (TEDS). Highlights - 2004. National Admissions to Substance Abuse Treatment Services*, DASIS Series: S-31, DHHS Publication No. (SMA) 06-4140, Rockville, MD: DHHS, 2006.

Thompson PM, Hayashi KM, Simon SL, Geaga JA, Hong MS, Sui Y, Lee JY, Toga AW, Ling W, London ED. Structural abnormalities in the brains of human subjects who use methamphetamine. *J Neurosci* 24:6028-6036, 2004.

Vanderschuren, L.J.M.J. and Everitt, B.J., Drug seeking becomes compulsive after prolonged cocaine self-administration. *Science* 305: 1017-1019, 2004.

Volkow ND, et al. Association of dopamine transporter reduction with psychomotor impairment in methamphetamine abusers. *Am J Psychiatry* 158(3):377-382, 2001.

Volkow ND, et al. Loss of dopamine transporters in methamphetamine abusers recovers with protracted abstinence. *J Neurosci* 21(23):9414-9418, 2001.

Wang G-J, et al. Partial recovery of brain metabolism in methamphetamine abusers after protracted abstinence. *Am J Psychiatry* 161(2):242-248, 2004.

CHAPTER 8: VOCABULARY LIST

Analgesia   *A deadening or absence of the sense of pain without loss of consciousness*

Bradycardia   *Slowness of the heart rate, usually fewer than 60 beats per minute in an adult human.*

Buprenorphine   *Brand names, Buprenex®, Suboxone®, Subutex®, it is a semi-synthetic opiate with partial agonist and antagoniost actions used in pain and addiction medicine.*

Delta opioid receptor   *Receptor subtype within the endogenous opioid system. Delta1 is responsible for analgesia and euphoria, delta2 only causes analgesia.*

Dextromethorphan   *An over-the-counter narcotic used most often as a cough suppressant.*

Dolophine   *(Methadone) Long-lasting synthetic opioid used in pain and addiction medicine.*

Gate Control Theory of pain   *A model to explain pain sensation created by Ron Melzack and Patrick Wall in the 1960's and still used today.*

Kappa opioid receptor   *Receptor subtype within the endogenous opioid system largely responsible for sedation and analgesia.*

Mu opioid receptor   *Receptor subtype within the endogenous opioid system responsible for euphoria, sedation, analgesia and, if over stimulated, respiratory depression.*

Nociception   *The physiological system by which one feels the sensation of pain.*

Nociceptors   *A sensory receptor that responds selectively to potentially damaging stimuli. Its stimulation results in pain sensation.*

Naloxone   *(Narcan®) reverses effects that are caused by narcotic drugs such as difficult breathing and coma. Narcotics may be used during surgery to help produce anesthesia and relieve pain, and naloxone can reverse these effects after surgery. Naloxone is also used to treat cases of opioid drug overdose.*

Naltrexone   *A modified version of naloxone but with a longer half-life. Naltrexone is a medication that blocks the effects of opioids. It competes with these drugs for opioid receptors in the brain and disallows activation. Thus, it is used in the treatment of opioid addiction. Naltrexone is also used as an anti-craving medicine in the treatment of alcoholism.*

Papaver somniferum   *The poppy plant, which is the source of naturally occurring opium.*

CHAPTER 8: OPIATES AND THE PHYSIOLOGY OF PAIN SENSATION

Opiates/Opioids

Opium has long been used throughout history for a wide variety of treatments. Literature from Greece, Rome and Egypt provide descriptive accounts of the use of the opium poppy to alleviate coughing, anxiety and pain, and as a general euphoriant. During the 1800s, medicine containing opium was popular, and Civil War soldiers were provided with morphine as an analgesic. The Harrison Narcotic Act in 1914 limited the free sales of narcotics, and the new law required people to obtain a physician's note in order to receive morphine.

Opium is an extract of the seedpods of the opium poppy, Papaver somniferum. Opium is a complex mixture of chemicals that contain sugars, proteins, fats, water, meconic acid, ammonia, sulphuric and lactic acids, plant wax, latex, gums, and most importantly, numerous alkaloids, most notably morphine (10%-15%), codeine (1%-3%). Papaverine (1%-3%) and noscapine (4%-8%) are also present, but have essentially no effect on the CNS, and are not usually considered to be non-narcotic opiates. Thebaine (1%-2%), though without analgesic effect, is of immense pharmaceutical worth. This is because it can be used to produce semi-synthetic opioid morphine analogues such as oxycodone (Oxycontin), hydromorphone (Dilaudid), hydrocodone (Vicodin), and buprenorphine (Suboxone, Subutex).

Drugs that are derived directly from opium are termed *opiates*. Examples: morphine and codeine

Drugs that are derived from synthetic routes or from derivatives of opiates are termed *opioids*. These are classified as 'Semi-Synthetic' or "Synthetic'. Examples are:

- *'Semi-Synthetic'*: Heroin, Codeine (commercially prepared codeine), hydrocodone, oxycodone, hydromorphone etc.

- *'Synthetic'*: meperidine, fentanyl, propoxyphene, pentazocine, butorphanol, methadone, etc.

Opioid Receptors

Several opioid receptor subtypes have been described and characterized. Analgesics are primarily used for their ability to reduce the perception of pain impulses by the Central Nervous System (CNS). Analgesic activity is mediated by opiate receptors in the CNS. Five major categories of opioid receptors are known: mu, kappa, sigma, delta, and epsilon .

Pain killing drugs occupy the same receptors as endogenous opioid peptides - enkephalins or endorphins – which are described in more detail below. Both the endogenous agonist and narcotic analgesics may alter the central release of neurotransmitters from afferent nerves sensitive to noxious stimuli such as pain. The actions of the narcotic analgesics commercially available can be defined by their activity at three specific opiate receptor types: mu (μ), kappa (κ), and delta (δ).

μ Receptors: Classic opioids like morphine bind here preferentially. Also, the endogenous opioids Beta-Endorphin and Leu-Enkephalin, exerts some of its effects here. They are believed to be responsible for most of analgesic properties of opiates, as well as for euphoria, sedation, constipation, respiratory depression and dependence.

κ Receptors: The endogenous opioid Dynorphin exerts some of its effects here.
These specifically respond to pain from non-thermal stimuli.

δ Receptors: These appear to be the preferential binding site for the endogenous pentapeptide Met-Enkephalin, as well as several synthetic peptides. They are probably more important in the periphery and contribute to analgesic effects.

Pure Agonists, Partial Agonists and Antagonists
An opioid agonist is a substance that binds to any of the several subtypes of opioid receptor and produces some action. An opioid antagonist is a substance that binds to receptor subtypes and inhibits an action. Opiates with an affinity for μ-receptors can be classified into **four** groups:

- Pure Agonists: These have high affinity for μ - receptors as well as strong intrinsic activity at said receptors. (e.g., heroin, morphine, and methadone)

- Partial Agonists: These drugs bind to the receptor but exert only a partial or even minimal action. Some of these have both agonist and antagonist activity at the μ - receptors (e.g., buprenorphine)

- Pure Antagonists: These bind to the opiate receptors but to do not exert any activity. All they do is to block the effects of agonists at μ - receptor sites by preventing any agonists from binding to the receptor. In dependent individuals, they precipitate withdrawal symptoms (e.g., naloxone, naltrexone)

- Mixed Agonist-Antagonists: These drugs act as agonists at one receptor whilst behaving as an antagonist at other receptors. (e.g., pentazocine, butorphanol, nalbuphine)

The Physiology of Pain Simply Explained
Pain often has a physical cause, an injury to the body outside of the nervous system. In these cases, pain is initiated by mechanical, thermal or chemical changes in non-nervous tissues; this causes activation of specific nerves which relay to spinal centers concerned with the detection of injury, and thence to the thalamus and cortex, as well as to the reticular system. This hard-wired injury detection mode for pain is called nociception, meaning detection of harm, while the nerves which detect the damage are called nociceptor nerves (nociceptors, for short).

Nociception is the term introduced almost 100 years ago by the great physiologist Sherrington (1906) to make a clear distinction between detection of a noxious event or a potentially harmful event and the psychological and other responses to it. Nociception is also known as *physiological pain*.

Common causes of nociceptive pain include traumatic injury (fractures, torn tissue and burns), degenerative conditions such as osteoarthritis, infections and inflammatory conditions such as abscesses or sunburn, and cancers causing tissue breakdown.

Nociceptors (pain receptors)
All nociceptors are free nerve endings that have their cell bodies outside the spinal column in the dorsal column and are named based upon their appearance at their sensory ends. These sensory endings look microscopically like the branches of small bushes. There are mechanical, thermal, and chemical nociceptors. They are found in skin and on internal surfaces. Deep internal surfaces are only weakly supplied with pain receptors and will propagate sensations of chronic, aching pain if tissue damage in these areas occurs.

Two main types of nociceptor, A delta (Aδ) and C fibers, mediate fast and slow pain respectively. Thinly myelinated type Aδ fibers, which transmit signals at a rate of about 40 mph to mediate fast pain. This type of pain is felt within a tenth of a second of application of the pain stimulus. It can be described as sharp, acute, stinging pain and includes both mechanical and thermal pain. Slow pain, mediated by slower, unmyelinated ("bare") type C pain fibers that send signals at a rate of about 3 mph, is an aching, throbbing, burning pain. Chemical pain is an example of slow pain. Nociceptors do not adapt to stimulus. In some conditions, excitation of pain fibers becomes greater as the pain stimulus continues, leading to a condition called hyperalgesia.

Transmission of Nociception (Pain) Signals in the Central Nervous System
There are 2 pathways for transmission of nociception in the CNS. These are the neospinothalamic tract (for fast pain) and the paleospinothalamic tract (for slow pain).

- Fast pain travels via type Aδ fibers to terminate on the dorsal horn of the spinal cord. Second order neurons are then activated and give rise to long fibers that cross the midline through the grey commisure then terminate on the thalamus. From there, third order neurons communicate with the somatosensory cortex.

- Slow pain is transmitted via slower type C fibres to other parts of the dorsal horns, in an area called the substantia gelatinosa. Second order neurons take off and terminate also in the dorsal horn. Third order neurons then join fibers from the fast pathway, crossing to the opposite side via the grey commisure, and traveling upwards. These neurons terminate widely in the brain stem, with one tenth of fibers stopping in the thalamus, and the rest stopping in the medulla, pons and tectum of the midbrain. Slow pain is not very localized.

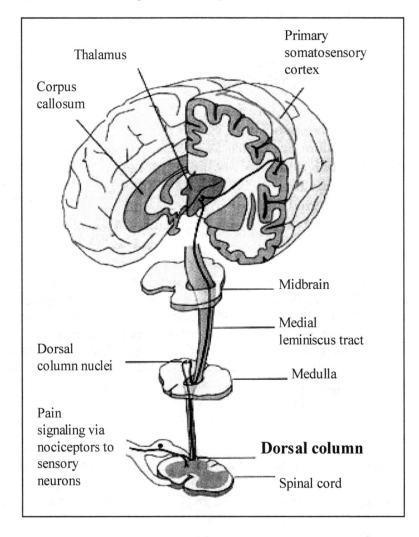

When the nociceptors are stimulated they transmit signals through sensory neurons in the spinal cord. These neurons release glutamate, a major exicitory neurotransmitter, that relays signals from one neuron to another. If the signals are sent to the thalamus, then pain enters consciousness, but in a dull poorly localized manner. From the thalamus, the signal can travel to the somatosensory cortex when the pain is experienced as localized and having more specific qualities.

The Gate Control Theory of Pain
The most influential theory that describes the sensation of pain, and still used today, was developed in 1965 to account for the clinically recognized importance of the mind and brain in pain perception. It is called the Gate Control Theory of Pain, and it was initially developed by Ronald Melzack (a psychologist) and Patrick Wall (an anatomist). The theory combines both a biomedical element and a psychological element that significantly helps to explain a rather complicated biobehavioral process.

In the gate control theory, the experience of pain depends on a complex interplay of the central and peripheral nervous systems as they each process pain signals in their own way. Upon injury, pain messages originate in nerves associated with the damaged tissue and flow along the peripheral nerves to the spinal cord and on up to the brain.

However, in the gate control theory, before they can reach the brain these pain messages encounter "nerve gates" in the spinal cord that open or close depending upon a number of factors (possibly including instructions coming down from the brain). When the gates are opening, pain messages "get through" more or less easily and pain can be intense. When the gates close, pain messages are prevented from reaching the brain and may not even be experienced.

Interneurons (I) are small nerve cells in the spinal cord that bridge the gap between larger neurons and function as "gatekeepers" for pain signals. If the pain carrying A-delta (Aδ) fibers are stimulated, they act on the interneurons, opening the gate to pain sensation. If however, the signals are coming from large C fibers, the pain signal is less intense and, upon reaching the brain, the pain sensation is much less intense.

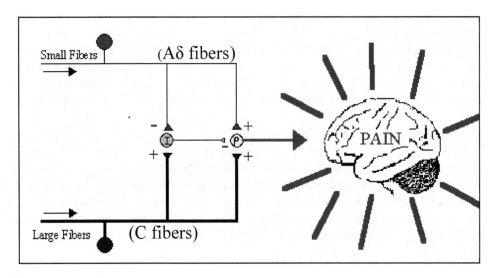

The peripheral nervous system

Sensory nerves bring information about pain, heat, cold and other sensory phenomena to the spinal cord from various parts of the body. As stated previously, there are basically two types of nerve fibers thought to carry the majority of pain messages to the spinal cord: Aδ nerve fibers ("fast" pain), and C-fibers ("slow" or "continuous pain")

After bumping an elbow or stubbing a toe, rubbing the area seems to provide some relief. This activates other sensory nerve fibers that are even "faster" than Aδ fibers, and these fibers send information about pressure and touch that reach the spinal cord and brain to override some of the pain messages carried by the Aδ and C-fibers.

The action of these other types of nerve fibers helps to explain why treatments such as massage, heat or cold packs, transcutaneous nerve stimulation, or even acupuncture are often effective in treating back pain. The nerve endings in the back are transmitted by special peripheral nerves first to the spinal cord and then up to the brain. These messages can be overridden by other signals in the manner described above. Treatments such as massage, heat, cold, TNS (transcutaneous nerve stimulation), or acupuncture can change a pain message due to some of these differences in nerve fibers.

The same principles apply in back pain. The nerve endings that detect pain are present in many structures in the back including the muscles and ligaments, the disks, the vertebrae, and the facet joints. When one of these parts is irritated, inflamed, or mechanically malfunctioning, the pain message will be transmitted by special peripheral nerves to the spinal cord and up to the brain. These messages can be over-ridden by other signals produced by the treatments listed previously.

TYPES OF PAIN

Neuropathic Pain

Neuropathic pain is caused by damage to or dysfunction of the nerves, spinal cord, or brain. Neuropathic pain may be felt as burning or tingling or as hypersensitivity to touch or cold. Causes include compression of a nerve (for example, by a tumor, by a ruptured intervertebral disk, or as occurs in carpal tunnel syndrome), nerve damage (for example, as occurs in a metabolic disorder such as diabetes mellitus), and abnormal or disrupted processing of pain signals by the brain and spinal cord. Processing of pain is abnormal in phantom limb pain and complex regional pain syndrome.

Phantom Limb Pain: Pain seems to be felt in an amputated part of the body, usually a limb. It differs from phantom limb sensation—the feeling that the amputated part is still there—which is much more common. Phantom limb pain cannot be caused by a problem in the limb. Rather, it must be caused by a change in the nervous system above the site where the limb was amputated. But the brain misinterprets the nerve signals as coming from the amputated limb. Usually, the pain seems to be in the toes, ankle, and foot of an amputated leg or in the fingers and hand of an amputated arm. The pain may resemble squeezing, burning, or crushing sensations, but it often differs from any sensation previously experienced. For some people, phantom limb pain occurs less frequently as time passes, but for others, it persists. Massage can sometimes help, but drug therapy is sometimes necessary.

Complex Regional Pain Syndrome: This chronic pain syndrome is defined as persistent burning pain accompanied by certain abnormalities that occur in the same area as the pain. Abnormalities include increased or decreased sweating, swelling, changes in skin color, damage to the skin, hair loss, cracked or thickened nails, muscle wasting and weakness, and bone loss. This syndrome typically occurs after an injury. There are two types:

- Type 1, which used to be called reflex sympathetic dystrophy, results from injury to tissues other than nerve tissue, as when bone is crushed in an accident or when heart tissue is damaged in a heart attack.
- Type 2, which used to be called causalgia, results from injury to nerve tissue.

Sometimes complex regional pain syndrome is made worse by activity of the sympathetic nervous system, which normally prepares the body for stressful or emergency situations—for fight or flight. For this reason, doctors may suggest treatment with a sympathetic nerve block. Physical therapy and drugs may also help.

Nociceptive Pain

Nociceptive pain is caused by an injury to body tissues. The injury may be a cut, bruise, bone fracture, crush injury, burn, or anything that damages tissues. This type of pain is typically aching, sharp, or throbbing. Most pain is nociceptive pain. Pain receptors for tissue injury (nociceptors) are located mostly in the skin or in internal organs. The pain almost universally experienced after surgery is nociceptive pain. The pain may be constant or intermittent, often worsening when a person moves, coughs, laughs, or breathes deeply or when the dressings over the surgical wound are changed.

Most of the pain due to cancer is nociceptive. When a tumor invades bones and organs, it may cause mild discomfort or severe, unrelenting pain. Some cancer treatments, such as surgery and radiation therapy, can also cause nociceptive pain. Pain relievers (analgesics), including opioids, are usually effective.

Psychogenic Pain

Psychogenic pain is pain that is mostly related to psychologic factors. When people have persistent pain with evidence of psychologic disturbances and without evidence of a disorder that could account for the pain or its severity, the pain may be described as psychogenic. However, psychophysiologic pain is a more accurate term because the pain results from interaction of physical and psychologic factors. Psychogenic pain is far less common than nociceptive or neuropathic pain.

Any kind of pain can be complicated by psychologic factors. Psychologic factors often contribute to chronic pain and may contribute to pain-related disability. In such cases, the pain, disability, or both usually have a physical cause, but psychologic factors exaggerate or enhance the pain, making it worse than what most people with a similar physical disorder experience. For example, people with chronic pain know it will recur and may become fearful and anxious as they anticipate the pain. These emotions make them more sensitive to pain. Sometimes doctors describe chronic pain that is worsened by psychologic factors as a chronic pain syndrome.

The fact that pain is caused or worsened by psychologic factors does not mean that it is not real. Most people who report pain are really experiencing it, even if a physical cause cannot be identified. Doctors always investigate whether a physical disorder is contributing to pain.

Pain complicated by psychologic factors requires treatment, often by a team that includes a psychologist or psychiatrist. Treatment for this type of pain varies from person to person, and doctors try to match the treatment with the person's needs. For most people who have chronic psychogenic pain, the goals of treatment are to improve comfort and physical and psychologic function. Doctors may make specific recommendations for gradually increasing physical and social activities. Drugs and nondrug treatments—such as biofeedback, relaxation training, distraction techniques, hypnosis, transcutaneous electrical nerve stimulation (TENS), and physical therapy—may be used. Psychologic counseling is often needed.

Pain Management

The body has the ability to produce its own natural analgesic substances (endorphins). These endogenous opiates (endorphins) include enkephalins, dynorphins, and β-endorphins.

There are three major classes of opiate receptors are widely distributed throughout the CNS. Enkephalins are active at the mu and delta opiate receptors, whereas dynorphin is active at the kappa receptor. The primary classes of opiate receptors may be further subdivided into distinct subtypes. The different receptor classes may modulate the activity of different types of nociceptive inputs. The three principle ways of relieving pain can be summarized by the following: 1) blocking the ability of a nerve to carry pain signals by interfering with the electrical impulses traveling through the nerve fiber; 2) blocking the action of the neurotransmitters that relay pain signals between nerves and; 3) enhancing the action of systems in the body that inhibit pain signals from being passed on.

With regard to medications, narcotic analgesics have a mechanism of action that includes targeting the body's endorphins systems and opiate receptors where they act as agonists or partial agonists/antagonists. Opiates such as morphine are potent agonists of the *mu* receptor. Opiates act at supra spinal levels (i.e., in the raphe nuclei) to suppress GABA-releasing interneurons that normally inhibit descending pathway activity. This disinhibitory mechanism serves to activate the descending pain suppression pathways. Opiates also exhibit analgesic activity at the level of the primary afferent synapse in the dorsal horn of the spinal cord. The superficial dorsal horn has a large number of enkephalin- and dynorphin-containing interneurons. Mu opiate receptors are located on the terminals of nociceptive afferents and the dendrites of postsynaptic dorsal horn neurons.

Opiate alkaloids and endogenous opioid peptides act presynaptically to suppress neurotransmitter release from sensory neurons. They also act postsynaptically to suppress the activity of the nociceptive dorsal horn neurons. That opioid receptors are ubiquitous throughout the CNS suggests that modulation of nociceptive data may occur at multiple sites, in addition to the aforementioned descending pathways and dorsal horn.

Pharmacotherapy Treatment of Opioid Addiction

Methadone in the Treatment of Opioid Addiction

Opioid addicts say that ingesting opiate drugs like heroin calms their nerves, satisfies their cravings and helps them relax. Scientists believe they now know why that might be. Ingesting opiate drugs produces major changes in the flow of "feel good" chemicals (i.e. dopamine in the MCLP) in the brain, both temporarily and long-term.

Heroin is a semisynthetic opiate derived from dried sap of the opium poppy. Also derived from poppy, though not synthesized, are morphine and codeine.

Heroin can be injected, smoked, swallowed or snorted. Intravenous injection produces the greatest intensity and most rapid onset of euphoria. Effects are felt within seconds. Even though effects for sniffing or smoking develop more slowly, beginning in 10 to 15 minutes, sniffing or smoking heroin has increased in popularity because of the availability of high-purity heroin and the fear of sharing needles. Also, users tend to mistakenly believe that taking heroin in ways other than IV use will not lead to addiction.

After ingestion, heroin rapidly crosses the blood-brain barrier. The blood-brain barrier is basically a layer of tightly packed cells that make up the walls of brain capillaries and prevent substances (i.e. toxins) in the blood from entering into the brain. These cells selectively filter out the molecules that are allowed to enter the brain, creating a more stable, nearly toxin-free environment. However, all psychoactive drugs freely pass the blood brain barrier and enter the brain.

While in the brain, heroin is converted to morphine, which rapidly binds to opioid receptors. Users tend to report feeling a "rush" or a surge of pleasurable sensations. The feeling varies in intensity depending on how much of the drug was ingested and how rapidly the drug enters the brain and binds to the natural opioid receptors. The rush is usually accompanied by a warm flushing of the skin, dry mouth, and a heavy feeling in the user's arms and legs. Following the initial effects, the user will be drowsy for several hours with clouded mental functioning and slow cardiac function. Breathing is slowed, and can possibly slow to the point of death.

Repeated use of heroin produces physical dependency, which means the development of tolerance to the drug's effects that necessitates ever larger amounts of the drug to achieve the same effect. A characteristic withdrawal syndrome upon abrupt cessation of use also develops. Withdrawal symptoms can begin within a few hours of last use and can include restlessness, body ache, muscle pain, insomnia, diarrhea, nausea, stomach cramps, vomiting, and hot/cold flashes. These symptoms peak between 24 and 48 hours after the last dose and subside after about a week, but may persist for up to a month. Heroin withdrawal is generally not fatal in an otherwise healthy adult, but can cause death to the fetus of a pregnant addict.

When purchased on the street, heroin is often adulterated with substances such as sugar, starch, powdered milk, strychnine and other poisons, or other drugs. These additives may not dissolve when injected in a user's system and can clog the blood vessels that lead to the lungs, liver, kidneys, or brain, infecting or even killing patches of cells in vital organs. In addition, many users do not know the heroin's actual strength or its true contents and are at risk of exposure to a tainted or contaminated quantity of heroin causing neurotoxic damage, drug overdose or even death.

Chronic heroin use can lead to medical consequences such as scarred and/or collapsed veins, bacterial infections of the blood vessels and heart valves, abscesses and other soft-tissue infections, and liver or kidney disease. Poor health conditions and depressed respiration from heroin use can cause lung complications, including various types of pneumonia and tuberculosis. Other long-term effects of heroin use can include arthritis and other rheumatologic problems and infection of blood borne pathogens such as HIV/AIDS and hepatitis B and C (which are contracted by sharing and reusing syringes and other injection paraphernalia). It is estimated that injection drug use has been a factor in one third of all HIV and more than half of all hepatitis C cases in the United States. Heroin use by a pregnant woman can result in a miscarriage or premature delivery. Heroin exposure *in utero* can increase a newborns' risk of SIDS (sudden infant death syndrome).

Research from the National Institute of Drug Abuse (NIDA) has shown that opioid dependent individuals will compulsively continue to use opioids despite adverse physical, emotional and life altering consequences because of at least two motivational factors: 1) the desire to self medicate the pain of narcotic withdrawal symptoms, and 2) the driving force of drug craving.

The primary goals of methadone treatment are to stabilize clients on a sufficient dose of methadone to both treat the symptoms of withdrawal and to block the behaviors of drug craving – two precipitating dynamics for relapse behaviors. Once stabilized, clients can then begin the process of recovery by gaining new skills from counseling that will enable them to regain a normal lifestyle.

As used in maintenance treatment, methadone is not a heroin substitute. It is important to understand that methadone does not actually "replace" or "substitute" for other opioids. That's why the terms replacement and/or substitution therapy are inaccurate and misleading. Instead, these medications are able to suspend withdrawal symptoms, decrease drug craving behaviors and block the actions from other opioid drugs such as heroin.

The pharmacological effects of methadone are markedly different from those of heroin. Injected, snorted, or smoked, heroin causes an almost immediate "rush" or brief period of euphoria that wears off quickly, terminating in a "crash." The cycle of euphoria, crash, and craving repeated several times a day leads to a cycle of addiction and severe behavioral disruption.

These characteristics of heroin use result from the drug's rapid onset of action and its short duration of action in the brain. An individual who uses heroin multiple times per day subjects the brain and body to marked, rapid fluctuations as the opiate effects come and go (figure 1). The individual also will experience an intense craving for more heroin to stop the cycle, fend off withdrawal and to reinstate the euphoria. Ultimately however, when tolerance to the drug has been established, the addicted person continues to use to avoid the pain of drug withdrawal and to feel relatively normal.

Methadone has a very gradual and slow onset of action compared with heroin. Because of this, patients stabilized on methadone do not experience the euphoric "rush" (figure 2). Methadone is metabolized more slowly than heroin and thereby allows the brain and body to avoid the stressful ups and downs caused by heroin. When on a stabilized dose during maintenance treatment, there is also a marked reduction of the desire and craving for heroin.

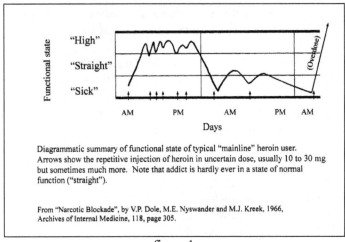

Diagrammatic summary of functional state of typical "mainline" heroin user. Arrows show the repetitive injection of heroin in uncertain dose, usually 10 to 30 mg but sometimes much more. Note that addict is hardly ever in a state of normal function ("straight").

From "Narcotic Blockade", by V.P. Dole, M.E. Nyswander and M.J. Kreek, 1966, Archives of Internal Medicine, 118, page 305.

figure 1

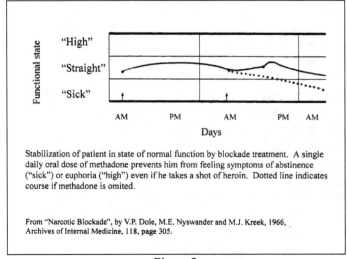

Stabilization of patient in state of normal function by blockade treatment. A single daily oral dose of methadone prevents him from feeling symptoms of abstinence ("sick") or euphoria ("high") even if he takes a shot of heroin. Dotted line indicates course if methadone is omited.

From "Narcotic Blockade", by V.P. Dole, M.E. Nyswander and M.J. Kreek, 1966, Archives of Internal Medicine, 118, page 305.

Figure 2

Essentially all physiological systems are affected by opiate addiction. A characteristic syndrome occurs when an opiate addict goes through withdrawal. This syndrome includes perspiration, tremor, gooseflesh, restlessness, myalgia, anorexia, nausea, vomiting, abdominal cramps, diarrhea, fever, hyperpnea, and hypertension. Persistent symptoms such as sleep disturbances, irritability, restlessness, and poor concentration can continue for months or longer after the drug use has stopped.

On one level, opioid dependency is an adaptation of the body to opiates. With repeated use, dependence develops when the body's various systems have adapted to the opioid where they require the drug to regulate a physiological balance.

Methadone, as used in the treatment of opioid addiction, has an affinity for *mu* opioid receptors in the brain where it blocks the withdrawal syndrome and diminishes craving behaviors which otherwise can lead to continued illicit drug use.

Of importance is the fact that at *mu* receptor sites, methadone will also block the effects of other opioid drugs including heroin. This means that even if a patient on methadone ingests heroin, the blocking effect will disallow any heroin action and the patient is prevented from what might have otherwise been a long and torturous relapse.

An Optimal Dose for Methadone Maintenance
There have been many research studies comparing various doses of methadone for maintenance treatment. Reports have consistently shown that patients receiving higher doses of methadone compared to those receiving lower doses have much better outcomes – where outcomes are defined in terms of abstinence from illicit opioid use, length of treatment stay, and overall improvement in the quality of life.

Essentially, all of the research on dosing has concluded that there is no evidence of lower doses being adequate for the vast majority of patients. Vincent Dole, one of the co-discoverers of methadone for the treatment of opioid addiction, stated, "There is no compelling reason for prescribing doses that are only marginally adequate. As with antibiotics, the prudent policy is to give enough medication to ensure success (figure 3).

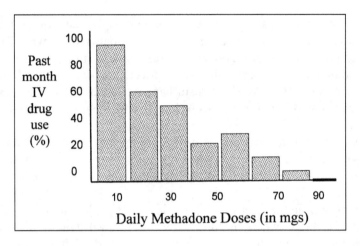

Figure 3

Payte (2002) noted, "Arbitrary dose ceilings have no foundation in science or clinical medicine. Programs with 'dose caps' can expect problems with accreditation." Furthermore, the U.S. federal regulations or addiction medicine associations do not endorse such "caps".

In terms of safety, a meta-analysis of methadone dosing studies found that patients having access to "high-dose maintenance" were actually at a greater reduced risk of fatal heroin overdose during treatment compared with those at lower doses. Remember, the goal of methadone is to stabilize the opioid addicted person so that withdrawal pain and drug craving behaviors are suspended. The optimal dose amount to initiate and maintain stabilization depends on individual patient needs.

Since 1965, methadone maintenance programs have proved to be the most effective treatment for opiate (e.g., heroin) addiction. Under medical supervision, a daily dose of 60-100 mg of methadone prevents withdrawal symptoms and drug craving behaviors, produces no euphoria, and allows patients the opportunity to return to a lifestyle free of the need for compulsive drug seeking and use. The effectiveness of methadone treatment has also been demonstrated extensively by remarkable reductions in criminal arrests, increases in employment, and stability of social relationships.

Buprenorphine
In 2002, the U.S. Food and Drug Administration approved buprenorphine for the treatment of opioid addiction. Buprenorphine is intended for the treatment of pain (Buprenex®) and opioid addiction (Suboxone® and Subutex®). Buprenorphine has a unique pharmacological profile. It produces the effects typical of both pure mu agonists (like morphine) and partial agonists (like pentazocine) depending on dose, pattern of use and population taking the drug. It is about 20-30 times more potent than morphine as an analgesic and, like morphine it produces dose-related euphoria, drug liking, pupillary constriction, respiratory depression and sedation. However,

acute, high doses of buprenorphine have been shown to have a blunting effect on both physiological and psychological effects due to its partial opioid activity. The addition of naloxone in the Suboxone® product is intended to block the euphoric high resulting from the injection of this drug by non-buprenorphine maintained narcotic abusers.

Buprenorphine has a high affinity for opioid receptors. It is a partial mu-receptor agonist as well as a kappa-receptor antagonist. Mu opioid receptors mediate the common opioid effects such as analgesia, sedation, euphoria and respiratory depression. As a partial mu receptor agonist, buprenorphine results in less sedation than full mu-opioid agonists such as methadone and morphine, while still decreasing cravings for other opioids and preventing opioid withdrawal. The clinical implication of the antagonist kappa receptor effect is not well understood, but it may result in buprenorphine having some mild antidepressant properties. As a partial agonist, buprenorphine has a "ceiling effect": there is a plateau to its opioid agonist effects at higher doses.

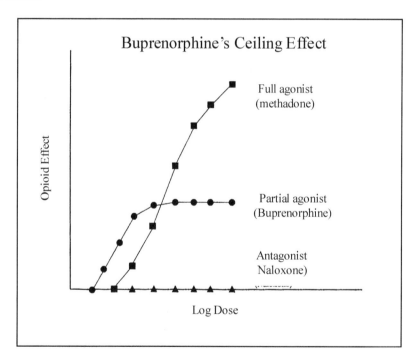

Buprenorphine has a higher affinity for and lower intrinsic activity at opioid receptors than full μ-opioid agonists such as methadone, oxycodone and heroin. Hence, buprenorphine displaces agonists from opioid receptors and may precipitate withdrawal in patients physically dependent on opioids. The effect of buprenorphine peaks at 1–4 hours after the initial dose. Buprenorphine is metabolized mainly by cytochrome P4503A4 and its half-life is 24–60 hours.

Compared with methadone, buprenorphine has a relatively lower risk of abuse, dependence, and side effects, and it has a longer duration of action. Because buprenorphine is a partial opioid agonist, its opioid effects, such as euphoria and respiratory depression, as well as its side effects reach a ceiling of maximum effect, unlike with methadone or heroin.

Adverse effects are similar to those of other opioids and include nausea, vomiting and constipation. It is important to note that buprenorphine may precipitate opioid withdrawal symptoms if it is administered before other opioid agonist effects have subsided. Respiratory depression (and death) have been reported in the context of intravenous polysubstance, usually benzodiazepine, abuse.

Buprenorphine vs. Methadone	
Buprenorphine	**Methadone**
Partial agonist and produces only a low level of euphoria.	Full agonist and can produce significant intoxication.
Has low dependence potential compared with full opioid agonists.	Potential to produce significant dependence. As tolerance increases, dose increases over time are required.
Abstinence leads to mild withdrawal symptoms.	Abstinence leads to marked withdrawal symptoms.
At high doses, there is a ceiling effect. The risk of fatal respiratory depression by overdose of buprenorphine by itself is minimal. But when combined with benzodiazepines (diazepam), alcohol and other CNS depressants, respiratory depression has been reported.	Risk of fatal overdose by respiratory depression.
Sublingual tablets are effectively absorbed. It is not orally active. Sublingual tablets can be crushed, easily dissolved and injected.	Orally active.

Buprenorphine will not replace methadone therapy. Rather, it is an important addition to the medications needed for the various types of opioid addicts. Methadone is still the "gold standard" in the treatment of many opioid addictions, particularly heroin. However, buprenoprphine gives the addiction medicine physician an additional option in treating opioid addiction, particularly in the treatment of addiction to long-acting prescription pain medications including Oxycontin or methadone.

CHAPTER 8: SELF-STUDY QUESTIONS

TRUE/FALSE

1. *Pain killing drugs occupy the same receptors as endogenous opioid peptides.*

2. *Two categories of opioid receptors are known: kappa and epsilon.*

3. *Nociception is also known as physiological pain.*

4. *Developed in 1965 to show the importance of the mind and brain in pain perception, the Gate Control Theory is still used today to explain a rather complicated biobehavioral process*

5. *Opiate alkaloids and endogenous opioid peptides act presynaptically to suppress neurotransmitter release from sensory neurons.*

6. *While in the brain, heroin is converted to morphine, which rapidly binds to opioid receptors.*

7. *The primary goals of methadone treatment are to stabilize clients on a sufficient dose of methadone to both treat the symptoms of withdrawal and to block the behaviors of drug craving – two precipitating dynamics for relapse behaviors.*

8. *The pharmacological effects of methadone are very similar to those of heroin.*

9. *Buprenorphine has a unique pharmacological profile. It produces the effects typical of both pure mu agonists (like morphine) and partial agonists (like pentazocine) depending on dose, pattern of use and population taking the drug.*

10. *As a partial agonist, buprenorphine has a "ceiling effect" meaning that there is a plateau to its opioid agonist effects at higher doses.*

* Answers to Self Study Tests are located on page 351

Chapter 8 References

Ball, J.C. and Ross, A. The Effectiveness of Methadone Maintenance Treatment. New York: Springer-Verlag. 1994.

Caplehorn, J.R.M. A comparison of abstinence-oriented and indefinite methadone maintenance treatment. *International Journal of the Addictions* 29(11): 1361-1375. 1994.

Dole VP, Nyswander ME, Kreek MJ. Narcotic blockade. *Arch Int Med.* 1966;118:304-309.

Doran CM, Shanahan M, Mattick RP, et al. Buprenorphine versus methadone maintenance: a cost-effectiveness analysis. *Drug Alcohol Depend* 2003;71(3):295-302.

Fischer B, Chin AT, Kuo I, et al. Canadian illicit opiate users' views on methadone and other opiate prescription treatment: an exploratory qualitative study. *Subst Use Misuse* 2002;37:495-522.

Hughes, J. Isolation of an endogenous compound from the brain with properties similar to morphine. *Brain Research* 1975 (a), 88: 295-308

Kandel E.R., Schwartz, J.H., Jessell, T.M. *Principles of Neural Science*, 4th ed. McGraw-Hill. 2000.

Kosten TR, George TP. The neurobiology of opioid dependence: implications for treatment. *Science & Practice Perspectives.* 2002;1(1):13-20.

Mattick, RP, Kimber J, Breen C, et al. Buprenorphine maintenance versus placebo or methadone maintenance for opioid dependence. [Cochrane review]. In: the Cochrane Library; Issue 2, 2003. Oxford: Update Software.

Melzack, R and Wall, P. Pain Mechanisms: A New Theory. *Science*: 150, 171-179. 1965.

Nestler, EJ, Malenka RC. The addicted brain. *Scientific American.* March 2004.

NIH (National Institutes of Health). Effective Medical Treatment of Opiate Addiction. NIH Consensus Statement. Bethesda, MD: National Institutes of Health; 1997 (Nov 17-19);15(6):1-38. (See also: *JAMA.* 1998;280:1936-1943.)

Payte JT, Zweben JE, Martin J. Opioid maintenance treatment. In: Graham AW, Schultz TK, Mayo-Smith MF, Ries RK, Wilford BB. Principles of Addiction Medicine. Chevy Chase, MD: *American Society of Addiction Medicine*; 2003: 751-766.

Simon, EJ. Opiates: Neurobiology. Lowinson, JH, Ruiz, P, Millman, RB, and Langrod, JG (editors), *Substance Abuse A Comprehensive Sourcebook*. Fourth Edition. Lippincott Williams & Wilkins. 2005.

Stanford, M, Avoy, D. Professional Perspectives on Addiction Medicine: Understanding Opioid Addiction and the Functionality of Methadone Treatment. *Santa Clara County Health & Hospital System*. 2007.

CHAPTER 9: VOCABULARY LIST

Δ^9-tetrahydrocannabinol (THC), the main psychoactive ingredient of cannabis.

Adiponectin Hormone secreted by adipose (fatty) tissue that seems to be involved in energy homeostasis; it enhances insulin sensitivity and glucose tolerance, as well as oxidation of fatty acids in muscle. Its blood concentration is reduced in obese people and those with Type II diabetes.

Amotivational Syndrome Characterized by impaired judgment, concentration and memory, along with apathy or loss of interest in pursuit of conventional goals

Cannabinoids Also, called phytocannabinoids, are those compounds commonly found in the marijuana plant of which there are over 60.

Cannabinoid receptors The chemistry of the ES is the endocannabinoids where they are released into synapse and bind to and activate distinct cannabinoid receptor. To date, 2 types of cannabinoid receptors have been identified; CB_1 and CB_2. CB_1 receptors are found primarily in the brain and the CB_2 receptors are located mainly in immune cells and in peripheral tissues of the body in adipocytes (or "fat cells") that are associated with lipid and glucose metabolism.

Cannabis sativa The marijuana plant.

Endocannabinoids Endocannabinoid, is a word condensed from two other words; endogenous: from within, and cannabinoid: substances resembling the components within the C. sativa plant. The two major endocannabinoids are arachidonoyl ethanolamide (anandamide) and 2-arachidonoyl glycerol (2-AG).

Endocannabinoid system (ES) is a physiological system consisting of cannabinoid receptors and corresponding chemical messengers that is believed to play an important role in regulating body weight, glucose and lipid metabolism, pain, movement, cognitive functioning and addiction.

Lipophilic

Having an affinity for, tending to combine with, or capable of dissolving in lipids.

Pyrolysis

Decomposition or transformation of a compound caused by heat.

Metabolic Syndrome

The Metabolic Syndrome is a cluster of conditions that occur together, increasing your risk of heart disease, stroke and diabetes. The main features of metabolic syndrome include insulin resistance, hypertension (high blood pressure, cholesterol abnormalities, and an increased risk for clotting. Patients are most often overweight or obese.

CHAPTER 9: MARIJUANA, CANNABINOIDS AND CANNABINOID-BASED MEDICINES

The therapeutic value of the cannabis plant has been referenced for approximately four millennia by a variety of sources and throughout different countries. While cannabis has been used medicinally for quite some time, it wasn't until rather recently that neuroscience research has discovered safer and more effective treatment possibilities. Only as recently as the 1990s, scientists found and were able to replicate receptor-proteins located on the surface of cells that are responsible for many of the actions of Δ^9-tetrahydrocannabinol (THC), the main psychoactive ingredient of cannabis. This new understanding has allowed scientists to develop a foundation for a cannabinoid pharmacology that can provide the way for a more efficient therapeutic direction way beyond medical marijuana and toward cannabinoid-based medicines.

The Institute of Medicine (IOM), in its seminal 1999 report, recognized the medical value of cannabinoids, the active compounds in the marijuana or cannabis plant, for several important indications. The IOM report only cautiously endorsed short-term interim studies of smoked marijuana for a few limited indications, stating instead that, "the future of medical marijuana lies in classical pharmacological drug development". Since then, as you will find out in this chapter, neuroscience research has shed new light on the function of the endogenous cannabinoid system. By using powerful new research tools, the varied functions of this system are being elucidated and the potential for the development of cannabinoid-based pharmacotherapies is now being described.

About the Cannabis Plant
The marijuana plant, referred to as Cannabis sativa (*C. sativa*), is both a widespread illegal drug of abuse and a recognized medicinal plant. One of the challenges for neuroscience was to isolate the active components of the plant associated with potential therapeutic uses and at the same time try to develop cannabinoid-based medicines without any adverse effects. After four decades of research, there is a much greater understanding about the pharmacology of plant-derived cannabinoid compounds (called phytocannabinoids) and how they relate to the endogenous cannabinoids within the human body.

Pharmacology of Marijuana: Constituents and chemical characteristics.
C. sativa contains more than 400 chemical compounds and over 60 various phytocannabinoids, some of which are bioactive - defined by their ability to target and activate specific receptors in the brain, the cannabinoid receptors. The best-known phytocannabinoid is Δ^9-tetrahydrocannabinol (THC), the most psychoactive phytocannabinoid and the one that probably mediates the addictive properties of *C. sativa a*. Delta-8-THC is similar in potency to THC but is present in only small concentrations. Cannabinol and cannabadiol are the other major cannabinoids present. The former is slightly psychoactive, but not in the amounts delivered by

191

smoking marijuana. The average content of THC in marijuana plants usually ranges from 0.3 percent to 4 percent based on the climate, soil and growing conditions, and handling after harvest, but values as high as 20 percent have been achieved in some preparations. THC is very highly lipid soluble. It binds to glass, diffuses into plastic, and is photolabile and susceptible to heat and oxidation.

Pyrolysis (burning) releases over 100 compounds which can be highly carcinogenic. While most research has concentrated on evaluating the molecular and biochemical mechanisms of THC that underlie actions of the cannabinoids, these other compounds also play a role in the acute and long-term consequences of marijuana use.

Smoking plant material is a very unique method of drug delivery into the system. First it provides rapid delivery of the drug into the bloodstream, such that the effects may be felt within minutes and last for 2 to 3 hours. Also, drug inhalation produces a different behavioral and physiological response than oral or even IV administration. Clinical psychopharmacology and toxicology illustrate this point all too well through studies of other plants that are smoked, such as tobacco and cocaine. When marijuana is smoked, THC in the inhaled smoke rapidly absorbs within seconds and is delivered to the brain quickly (as one would expect from a very lipophilic substance). Oral ingestion of THC is quite different than smoking. Some marijuana users prepare teas and other liquid solutions, and sometimes bake the marijuana in cookies to ingest the substance orally. However, maximum THC and blood cannabinoid levels are only reached after 1 to 3 hours. Thus, onset of the psychoactive effects is much slower after oral ingestion.

Cannabis Naturally In the Human Body?
Well, sort of. In the way the body has its own natural morphine (endorphins) that is similar in chemistry to morphine from the opium plant; the body also has its own versions of chemical agents of the cannabis plant, called *endocannabinoids*. These chemical messengers help regulate processes of brain and body functions. Since science has now developed a more sophisticated understanding of the endocannabinoids, new medicines can be developed to treat a variety of health conditions including obesity, Type 2 diabetes, non-morphine analgesics, and addiction medicines, to name a few. In the not so distant future, it is plausible to expect that neuroscience research will discover novel medicinal ways to facilitate changes within the endocannabinoid system that can further help treat other conditions, from addiction and alcoholism, to epilepsy, pain, anxiety, and depression. In the 1990s, the discovery of specific cellular receptors of THC revealed a whole endogenous signaling system now referred to as the *endocannabinoid system* (figure below).

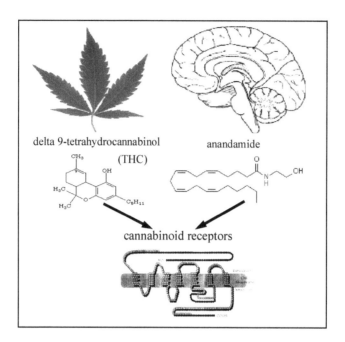

delta 9-tetrahydrocannabinol (THC)

anandamide

cannabinoid receptors

Endocannabinoids

The Endocannabinoid System (ES) is a physiological system consisting of cannabinoid receptors and corresponding chemical messengers that is believed to play an important role in regulating body weight, glucose and lipid metabolism, pain, movement, cognitive functioning and even addiction. The word, *endocannabinoid,* is a word condensed from two other words; *endogenous*: from within, and *cannabinoid*: substances resembling the components within the *C. sativa* plant. The two major endocannbinoids are arachidonoyl ethanolamide (anandamide) and 2-arachidonoyl glycerol (2-AG). As their chemical names suggest, both are derived from arachidonic acid, which is also the precursor for the prostaglandins, which allows one to see the potential role of the ES in pain and inflammation treatments.

Cannabinoid Receptors

Basically, the chemistry of the ES is the endocannabinoids where they are released into synapse and bind to and activate distinct cannabinoid receptor. To date, 2 types of cannabinoid receptors have been identified; CB_1 and CB_2. CB_1 receptors are found primarily in the brain and the CB_2 receptors are located mainly in immune cells and in peripheral tissues of the body in adipocytes (or "fat cells") that are associated with lipid and glucose metabolism.

It is the CB_1 receptor that is presumed to mediate all the CNS effects of the cannabinoids. The number of CB_1 receptors in the brain is large, comparable to the numbers of receptors for the monoamines, serotonin and dopamine. The large number of CB_1 receptors, called *receptor reserve*, tells us how a partial agonist like THC is able to produce a response. Namely, the more receptors in the system, the greater the likelihood of an activator-inhibitor interaction. Signal transduction studies have revealed that THC is not a very strong partial activator.

The distribution of CB_1 receptors within the brain is rather heterogeneous, with the largest concentrations found in basal ganglia, cerebellum, hippocampus, and the cerebral cortex. CB_1 receptor activation is particularly expressed in an area of the brain called the nucleus accumbens, a small subcortical area believed to be important in motivational processes that mediate the incentive value of food, and which may also play an important part in the establishment and maintenance of drug addiction.

CB1 receptors are also integral in initiating food intake and, when activated, will stimulate the ingestion of food. Research indicates that endocannabinoids may play a role in appetite control. This is achieved by modulating the expression and release of appetite suppressing and appetite stimulating neurotransmitters in the hypothalamus region of the brain.

The CB2 receptor is not expressed in the brain. It was originally detected in macrophages and is particularly abundant in immune tissues, where the largest concentrations have been detected in B-cells and natural killer cells. The functions of the CB2 receptor in the immune system are less clear. Most of the research studies seemed to suggest that the cannabinoids are primarily immunomodulatory in nature. That is, depending on dosage, some immune cells are suppressed while others are stimulated.

General Effects of Marijuana
Since marijuana inhalation exposes the user to many potentially psychoactive compounds in addition to THC, the subjective effects of marijuana vary somewhat among individuals. The behavioral response to marijuana can be a function of dose, setting, experience, expectation of the user, cannabinoid content, and peripheral compounds that are produced as the marijuana is burned. Nevertheless, several behavioral effects are attributed to marijuana use, which are generally dose-dependent

Marijuana generally produces a *bi-phasic psychic reaction:* the euphoric *stimulant phase* and the sedative *depressive phase.* During the initial stimulant phase, short-term memory is impaired and appetite is usually suppressed. Users can easily lose their train of thought. Also during this phase, THC acts like a sympathomimetic, which can induce a panic reaction with symptoms of anxiety and paranoia.

Following the stimulant phase, drowsiness, lethargy and *anergy* (low energy) are common. Like drugs in the sedative-hypnotic class, REM sleep is inhibited and thus restful restoration is compromised. Unlike sedatives however, there is no REM rebound from THC use. During the depressive phase, appetite is often increased and at extremely high doses (greater than 12 mg), marijuana can produce memory impairment, confusion, disorientation and even delirium.

Some studies have documented impairment of a variety of cognitive and performance tasks involving memory, perception, learning, reaction time and motor coordination. The short term damage from marijuana use can also result in dysphoria, disorientation and panic attacks. Recent findings also indicate that long-term use of marijuana produces changes in the brain similar to those seen after long-term use of other major drugs of abuse. Mild cross-tolerance to effects of marijuana will occur in some individuals tolerant to CNS depressants including alcohol and opiates. An amotivational syndrome, characterized by impaired judgment, concentration and memory, along with apathy or loss of interest in pursuit of conventional goals, has been described in the literature. Evidence shows that this syndrome is a result of chronic high-dose use.

Scientists have found that the positive or negative sensations resulting from smoking marijuana are also influenced by heredity. A recent study demonstrated that identical male twins were likely to report similar responses to marijuana use. This indicates a genetic basis for their sensations, since identical twins share all of their genetic codes. Also, environmental factors have been implicated in their contribution to the overall effects experienced from marijuana use. However, it was discovered a shared family environment had no detectable differences between certain subjects' response to marijuana.

Physiological Effects
While marijuana produces euphoria in humans, in general, animals do not self-administer THC in controlled studies. Cannabinoids generally do not lower the threshold of electrical stimulation needed for animals to stimulate the brain reward system, as do other drugs of abuse. Although, one series of studies involving the inbred Lewis rat does show that THC not only lowers the threshold for electrical self-stimulation but also enhances the release of dopamine in the nucleus accumbens. Also, the endogenous opioids were able to regulate this response. The fact that these results have been observed in an inbred strain of rats indicates an inherited variation related to the mechanism of THC.

Researchers have found that THC changes the way in which sensory information gets into and is acted on by the hippocampus. This is a component of the brain's limbic system crucial for learning, memory, and integrating sensory experiences with motivations. Investigations have shown that neurons in the information processing system of the hippocampus and the activity of the nerve fibers are suppressed by THC. In addition, researchers have discovered that learned behaviors, which depend on the hippocampus, also deteriorate.

Pulmonary Effects

The pulmonary effects of smoked marijuana include transient bronchodilation after acute exposure. Chronic bronchitis and pharyngitis have been associated with repeated exposure, with an increased frequency of pulmonary illness. With chronic smoking, large-airway obstruction is evident on pulmonary function tests, and cellular inflammatory histopathological abnormalities appear in bronchial epithelium. These effects appear to be both similar and additive to those produced by tobacco smoking.

Marijuana smoke can be divided into two phases: the gas phase and the particulate or tar phase. Marijuana smoke contains several irritants and toxic agents like carbon monoxide, ammonia, hydrogen cyanide, acetone, acetaldehyde and toluene. During the gas phase, a number of these known carcinogens, including benzene and various *nitrosamines,* have been detected.

Marijuana smoke also contains several poly-nuclear hydrocarbons such as benzoanthracene, benzopyrene, and a variety of naphthalenes, which are known carcinogens. During the particulate phase, the toxins from marijuana smoke delivered to the respiratory tract are approximately four times greater than those in tobacco smoke. Marijuana smokers, when compared to non-marijuana smokers, have more respiratory illness.

Immune System

THC and other cannabinoids have immunosuppressant properties, which impair immune system responses. Much literature outlines the results of experiments with animal tissue in-vivo and in-vitro model systems. THC and other cannabinoids suppress antibody formation, cytokine production, leukocyte migration and natural killer-cell activity, which protect the body from invasion Cannabinoids decrease host resistance to infection from bacterial and viral infection in animals. Marijuana smokers show impaired immune function: for example, decreased leukocyte blastogenesis in response to mitogens. These immune system effects of THC and other cannabinoids makes marijuana's medical use extremely risky. However, conclusive evidence for increased malignancy or enhanced HIV acquisition, or the development of AIDS, has not yet been associated with marijuana use.

Heart Rate and Blood Pressure Effects

A consistent and sudden sympathomimetic effect of marijuana is a 20-100% increase in heart rate, lasting up to 3 hours. Marijuana also induces a dose-dependent tachycardia and orthostatic hypotension during the initial stimulant phase of the behavioral syndrome.

Research indicates that smoking marijuana with cocaine use has the potential to cause severe increases in heart rate and blood pressure beyond that of each drug by itself. In one study, experienced marijuana and cocaine users were given marijuana alone, cocaine alone, and then a combination of both. Each drug alone produced cardiovascular effects; but when they were combined, the effects were greater and lasted longer. The heart rate of the subjects in the study increased 29 beats per minute with marijuana alone and 32 beats per minute with cocaine alone. However, when the drugs were used together, the heart rate increased an average of 49 beats per minute, and the increased rate persisted for a longer time. In some situations, an individual may smoke marijuana and inject cocaine in addition to physically stressful activities, which may significantly increase an overload on the cardiovascular system.

Effects of Heavy Marijuana Use on Learning and Social Behavior

A study of college students has shown that critical skills related to attention, memory, and learning are impaired among people who use marijuana heavily, even after discontinuing its use for at least 24 hours. Researchers compared 65 "heavy users," who had smoked marijuana a median of 29 of the past 30 days, and 64 "light users," who had smoked a median of 1 of the past 30 days. After 19-24 hours of closely monitored abstinence from marijuana and other drugs including alcohol, the undergraduates were given several standard tests measuring aspects of attention, memory, and learning. Compared to the light users, heavy marijuana users made more errors and had more difficulty sustaining attention, shifting attention to meet the demands of changes in the environment, and in registering, processing, and using information.

The findings suggest that greater impairment among heavy users is likely due to an alteration of brain activity produced by marijuana. Longitudinal research also indicates frequent use among young people below college age who have lower achievement, more deviant behavior, higher delinquency and aggression, poorer relationships with parents, and more associations with drug-using peers.

Pregnancy

All drugs of abuse can damage a mother's health during pregnancy, a time when she should take special care of herself. Drugs also interfere with proper nutrition and rest, which will hinder immune system functioning. Some studies have found that babies born to mothers who used marijuana during pregnancy were smaller than those born to mothers who did not use the drug. In general, smaller babies are more likely to develop health problems.

A nursing mother who uses marijuana also passes some of the THC to the baby through her breast milk. Research indicates that the use of marijuana by a mother during the first month of breast-feeding can impair the infant's motor development (control of muscle movement) and have other damaging effects.

Abuse Potential – Tolerance and Withdrawal

As you have already read, a drug contains abuse potential if it targets and activates dopamine within the brain mesocorticolimbic pathway (MCLP) where behaviors of compulsive and continued drug craving, seeking, and use, occur despite negative health and social consequences. Marijuana meets this criterion. More than 120,000 people seek treatment per year for primary marijuana addiction. In addition, animal studies suggest marijuana causes physical dependence.

Tolerance readily develops (after a day or two) to the behavioral and pharmacological effects of THC in both human and animal experimental models. In humans, tolerance develops to mood, memory, cardiovascular and autonomic effects. The mechanism of this tolerance is thought to be a desensitization of the THC receptor, perhaps by some alterations in its interaction with the second messenger. After exposure is stopped, tolerance is lost with similar rapidity.

Marijuana cessation does not give rise to an intense withdrawal syndrome at continuous low doses (less than 4 mg). However, since THC is very lipophilic, its slow rate of excretion may mask the extent and intensity of delayed withdrawal symptoms. In contrast, subjects using high doses several times a day for a few weeks do exhibit withdrawal reactions consisting of irritability, sleep disturbances, nausea, vomiting, diarrhea, tremors, sweating, and anorexia. These symptoms are generally associated with drug craving. Several studies reported by NIDA have demonstrated that daily users of marijuana who quit for as few as three days display numerous withdrawal symptoms, including cravings, irritability, restlessness, headaches, loss of appetite, and depression.

As with all drugs, the relative intensity of the withdrawal syndrome is dependent on the quantity, frequency, and duration of drug use. While a severe syndrome of physical dependence is not usually associated with cannabis withdrawal, the probability of developing some form of craving is great. The mechanism for these various withdrawal effects is unknown, but it is likely related to the unmasking of the desensitized receptors on drug cessation.

Medical Marijuana: Toward Cannabinoid-Based Medicines
The controversy over the issue of "medical marijuana" is actually all but over since medical research has made significant advances about the science of cannabinoid-based medicines. Synthetic analogs and other drugs acting on the human body's endogenous cannabinoid system are beginning to provide a myriad of potential therapeutic benefits attributed to marijuana, without the smoke, the contaminants, and the variable potency.

As previously stated, according to the research data, acutely, marijuana increases heart rate, and blood pressure may decrease on standing. Intoxication is associated with deficits in short-term memory, attention, motor skills, and reaction time. Heavy users can experience apathy, decreased motivation, and impaired cognitive performance. Chronic marijuana use is associated with development of tolerance to some effects and the appearance of a withdrawal syndrome characterized by restlessness, irritability, agitation, insomnia, sleep disturbances, anorexia, and nausea. Of comparable or greater concern, are the potential adverse effects of cannabinoids and marijuana smoke on the immune, respiratory, cardiovascular, and reproductive systems, and the potential for enhancing carcinogenesis. Like tobacco, chronic marijuana smoking is associated with lung damage, increased symptoms of chronic bronchitis, and possibly increased risk of lung cancer.

Just as nicotine is not tobacco, or taxol is not yew tree bark, and digoxin is not foxglove, cannibinoids are not marijuana. Neuroscience research has cast new light on the function of the human endogenous cannabinoid (EC) system and how cannabinoid-based medicines will be of significant therapeutic value in the not-so-distant future. By using powerful new research tools, the varied functions of the EC system are being elucidated and the potential for the development of novel new medications is now being described. And, as the reader will discover, we are clearly moving beyond the limitations and problems associated with medical marijuana and moving toward cannabinoid-based medicines.

Cannabinoid-Based Medicines
Significant advances came when scientists discovered ways to more efficiently modify endocannabinoid activity indirectly, thereby avoiding abuse potential and unwanted side effects associated with THC. The most current pharmacological methods either decrease endocannabinoid activity by blocking the receptors where they exert their effect, or increase the action of endocannabinoids by inhibiting their breakdown, usually by blocking the enzymes that deactivate them.

As research progresses, scientists will be able to develop better approaches that will use the potential of the endocannabinoid system to treat more diseases and conditions. Cannabinoid-based medicines will more than likely act through the activity-inhibition mechanisms at selective cannabinoid receptor sites, through reuptake inhibition, and/or by targeting the degrading enzymes responsible for endocannabinoids.

In addition to appetite stimulation and suppression of nausea and vomiting, possible therapeutic uses of cannabinoid receptor agonists would include treatment of:

- postoperative pain, cancer pain, and neuropathic pain

- inflammatory disorders

- metabolic syndrome (obesity, high blood pressure, increased triglycerides, Type 2 diabetes)

Of all these potential indications, analgesia has probably received the most research attention. There is an increasing amount of evidence showing that the cannabinoid receptor system is an analgesic system. Research into pain medicines is allowing scientists to measure the specific effects of cannabinoids on various pain pathways. This system appears quite distinct from the endogenous opioid system, which indicates there are different types of pain and that certain pain types not responsive to opioid drugs might be better treated with cannabinoid-based medicines. While there is no drug as of yet with a selective pharmacologic profile, there are several distinct chemical classes of compounds known to interact with the CB_1 receptor.

A Growing Formulary of Cannabinoid-Based Medicines

In the 1970s, Pfizer pharmaceutical company launched a cannabinoid research program that resulted in the development of a cannabinoid analog, *levonantradol*, which was 1,000 times more potent than THC. Clinical trials showed efficacy for postoperative pain and chemotherapy-associated nausea and vomiting; however, side effects (sleepiness, dysphoria, dizziness, thought disturbance, and hypotension) were judged to be excessive, and the project was discontinued.

Approved in 1985 by the Food and Drug Administration, **Marinol** (dronabinol), a synthetic oral preparation of THC encapsulated with sesame oil, was introduced for the treatment of chemotherapy-associated nausea and vomiting. Marinol was later approved for management of AIDS-associated wasting and anorexia. It is also being studied for possible benefit in alleviating mood and behavioral changes associated with Alzheimer's disease. Marinol's usefulness is limited by the fact that it is poorly absorbed by the human body and its delayed onset of action. Peak blood levels are not reached until 2–4 hours after dosing. In cases of intractable vomiting, the idea of swallowing anything, let alone a medicine pill, is not very realistic. Unimed Pharmaceuticals, which manufactures Marinol, and Roxane Laboratories, which jointly markets Marinol, are currently studying new aerosol, nasal spray, and sublingual formulations that may achieve a more rapid onset of action.

Developed by GW Pharmaceuticals, **Sativex** is a cannabis plant extract indicated for relief of symptoms of multiple sclerosis (MS) and for treatment of severe neuropathic pain. Sativex is administered by means of a spray into the mouth rather than smoked. The spray is composed primarily of Δ^9-tetrahydrocannabinol (*Tetranabinex*) and cannabidiol (*Nabidiolex*), a nonpsychoactive cannabinoid with additional beneficial effects. Both are extracts of chemically and genetically characterized *Cannabinis sativa L.* plants and are delivered in a 2.7-mg/25-mg ratio, with each application being under the tongue or on the inside of the cheek. Although the mechanism of action is unclear, the product is thought to exert its action by acting on cannabinoid receptors distributed throughout the central nervous system and in immune cells.

In 2005, Health Canada began using Sativex as a buccal spray for adjunctive analgesic treatment in adult patients with advanced cancer who experience moderate to severe pain during the highest tolerated dose of strong opioid therapy for persistent background pain.

Clinical trials data from a double-blind parallel group study showed that the addition of cannabinoid-based treatment to existing opioid and other analgesic medication significantly improved pain relief relative to placebo in patients with cancer pain not responding adequately to strong opioids. Furthermore, more than 40% of patients were able to achieve a clinically important reduction in pain.

In 2006 in the United Kingdom, **rimonabant** (Acomplia) was approved for use and is the first drug to target the endocannabinoid pathway by inhibiting the actions of anandamide and 2-archidonyl-glycerol on CB_1 receptors. Rimonabant blocks the central effects of the endocannabinoid pathway involved in obesity and weight control. Blockade of CB_1 receptors leads to a decrease in appetite and also has direct actions in adipose tissue and the liver to improve glucose, fat and cholesterol metabolism so improving insulin resistance, triglycerides and high-density lipoprotein cholesterol (HDL-C) and in some patients, blood pressure.

The Rimonabant in Obesity (RIO) trials have shown that the drug induces weight loss >5% in 30–40% of patients and >10% in 10–20% above both a dietary run-in and long-term hypocaloric management over a 2 year period with a low level of drug-related side effects. Rimonabant therapy is associated with an extra 8–10% increase in HDL-C and a 10–30% reduction in triglycerides and improvements in insulin resistance, glycemic control in patients with diabetes. Therefore, rimonabant has major effects on both the metabolic syndrome and cardiovascular risk factors thus has the potential to reduce the risks of type 2 diabetes and cardiovascular disease.

Appoved in in 1985 and marketed in 2006, **Nabilone** (Cesamet®)is a synthetic cannabinoid with antiemetic properties which is used for the treatment of chemotherapy-induced nausea and vomiting that has not responded to conventional antinauseants. It is also approved for use in treatment of anorexia and weight loss in patients with AIDS. Unlike Marinol, Nabilone is not derived from the cannabis plant.

Additional Cannabinoid-Based Medicines: Looking To the Not So-Distant Future

Obesity and Metabolic Disorders
Obesity has reached global epidemic proportions with more than 1 billion adults overweight and at least 300 million of them recognized as clinically obese. Obesity is widely recognized as a major contributor to the global burden of chronic disease and disability and appears on the WHO list of Top 10 global health risks.

The combination of a sedentary lifestyle and a calorie-dense diet tends to disrupt the body's energy balance system, leading to obesity and the chronic over activity of the endocannabinoid system (EC). Furthermore, research is showing how some chronic pathologic states, including obesity, lead to on-going over stimulation of the synthesis of endocannabinoids (or under-stimulation of their breakdown), resulting in over activation of the CB_1 receptors, which maintains or exacerbates the symptoms of these disorders.

In these situations of over activity, the EC system is working beyond its normal range and the over stimulation seems to promote fat storage and is associated with insulin resistance, glucose intolerance, elevated triglycerides and low HDL cholesterol levels, all of which are risk factors for cardiovascular disease. CB_1 receptor blockade can modulate this overactive EC system resulting in the restoration of balance.

Blocking the CB_1 receptor eliminates the part of obesity that is controlled by the EC System such as increased appetite, excessive hunger and food intake. It also increases adiponectin levels, which is thought to result in increased fat metabolism and an improvement in glucose metabolism (see figure below). This may result in reducing cardiovascular risk factors through weight loss and an improvement in metabolic risk factor profile.

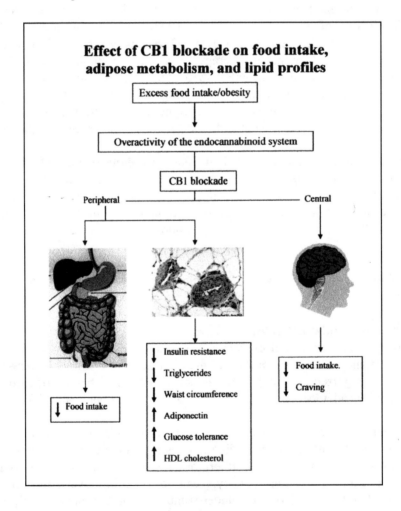

Endocannabinoids and Addiction
As was previously discussed, the endocannabinoid (EC) system is a physiological system that assists in the body's overall maintenance of homeostasis and energy

balance. The system plays an integral role in regulating body weight, glucose levels, lipid metabolism, pain, movement, and cognitive functioning. Science is also discovering the role of the EC system in drug addiction and how its activation may contribute to the reinforcing and rewarding properties of drugs having abuse potential. More importantly, the implications of this research have a focus on how the EC system can be important in the treatment of drug addiction through anti craving properties and relapse prevention mechanisms.

Although the use of psychoactive drugs begins as a voluntary behavior, in addicted individuals it becomes as uncontrollable as the compulsive, ritualized acts that afflict obsessive-compulsive disorder patients. The overpowering nature of drug addiction and the associated changes in brain structure and function have led to conceptualization of this condition as a chronic disease of the central nervous system. Like other chronic brain diseases, drug addiction goes through recurrent cycles of symptoms remission and relapse, which can be readily triggered when abstinent addicts are confronted with reminders of their drug habit ('conditioned cues') or with emotional distress. The prevention of such relapses is, of course, one of the primary goals of addiction treatment.

Drug Relapse and the Dopamine−Endocannabinoid Connection
Relapsing behaviors are related to an increased activity of the brain's mesocorticolimbic dopamine system—a neural pathway for reward and reinforcement thought to be activated in behaviors such as eating and mating, and to underlie the rewarding properties of many psychoactive drugs.

Some research studies have shown how elevated dopamine levels produced by cocaine or cocaine-associated cues elicit the release of endocannabinoids, which cause relapse. It seems that cocaine or cocaine-associated cues elevate endocannabinoid levels, which cause relapse by enhancing dopamine release. These studies have shown that blockade of CB_1 receptors prevents associative-conditioning relapses to cocaine seeking. Because cannabinoid agonist mechanisms have no effect on cocaine self-administration, these findings suggest that cannabinoid receptors must be selectively involved in triggering cocaine craving during abstinence, rather than in mediating the primary effects of the drug. These findings are of great therapeutic significance and pave the way for a new direction of addiction medicines by blocking CB_1 receptors.

Cannabinoid Receptors in Nicotine Addiction
Almost one billion men and 250 million women in the world smoke tobacco. Tobacco use, particularly smoking, remains the leading preventable cause of death in the world. Nicotine is the chemical within tobacco smoke that causes addiction. In the US, it has been estimated that 70 percent of smokers want to quit, but only 2.5 percent per year succeed in quitting smoking permanently.

It has been demonstrated that chronic nicotine consumption results in persistent over-stimulation of the EC system in animals. Dopamine release into the nucleus accumbens is part of the neurochemistry underlying the motivation to consume nicotine. The chronic consumption of nicotine permanently over-stimulates the EC system in the nucleus accumbens, with subsequent reinforcement of dopamine release and continued reinforcement of nicotine abuse. Blockade of CB_1, and thereby impairing the release of dopamine in the nucleus accumbens, tends to reduce the motivation to use nicotine.

Cannabinoid Receptors in Cocaine Addiction
Several neurobehavioral studies have demonstrated that the central mechanism involved in cocaine relapse is closely linked to the sites where marijuana has its effect, suggesting that cannabinoid receptor antagonists might be useful as anti-craving agents.

One large study used the rat reinstatement model to test whether cannabinoid receptors—the target of marijuana's psychoactive component, THC—have a role in cocaine relapse. They have shown that a cannabinoid agonist can precipitate relapse, whereas a cannabinoid antagonist can prevent relapse-induced by cocaine or cocaine-associated cues, but not relapse induced by stress.

Cannabinoid Receptors in Heroin Addiction
As with other drugs of abuse, heroin use is characterized by a high incidence of relapse following detoxification that can be triggered by exposure to conditioned stimuli previously associated with drug availability. Recent findings suggest that cannabinoid CB_1 receptors modulate the motivational properties of heroin-conditioned stimuli that induce relapse behaviors. These findings provide new insights into the neural mechanisms through which CB_1 receptors modulate the motivational properties of heroin-associated cues inducing relapse and provide a basis for the development of cannabinoid based as an additional arsenol of medicines for the treatment of opioid addiction.

Cannabinoid Receptors in Alcohol Addiction
Just over the past several years, some remarkable advances have been made towards understanding the role of the EC system in the development of alcohol tolerance and alcohol-drinking behaviors. These studies have provided strong evidence that CB_1 receptors and the EC system serve as an attractive therapeutic target for the treatment of alcohol tolerance and alcohol-related disorders. The data reviewed here provide convincing evidence that alcohol tolerance involves the down regulation of the CB_1 receptor and its function. The observed neuroadaptation may be due to increased accumulation of the endocannabinoids anandamide and 2-AG. Research has shown that treatment with a CB_1 antagonist led to reduced consumption of alcohol in animal studies. Furthermore, activation of the same endogenous cannabinoid systems by the CB_1 receptor agonist actually promoted alcohol craving, which may be related to the change in the levels of dopamine in the nucleus accumbens.

These observations suggest the involvement of the CB$_1$ receptors in controlling voluntary alcohol consumption and the involvement of the endocannabinoid system in the development of alcohol tolerance. These studies will lead to the development of endocannabinoid drugs, which will help to reduce both alcohol intake and alcohol craving. Consistent results from a variety of research studies suggest that a cannabinoid antagonist drug is useful as a potential therapeutic agent in alcohol dependence.

CHAPTER 9: SELF-STUDY QUESTIONS

TRUE/FALSE

1. *The Endocannabinoid System (ES) is a physiological system consisting of cannabinoid receptors and chemical messengers that is believed to play an important role in regulating sleep.*

2. *To date, 3 types of cannabinoid receptors have been identified; CB_1 and CB_2 and anandamide.*

3. *There is an increasing amount of evidence showing that the cannabinoid receptor system is an analgesic system*

4. *Daily users of marijuana who quit for as few as three days display numerous withdrawal symptoms, including cravings, irritability, restlessness, headaches, loss of appetite, and depression.*

5. *The combination of a sedentary lifestyle and a calorie-dense diet tends to disrupt the body's energy balance system, leading to obesity and the chronic over activity of the endocannabinoid system.*

6. *Blockade of CB_1, and thereby impairing the release of dopamine in the nucleus accumbens, tends to reduce the motivation to use nicotine.*

7. *Several neurobehavioral studies have demonstrated that the central mechanism involved in cocaine relapse is closely linked to the sites where marijuana has its effect, suggesting that cannabinoid receptor antagonists might be useful as anti-craving agents.*

8. *Recent findings suggest that cannabinoid CB_1 receptors modulate the motivational properties of heroin-conditioned stimuli that induce relapse behaviors.*

9. *Just over the past several years, some remarkable advances have been made towards understanding the role of the EC system in the development of alcohol tolerance and alcohol-drinking behaviors*

10. *Research findings suggest the involvement of the CB_1 receptors in controlling voluntary alcohol consumption and the involvement of the endocannabinoid system in the development of alcohol tolerance.*

* Answers to Self Study Tests are located on page 351

Chapter 9 References

Alvarez-Jaimes, Polisand, L. I., and Parsons' L.H.. Attenuation of Cue-Induced Heroin-Seeking Behavior by Cannabinoid CB1 Antagonist Infusions into the Nucleus Accumbens Care and Prefrontal Cortex, but Not Basolateral Amygdala. *Neuropsychopharmacology* (2008) **33**, 2483–2493.

Bayewitch M, Rhee RH, Avidor-Reiss T, Brewer A, Mechoulam R, Vogel. (-)-Delta-(9)-Tetrahydro-cannabinol antagonizes the peripheral cannabinoid receptor-mediated inhibition of adenylyl cyclase. *J Biol Chem.* 271:9902-9905. (1996).

Basavarajappa, B. S., Cooper, T. B. and Hungund, B. L. (1998a) Chronic ethanol administration down-regulates cannabinoid receptors in mouse brain synaptic plasma membrane. *Brain Research* **793**, 212–218

D'Souza, D.C., Ranganathan, M., Braley, G., Gueorguieva, R., Zimolo, Z., Cooper, T., Perry, E., and Krystal, J. Blunted Psychotomimetic and Amnesic Effects of Δ^9-Tetrahydrocannabinol in Frequent Users of Cannabis. *Neuropharmacology* 1-12. (2008).

Dale, L. Anthenelli R. Rimonabant as an Aid to Smoking Cessation in Smokers Motivated to Quit. ACC Abstract. (2004).

Devane WA. New dawn of cannabinoid pharmacology. *TiPs.;*15:40-41. (1994).

Devane WA, Manus L, Breuer A, Pertwee RG, Stevenson LA, Griffin G, Gibson D, Mandelbaum A, Etinger A, Mechoulam R. Isolation and structure of a brain constituent that binds to the cannabinoid receptor. *Science.* 258:1946-1949. (1994).

Di Marzo V, Goparaju SK, Wang L, Liu J, Batkai S, Jarai Z, Fezza F, Miura GI, Palmiter RD, Sugiura T, Kunos G. Leptin-regulated endocannabinoids are involved in maintaining food intake. *Nature.* 12;410(6830):822-5. (2001).

Fowler, CJ. The cannabinoid system and its pharmacological manipulation--a review, with emphasis upon the uptake and hydrolysis of anandamide. *Fundam. Clin. Pharmacol.* 20(6):549-62. (2006).

Hungund, B. L. and Basavarajappa, B. S. Are anandamide and cannabinoid receptors involved in ethanol tolerance? a review of the evidence. *Alcohol and Alcoholism* **35**, 126–133. (2000).

Kirkham TC. Endogenous cannabinoids: a new target for the treatment of obesity. *Am J Regul Integr Comp Physiol.* **284**. (2003).

Lemberger, L. Nabilone: A synthetic cannabinoid of medicinal utility. In Marihuana and Medicine; Nahas, G. G., Sutin, K. M., Harvey, D. J., Agurell, S., Eds.; *Humana Press:* Totowa, NJ; pp. 561–566. (1999).

Maresz K, et al. Direct suppression of CNS autoimmune inflammation via the cannabinoid receptor CB(1) on neurons and CB(2) on autoreactive T cells. *Nat. Med.* 13(4):492-7. (2007).

Mechoulam R, Ben-Shabat S, Hanus L, Ligumsky M, Kaminski NE, Schatz AK, Gopher A, Almog S, Martin BR, Compton DR, Pertwee RG, Griffin G, Bayewitch M, Barg J, Vogel Z. Identification of an endogenous 2-monoglyceride, present in canine gut, that binds to cannabinoid receptors. *Biochem Pharmacol.* 50:83-90. (1995).

Obesity and Overweight. *World Health Organization.* (2004).

Pacher P, Sa´ndor B, Kunos G. The Endocannabinoid System as an Emerging Target of Pharmacotherapy. *Pharmacol. Rev.* 58(3):389-462. (2003).

Pertwee RG. Cannabinoid receptors and pain. *Prog Neurobiol.* 63:569-611. (2001).

Pertwee, RG., Inverse agonism and neutral antagonism at cannabinoid CB1 receptors. *Life Sci.* 76: 1307-1324 (2005).

Piomelli, D., Giuffrida, A., Rodríguez de Fonseca, F. & Calignano, A. The endocannabinoid system as a target for therapeutic drugs. *Trends Pharmacol. Sci.* **21**, 218–224 (2000).

Shaham, Y., Erb, S. & Stewart, J. Stress-induced relapse to heroin and cocaine seeking in rats: A review. *Brain Res. Rev.* **33**, 13–33 (2000).

Stanford M, Avoy D. Professional Perspectives on Addiction Medicine: Beyon Medical Marijuana: Toward Cannabinoid-Based Medicines. *Santa Clara County Health & Hospital System.* 2009.

Van Gaal L. The RIO-Europe Study: Use of a Selective CB1 Receptor Blocker (Rimonabant) in the Management of Obesity and Related Metabolic Risk Factors. ESC Abstract. (2004).

Welch, S. The Neurobiology of Marijuana. Lowinson, JH, Ruiz, P, Millman, RB, and Langrod, JG (editors), *Substance Abuse A Comprehensive Sourcebook.* 4th Edition. Lippincott Williams & Wilkins. 2005

Zajicek JP, Sanders HP, Wright DE, Vickery PJ, Ingram WM, Reilly SM, Nunn AJ, Teare LJ, Fox PJ, Thompson AJ. Cannabinoids in multiple sclerosis (CAMS) study:

safety and efficacy data for 12 months follow up. *J. Neurol. Neurosurg. Psychiatry.* 76(12):1664-9. (2005).

CHAPTER 10: VOCABULARY LIST

Acetylcholinesterase   The enzyme that degrades acetylcholine and increases acetylcholine activity.

Adrenergic hallucinogens   *Those drugs that act at the norepinephrine (NE) receptor sites,and includes mescaline and peyote.*

Anesthetic hallucinogens   *Also referred to as dissociative anesthetics, is a class of hallucinogens that includes Ketamine and phencyclidine.*

Anticholinergic syndrome   *A clinical syndrome resulting from antagonization of acetylcholine at the muscarinic receptor resulting in the inhibition of the transmission of parasympathetic nerve impulses. The central anticholinergic signs and symptoms include altered mental status, disorientation, delirium, agitation, somnolence, The peripheral anticholinergic syndrome includes hyperthermia, mydriasis, dry mucosa membranes, dry, hot and red skin, peripheral vasodilatation, tachycardia, and urinary retention.*

Anticholinergic hallucinogens   *Acetylcholine antagonist drugs, including atropine and scopolamine that are found in the plants of mandrake, datura (Jimson weed), henbane, belladonna and the poisonous mushroom, amita muscaria that block cholinergic muscarine receptors. Blockade of these by atropine or scopolamine leads to restlessness and mental excitement, and can improve the rigidity and tremor characteristic of Parkinson's disease. Large doses of atropine can cause hallucination.*

Atropine   *Atropine is extracted from plants of the family Solanaceae and is a competetive antagonist for the muscarinic acetylcholine receptor. It is classified as an anticholinergic drug.*

Bufotenine   *Bufotenine is a tryptamine related to the neurotransmitter serotonin. It is a poisonous hallucinogen obtained from the skin glands of toads of the genus Bufo marinus and also in seeds of the tree Piptadenia peregrina.*

Catechol hallucinogens   *Mescaline, from the peyote cactus, and synthetic derivatives of the amphetamines (i.e. MDA and MDMA) represent the catechol hallucinogens. They have psychological effects quite similar to those of the indole types.*

Datura
Datura stramonium (Jimson weed), contains the main active chemicals scopolamine, atropine, and hyoscamine. Scopolamine and atropine are anticholinergic deleriants.

Deadly Nightshade
Atropa belladonna, has leaves and berries that are highly toxic and hallucinogenic. The plant extract contains the alkaloids atropine, scopolamine,

Dissociative State
Hallucinogens and dissociative drugs are both categories of drugs that alter a persons' state of mind and mood. Hallucinogens can cause a person to hallucinate--that is to see, hear, or feel things that aren't actually real. Hallucinogens include LSD, Mescaline (Peyote), Psilocybin, and Psilocyn (Mushrooms). Dissociative drugs, such as Ketamine or PCP, alter a person's state of mind and mood but do not cause a person to hallucinate. Dissociative drugs cause a dissociative state, where the person detaches, or dissociates, from his or her surroundings.

Henbane
Plant (Hyoscyamus niger) of the nightshade family, yields three drugs: atropine, scopolamine, and hyoscyamine.

Ketamine
Ketamine hydrochloride is a synthetic chemical in the 'dissociative anaesthetic' class. It is parenterally administered anesthetic that produces catatonia, profound analgesia, increased sympathetic activity, and little relaxation of skeletal muscles. As a club drug, also known as Special K, Vitamin K or Cat Valiums. Ketamine is used recreationally primarily as a snorted white powder and for therapeutic and psychedelic use it is often injected intra-muscularly (IM). Its effects range (at lower doses) from mild inebriation, dreamy thinking, stumbling, clumsy, or 'robotic' movement, delayed or reduced sensations, vertigo, sometimes erotic feelings, increased sociability, and an interesting sense of seeing the world differently to (at higher doses) extreme difficulty moving, nausea, complete dissociation, entering complete other realities, classic Near Death Experiences (NDEs), compelling visions, and black outs.

LSD
Lysergic acid diethylamide (LSD), also known as "acid," belongs to a class of drugs known as hallucinogens, which distort perceptions of reality. LSD is the most potent mood-

and perception-altering drug known: doses as small as 30 micrograms can produce effects lasting six to 12 hours.

Mandrake   A southern European plant (Mandragora officinarum) having greenish-yellow flowers and a branched root. This plant was once believed to have magical powers because its root resembles the human body. The root of the plant contains the cholinergic hallucinogen alkaloid, hyoscyamine.

Mescaline   Hallucinogen, the active substance in the flowering heads of the peyote cactus. An alkaloid related to epinephrine and norepinephrine, mescaline is usually extracted from the peyote. When it is taken as a drug, its hallucinogenic effects begin in two to three hours and may last over 12 hours; the hallucinations vary greatly among individuals and from one time to the next, but they are usually visual rather than auditory. Side effects include nausea and vomiting.

Muscarine   A highly toxic alkaloid related to the cholines and having neurologic effects, isolated from certain mushrooms, especially Amanita muscaria. Muscarine mimics the action of the neurotransmitter acetylcholine at muscarinic receptors. Muscarine poisoning is characterized by increased salivation, sweating and tearflow (lacrimation). With large doses, these symptoms may be followed by abdominal pain, severe nausea, blurred vision, and labored breathing. The specific antidote is atropine.

Serotonergic hallucinogens   The indolealkylamines, including LSD, psilocybin, and dimethyltryptamine (DMT) that bear a structural resemblance to the neurotransmitter 5-hydroxytryptamine (serotonin).

CHAPTER 10: HALLUCINOGENIC DRUGS

Chemicals that alter or distort reality are known by several names including psychedelics, psychotomimetics and hallucinogens. The hallucinogenic drugs distort the perception of space and time, and produce exaggerated sensory phenomena in vision, hearing, and touch. The subjective effects associated with psychedelic drugs are strongly determined by a number of factors such as setting, expectations, user's personality and dose. In some cases, adverse psychiatric effects occur including "bad trips", panic reactions and even psychotic episode during intoxication. While these psychoactive drugs can have adverse consequences, their dependence potential, as measured by their reinforcing properties and neuroadaptive response, is low compared to other drugs. Somatic signs reflecting sympathetic arousal include dilated pupils, higher body temperature, increased heart rate and blood pressure, sweating, loss of appetite, sleeplessness, dry mouth, and tremors. Nausea and vomiting may occur, and are particularly prevalent with certain hallucinogens such as mescaline. Psychedelic use has undergone cycles of popularity, especially during the 1960s, which serves as an example of how extrinsic societal factors can affect drug use, in addition to the intrinsic pharmacological actions of a drug.

FIVE MAJOR CLASSES OF HALLUCINOGENS

1. Serotonergic (Indole) hallucinogens, including LSD, psilocybin (mushrooms), morning glory seeds, bufotenine and ibogaine

2. Adrenergic (Catechol) hallucinogens, including mescaline

3. Anticholinergic hallucinogens, including atropine and scopolamine

4. Cholinergic hallucinogens, including muscarine and physostigmine

5. Anesthetic hallucinogens, including Ketamine and phencyclidine

---

Serotonergic Hallucinogens
LSD (d-lysergic acid diethylamide) is the prototypical drug of the hallucinogen class. LSD was discovered in 1938 by Dr. Albert Hofmann who was in search of a substance that might create a "model psychosis" in lab animals to study the basis for certain mental disorders. It is manufactured from lysergic acid, which is found in ergot, a fungus that grows on rye and other grains. LSD is classified under Schedule I of the Controlled Substances Act, which includes drugs with no medical use and/or high potential for abuse.

LSD, commonly referred to as "acid," is sold on the street in tablets, capsules, and, occasionally, liquid form. It is odorless, colorless, and tasteless and is usually taken by mouth. Often LSD is added to absorbent paper, such as blotter paper, and divided into small decorated squares, with each square representing one dose. The Drug Enforcement Administration reports that the strength of LSD samples obtained currently from illicit sources range from 20 to 80 micrograms per dose. This is considerably less than the levels reported during the 1960s and early 1970s, when the dosage ranged from 100 to 200 micrograms, or higher, per unit. The effects of LSD are unpredictable. They depend on amount taken, the user's personality, mood, and expectations, and the surroundings in which the drug is used. Usually, the first effects of the drug occur within 30 to 90 minutes.

Sensations and feelings change much more dramatically than other physical signs. The user may feel several different emotions at once or swing rapidly from one emotion to another. If taken in a large enough dose, the drug produces delusions and visual hallucinations. The user's sense of time and self changes. Sensations may seem to "cross over," giving the user the feeling of hearing colors and seeing sounds, a condition called synesthesia. These changes can be frightening and can cause panic reactions.

Users refer to their experience with LSD as a "trip" and to acute adverse reactions as a "bad trip." These experiences are long and typically they begin to clear after about 12 hours. Some users experience severe terrifying thoughts and feelings, fear of losing control, insanity or despair while using LSD. Some fatal accidents have occurred during states of LSD intoxication.

LSD's psychedelic properties, being an indole hallucinogen, are a result of its actions on the serotonin neurotransmitter system. LSD is thought to stimulate the various receptor subtypes for serotonin, and has particular potency in activating the serotonin autoreceptor. To date, no evidence confirms that LSD supports self-administration in animal studies and there is no known lethal dose level for LSD. A similar activation of the serotonin system is seen with MDMA, a derivative of amphetamine and has both dopamine and serotonin stimulating properties. Unlike LSD, MDMA stimulates serotonin neurotransmission by blocking its reuptake into the presynaptic terminal. This action on serotonin gives MDMA psychedelic properties in addition to its amphetamine-like stimulating properties.

There is no evidence that a withdrawal syndrome is associated with termination of chronic hallucinogen use. The phenomenon of flashbacks, in which the perceptual changes associated with LSD spontaneously appear after drug cessation, are reported to occur in about 23 percent of regular users. It is still unclear whether flashbacks represent a withdrawal syndrome and are related to, or predictive of, hallucinogen dependence.

Most users of LSD voluntarily decrease or stop its use over time. LSD is not considered an addictive drug since it does not produce compulsive drug-seeking behavior as does cocaine, amphetamine, heroin, alcohol, and nicotine. However, like many addictive drugs, LSD produces tolerance, so some users who take the drug repeatedly must take progressively higher doses to achieve the state of intoxication that they had previously achieved. This is an extremely dangerous practice, given the unpredictability of the drug.

Rapid tolerance (called tachyphylaxis) develops soon with LSD and other psychedelics when they are repeatedly administered, and the extent of the tolerance is greater than with other drugs such as PCP or alcohol. The mechanism of LSD tolerance is unclear. Since LSD stimulates serotonin receptors and a typical response of receptors to continued activation is a desensitization process, it is possible that serotonin receptor desensitization plays a role.

Psilocybin and psilocin are naturally occurring substances found in a variety of mushrooms but the species, Psilocybe mexicana, contains the highest content of psilocybin. Psilocybin was first isolated from its natural source in the 1950s and then synthesized in the lab in 1961 by Dr. Albert Hoffman of LSD fame. Psilocybin is used primarily by oral ingestion of either the fresh or dried mushroom where it is well absorbed from the gastrointestinal (GI) tract. Initial effects can include nausea and vomiting due to the drug's rapid absorption from the GI tract. Psilocybin is serotonin-like and thus its hallucinogenic actions are related to its actions on brain serotonin systems.

An average 4mg dose can initiate the process of drug action characterized by physical and mental relaxation and some perceptual distortions. With increasing doses, hallucinations may take place. Autonomic effects are minimal and usually include mydriasis, elevated blood pressure and increased heart rate. The behavioral toxicity with psilocybin is similar to that observed with LSD, and includes symptoms of increased body temperature, anxiety, panic states, paranoia and depersonalization. There is no evidence that physical dependency is associated with psilocybin abuse and it is cross-tolerant with some of the other hallucinogens including LSD.

The psychoactive ingredient of the morning glory vine (ipomoea violaceae), is lysergic acid amide and it is only about one-tenth as active as LSD. Lysergic acid amide, not being very hallucinogenic at low doses, can easily induce anxiety, depression, • headache, nausea, and vomiting. As such, even though it is a common plant around the United States, its abuse potential is low due to the many adverse reactions it produces. However, since it is serotonin-based, it is classified as an indole or serotonergic hallucinogen.

Bufotenine
Bufotenine is a serotonergic hallucinogen which, like many of the naturally occurring substances, has a long history of use in ritual and ceremony throughout various

cultures. It is found within the glands of certain toad species (Bufo marinus) and also in seeds of the tree Piptadenia peregrina.

During the 1950's, bufotenine experiments were conducted where subjects reported tingling sensations at low doses, along with nausea and breathing difficulties. These symptoms increased with higher doses, and as circulation became more and more compromised, discoloration of the lips and faces occurred. Apparently, these studies also showed that at greater dose ranges, the subject's faces turned a deep purple color. Typical of all serotonergic hallucinogens, side effects of bufotenine include increased heart rate, elevated blood pressure and body temperature. Additionally, bufotenine also produces impairments in gait and muscle coordination, catalepsy and minor paralysis.

Ibogaine is a substance found in the iboga plant *(Tabernanthe iboga)* which grows in Western Africa. Ibogaine can produce sympathomimetic reactions in addition to being an hallucinogen. Its exact mechanism of action is not known. Interestingly, it was recently discovered that ibogaine may have a treatment role as an anti-craving medicine in that it seems to reduce the craving associated with drug dependence, especially fore heroin and cocaine.

Adrenergic Hallucinogens
Like psilocybin, mescaline is a naturally occurring hallucinogen. Mescaline is the chief psychoactive ingredient of peyote cactus *(peyotl)* common to Southwest United States and Mexico. Most of the plant grows underground with only a small top being visible above ground. This top, or crown, is cut into small pieces and dried into "mescal buttons" which are then ingested orally.

A dose of 3 mg/kg will produce euphoria whereas a dose of 5 mg/kg will produce active hallucinations lasting 6 to 12 hours. Mescaline does not get metabolized (biotransformed) in the liver, and the far majority of the drug gets excreted unchanged by the kidney. The absence of liver biotransformation probably accounts for the drug's long duration of action. As an adrenergic substance, mescaline will produce all of the classic sympathomimetic effects including pupillary dilation, increased heart rate and blood pressure, elevated body temperature, EEG arousal and tremors. Toxic doses (greater than 500 mg) can produce convulsions and death due to respiratory depression.

The CNS effects of mescaline produce a profound sensory and psychic alteration much like LSD. Toxic doses can produce a psychotic reaction with paranoia, delusions and extreme panic states. However, the low potency of mescaline, as compared with other hallucinogens, makes the occurrence of behavioral toxic overdose very rare. As with many of the other hallucinogens, physical dependence is not seen although tolerance does develop slowly with repeated use.

Mescaline is cross-tolerant to both LSD and psilocybin, although it seems odd that an adrenergic substance like mescaline could produce cross-tolerance to serotonergic compounds. However, even though mescaline contains a catechol structure, and therefore is an adrenergic substance, it must also affect serotonin nerve fibers to produce some of its hallucinogenic properties; this is probably the connection it has with LSD and psilocybin.

Anticholinergic Hallucinogens
There are two principal psychoactive substances that act as antagonists within acetylcholine systems, atropine and scopolamine. These chemicals produce their effects by essentially blocking certain cholinergic (muscarine) receptor sites in the brain. Atropine and scopolamine come from plants including deadly nightshade (Atropa belladonna), mandrake (Mandragora officinarum), henbane and datura (Datura stramonium). Because atropine and scopolamine block actions within the acetylcholine system, their effects include an anticholinergic syndrome of sorts. The substances are absorbed through the gastrointestinal tract and are distributed through the brain and body. Blocking of the muscarinic postsynaptic receptors produces an inhibition of secretion of various body fluids. Low perspiration and dry mouth are characteristic of this effect. Other symptoms of anticholinergic effects include tachycardia (racing heart), extreme elevation of body temperature, and dilated (widening) pupils.

The toxic behavioral effects of anticholinergic hallucinogens include delirium, confusion, drowsiness, impaired concentration and other symptoms resembling a toxic psychosis. These drugs do not produce sensory effects, and therefore are not popular recreational drugs. Medicine has had a lengthy history of applying therapeutic dose ranges of these substances for a variety of conditions. For example, because scopolamine blocks cholinergic-muscarinic receptors, it can causes dryness in the nose, throat and mouth and thus has a role in treating cold and flu symptoms as a decongestant.

Because atropine also antagonizes acetylcholinesterase inhibitors (AChE-I), it is sometimes used in hospital emergency rooms to counter potentially fatal reactions to AChE poisons such as insecticides, if accidentally ingested. Atropine is also used sometimes by ophthalmologists in eye drops to keep pupils dilated during the eye exam. The muscles in the eye that regulate pupil size in response to light become relaxed and therefore, in the presence of a bright flashlight directed in the eyes, remain relaxed and dilated.

Cholinergic Hallucinogens
Like the anticholinergic hallucinogens, the cholinergic substances come from natural sources and also have a long history of use by many different cultures for different purposes in rituals and healing. Cholinergic hallucinogens are agonists within acetylcholine (ACh) systems where they stimulate cholinergic postsynaptic receptors. As you recall from previous sections, activation of the ACh system produces both peripheral and central effects.

Peripherally, ACh governs the autonomic parasympathetic system controlling pupil and bronchial constriction, muscle contraction (perhaps to the extent of paralysis) and hypotension. Centrally, extreme activation of ACh systems produces effects of delirium, disorientation, mental confusion, ataxia, depression, convulsions, paralysis and coma.

Two plant species are the principal sources for the cholinergic hallucinogens; the fly agaric mushroom (Amanita muscaria) and the calabar bean (Physostigma venenosum). The active ingredient in the fly agaric mushroom is muscarine, a potent ACh agonist (because it acts on muscarinic receptors and hence its name reference). Muscarine is a direct-acting agent that stimulates certain ACh receptors in the body. Direct stimulation of muscarinic receptors produces tremors, excitement, agitation and delirium. Agitation can cause hallucinations, and following the experience, the user will fall into a deep sleep. Peripheral actions of ACh agonists of this type include profuse sweating, salivation, pupil constriction, decreased heart rate and blood pressure, and muscle spasms.

The other ACh agonist, physostigmine, increases cholinergic activity not directly (like muscarine), but inhibits an enzyme that degrades acetylcholine, called acetylcholinesterase (AChE). The effects, however, are the same as with muscarine in that there is a resultant increase in ACh activity in the brain and body.

Anesthetic Hallucinogens
Phencyclidine (PCP) is representative of a unique class of abused drugs that includes the anesthetic Ketamine. PCP was developed as an injectable anesthetic in the 1950s. However, phencyclidine anesthesia is quite dissimilar to that produced by typical anesthetics. It produces a dissociative state in which patients are generally unresponsive and perceive no pain. Patients are amnesic for the surgery and CNS depression seen with other general anesthetics is absent. The delirium that often occurs on emergence from PCP anesthesia curtailed PCP's use as an anesthetic in humans. It is still sometimes used as a veterinary anesthetic, but is no longer marketed in the United States.

At sub-anesthetic doses, PCP produces behavioral effects common to several other drugs including amphetamines, barbiturates, opiates, and psychedelics. Given its wide range of behavioral effects, PCP's broad neurochemical action in the brain is not surprising. PCP antagonizes the actions of the excitatory amino acid neurotransmitter glutamate at the N-methyl-D-aspartate (NMDA) receptor, one of the receptor subtypes for glutamate. Glutamate is found throughout the brain and increases the flow of calcium (Ca+) ions into cells to cause excitatory actions.

The NMDA receptor controls the Ca+ ion channel acted on by glutamate and binding of PCP to the receptor blocks calcium entry into the cell. It is likely that the diverse behavioral effects of PCP are due to the fact that glutamate is widely distributed in the brain and regulates the activity of a number of other neurotransmitter systems. PCP also affects brain dopamine systems in ways similar to amphetamine.

The subjective effects of PCP administration can vary dramatically depending on a user's personality, who may experience vastly different reactions during different drug-taking episodes. In most cases, low doses produce euphoria, feelings of unreality, distortions of time, space and body image, and cognitive impairment. Higher doses produce restlessness, panic, disorientation, paranoia, and fear of death. As with its use as an anesthetic, PCP often causes amnesia to occur beginning immediately after the drug is taken until its effects begin to wear off. PCP is often associated with violent behavior in users but laboratory studies indicate that it does not increase aggressive behavior in animals. The violence often associated with PCP use is likely to be due to a combination of its ability to block pain and its stimulant and hallucinogenic actions.

In animal studies, PCP has been shown to be a highly effective reinforcer. From clinical reports of human PCP use and from animal studies, route of administration appears to affect the self-administration rate. Intravenously delivered PCP has been established as a reinforcer in rats, dogs, and primates. Oral PCP is rapidly established as a reinforcer in primates but not in rats. In humans, the most common route of administration of PCP is smoking.

The mechanism of action of PCP's reinforcing effects remain unclear. Part of PCP's behavioral effects are similar to dopamine-stimulating drugs like amphetamine and its administration potentiates the sedating properties of alcohol and barbiturates. As previously mentioned, PCP blocks the action of glutamate at the NMDA receptor. All of these actions may be relevant to the production of its reinforcing effects.

Animals who received repeat PCP administration have shown to develop tolerance to many of its effects. The magnitude of the tolerance, however, is less than what is seen with most other drugs of abuse. Systematic studies of PCP tolerance in humans have been few, but chronic PCP users report that after regular use they increase the amount of PCP smoked by at least twice. Some evidence from animal studies also suggests that sensitization may develop to PCP under certain conditions.

A withdrawal syndrome occurs in animals that have been chronically administered PCP. It is characterized by signs of CNS hyperexcitability such as twitches, tremors and susceptibility to seizures. A PCP withdrawal syndrome in humans is observed upon cessation of drug use. Symptoms of depression, confusion, disorientation, memory deficits, drug craving, increased appetite, and increased need for sleep have been reported to occur between 1 week and up to 8 months after termination of chronic PCP use. It is not clear why the long duration of post-acute withdrawal symptoms occur in some individuals.

Ketamine (Ketalar, Ketaject) once was a widely used chemical agent for outpatient procedures but is severely restricted now because of the drug's psychotomimetic actions. It is a dissociative anesthetic which means that when administered, it leaves the patient semiconscious and in an analgesic state where any discomfort that may be experienced is not "associated" with the body. The site where ketamine binds is the sigma opioid receptor within the opioid peptide system. The substance is also a noncompetitive antagonist at the glutamate - NMDA receptor. As you recall from previous reading, blockade of the NMDA receptors produces a variety of actions in the CNS.

Because PCP is its parent compound, ketamine produces similar effects as those already described for PCP. Interestingly, ketamine has become one of the several illegal club drugs that are abused by a younger group. As an abused drug in this class of club drugs, it has a street name of "K", or "Special K'. In this context, ketamine (usually stolen from a medical clinic or pharmaceutical company and distributed on the street), is prepared in a liquid form for injection or in a powder form for snorting.

Salvia Divinorum
Salvia Divinorum is a perennial herb in the mint family native to certain areas of the Sierra Mazateca region of Oaxaca, Mexico. It is one of 500 species of Salvia in the New World similar to the sage plant. The plant grows in large groupings to well over 3 feet in height. Its large green leaves, hollow square stems and flowers are its characteristic features. S. Divinorum is one of several vision-inducing plants employed by the Mazatec Indians.

There has been a recent interest among young adults and adolescents to re-discover ethnobotanical plants that can induce changes in perception, hallucinations, or other psychologically-induced changes. Since S. Divinorum, or any of its active ingredients are not specifically listed in the Controlled Substances Act, some on-line botanical companies and drug promotional sites have advertised Salvia as a legal alternative to other plant hallucinogens like mescaline. The plant material is smoked for the induction of "mystical" or hallucinogenic experiences.

Salvia is being smoked to induce hallucinations, the diversity of which is described by its users to be similar to those induced by ketamine, mescaline, or psilocybin. It is being widely touted on internet sites aimed at young adults and adolescents eager to experiment with these types of substances.

Salvinorin A the active component of S. Divinorum, is most effective when vaporized and inhaled. Chemically, Salvinorin A is a neoclerodane diterpene, a psychotropic terpenoid. The grouping of psychoactive plants containing terpenoid essential oils includes Salvia Divinorum, Wormwood (Absinthe), and Cannabis Sativa (tetrahydrocannabinols, THC). Divinorin A was chemically characterized by Valdes et al., in 1984, however Ortega et al., (1982) had previously characterized the same substance and called it Salvinorin A and thus, out of convention, the psychoactive substance should be called Salvinorin A. A dose of 200 to 500 micrograms produces profound hallucinations when smoked. Its' effects in the open field test in mice and loco motor activity tests in rats are similar to mescaline. Salvinorin A's action in the brain are not well elucidated. However, recent tissue testing (in vitro assays) have suggested that Salvinorin A may act at the kappa opiate receptor site, but functional assays are lacking to determine the exact mechanism of action of this drug substance.

CHAPTER 10: SELF-STUDY QUESTIONS

TRUE/FALSE

1. *Chemicals that alter or distort reality are known by several names including psychedelics, psychotomimetics and hallucinogens.*

2. LSD *is the prototypical drug of the sedative class.*

3. *To date, no evidence confirms that LSD supports self-administration in animal studies and there is no known lethal dose level for LSD.*

4. *Unlike LSD, MDMA stimulates endorphin neurotransmission by blocking receptor sites.*

5. *LSD is considered an addictive drug since it produces compulsive drug-seeking behavior as does cocaine, amphetamine, heroin, alcohol, and nicotine.*

6. *Mescaline is cross-tolerant to both LSD and psilocybin, although it seems odd that an adrenergic substance like mescaline could produce cross-tolerance to serotonergic compounds.*

7. *Belladonna, mandrake, henbane, and datura (Jimson weed) are all plants that contain the chemicals atropine and scopolamine which essentially block cholinergic muscarine receptor sites to produce their psychoactive effects.*

8. *The toxic behavioral effects of anticholinergic hallucinogens include delirium, confusion, drowsiness, impaired concentration and other symptoms resembling a toxic psychosis.*

9. *The CNS effects of mescaline produce a profound sensory and psychic alteration much like cocaine.*

10. *Two plant species are the principal sources for the cholinergic hallucinogens; the fly agaric mushroom (Amanita muscaria) and the calabar bean (physostigma venenosum).*

* Answers to Self Study Tests are located on page 351

Chapter 10 Selected Readings

Aghajanian, GK. Serotonin and the Action of LSD in the Brain. *Psychiatr Ann* 1994;24;137-141.

Andrew, W, and Rosen, W. *From Chocolate To Morphine:Everything You Need To Know About Mind-Altering Drugs.*New York, Houghton Mifflin Company. 1993.

Jacobs, BL. How Hallucinogenic Drugs Work. *Am Sci* 1987;75;386-392.

Lewin, L. *Phantastica, Narcotic and Stimulating Drugs.* New York: E. P. Dutton, 1964.

Masters, R. E. L., and Jean Houston. *The Varieties of Psychedelic Experience.* New York: Holt, Rinehart & Winston, 1966. Reprint, London: Anthony Blond, 1967.

Pechnik, RN, and Ungerleider, JT. *Hallucinogens.* In: Lowinson, JH, Ruiz, P, Millman, RB, and Langrod, JG (editors), *Substance Abuse A Comprehensive Sourcebook.* Fourth Edition. Lippincott Williams & Wilkins. 2005.

Siegel, RK. *The Natural History of Hallucinogens.* In: Jacobs, BL, ed. *Hallucinogens: Neurochemical, Behavioral, and Clinical Perspectives.* Raven Press. 1984: 1-18.

Spengos, K, Schwartz, A, Hennerici, M. Multifocal Cerebral Demyelination After Magic Mushroom Abuse. *J Neuro* 2000; 247;224-225.

Stafford, P. *Psychedlics.* Ronin Publishing. 2003.

CHAPTER 11: VOCABULARY LIST

Aliphatic nitrites *Organic inhalants like cyclohexyl nitrite, amyl nitrite and butyl nitrite (now illegal).*

Gases *Household or commercial inhalants including propane, aerosols and sprays.*

Peripheral neuropathy *Peripheral neuropathy, in its most common form, causes pain and numbness I the hands and feet. The pain typically is described as tingling or burning, while the loss of sensation often is compared to the feeling of wearing a thin stocking or glove.*

Inhalants *Inhalants are a diverse group of volatile substances whose chemical vapors can be inhaled to produce psychoactive (mind-altering) effects. While other abused substances can be inhaled, the term "inhalants" is used to describe substances that are rarely, if ever, taken by any other route of administration. A variety of products common in the home and workplace contain substances that can be inhaled to get high; however, people do not typically think of these products (e.g., spray paints, glues, and cleaning fluids) as drugs because they were never intended to induce intoxicating effects. Yet young children and adolescents can easily obtain these extremely toxic substances, and are among those most likely to abuse them.*

Kaposi's sarcoma *Kaposi's sarcoma is a form of skin cancer that can involve internal organs. It is most often found in patients with acquired immunodeficiency syndrome (AIDS) and can be fatal.*

Solvents *A group of inhalants including paint thinners, gas, glues, and various household or industrial cleaners.*

CHAPTER 11: INHALANTS

The inhalants are a diverse group of substances that include glues, aerosols, refrigerants, cleaning fluids, cements, lighter fluid, marker pens, gasoline, volatile anesthetics, fingernail polish, bottled fuel gas, "White Out" correction fluid, paint, paint remover, and room deodorizers. These agents are generally sniffed or "huffed" orally from a bag or directly from the container. Inhalants are breathable chemical vapors that produce psychoactive effects. Although people are exposed to volatile solvents and other inhalants in the home and in the workplace, many do not think of inhalable substances as drugs because most of them were never meant to be used in that way.

Young people are likely to abuse inhalants, in part because inhalants are readily available and inexpensive. Sometimes children unintentionally misuse inhalant products that are found around the house in household products. Parents, therefore, should see that these substances are monitored closely so that they are not inhaled by young children.

In general, the effects of inhalants are similar to those of alcohol and other sedative-hypnotics. Very little research has been done to investigate the mechanism of action for these drugs. At low doses, the inhalants produce a generalized relaxed sensation with light-headedness and a mild euphoria. At increasing doses, ataxia and slurred speech develop. At still higher doses, psychotic behaviors, hallucinations and even seizures can occur. The effects last for about 30 minutes but are often increased by repeat ingestion of more of the drugs.

Inhalants fall into three categories: solvents, gases and nitrates. Industrial or household solvents include paint thinners, degreasers (dry-cleaning fluids), gasoline, glues, art supplies, and office supplies like correction fluid, felt-tip-marker fluid, and electronic contact cleaners. Gases used in household or commercial products include cigarette lighters and propane tanks, whipping cream aerosol (whippets), refrigerant gases, household aerosol propellants and other associated solvents such as spray paints, hair or deodorant sprays, and fabric protector sprays. Also included in this category are medical anesthetic gases such as ether, chloroform, halothane, and nitrous oxide (laughing gas). Aliphatic (organic) nitrites include cyclohexyl nitrite, which is available to the general public; amyl nitrite, which is available only by prescription; and butyl nitrite, which is now an illegal substance.

Sniffing highly concentrated amounts of the chemicals in solvents or aerosol sprays can directly induce heart failure and death. This is especially common from the abuse of fluorocarbons and butane-type gases. High concentrations of inhalants also cause death from suffocation by displacing oxygen in the lungs (and thus in the central nervous system) so that breathing ceases. Other irreversible effects caused by inhaling specific solvents can be permanent. Hearing loss can be caused by toluene (paint sprays, glues, dewaxers) and trichloroethylene (cleaning fluids, correction fluids). Peripheral neuropathies (limb spasms) can result from taking hexane (glues and gasoline) and nitrous oxide (whipping cream or gas cylinders).

Central nervous system brain damage can also result from toluene (paint sprays, glues and dewaxers). Finally, bone marrow damage can be caused by sniffing gasoline (benzene).

There are also serious but potentially reversible effects. Liver and kidney damage can result from substances containing toluene and chlorinated hydrocarbons (correction fluid and dry cleaners). Blood oxygen depletion can be very hazardous, caused by organic nitrites ("poppers," "bold" and "rush") and methylene chloride (varnish removers and paint thinners).

Death from inhalants is usually caused by a very high concentration of fumes. Deliberately inhaling from an attached paper or plastic bag or in an enclosed area greatly increases the chances of suffocation. Even when using aerosol or volatile products for their legitimate purposes (painting or cleaning), it is wise to do so in a well-ventilated room or better yet, outdoors.

Amyl and butyl nitrites have been associated with Kaposi's sarcoma (KS), the most common cancer reported among AIDS patients. Early studies of KS showed that many people with KS had used volatile nitrites. Researchers are continuing to explore the hypothesis of nitrites as a factor contributing to the development of KS in HIV-infected people.

Sustained chronic use of inhalants can lead to pathology including kidney, liver, and bone marrow suppression following benzene and chlorinated hydrocarbon exposure; cardiotoxic effects following haolgenated hydrocarbon exposure, lead encephalopathies in gasoline inhalation, neurodegenerative changes in toluene users, and peripheral neuropathies in hexane users. Death is a rare occurrence presumably due to the short half-lives of the inhalants.

ABUSED INHALANT SUBSTANCES	
Product	**Chemical Ingredients**
Aerosals Spray paint, hair sprays, deodorants, medical sprays, asthma mists	Toluene, butane, propane, fluorocarbons, hydrocarbons
Adhesives Model airplane glue, rubber cement, polyvinylchloride cement	Toluene, ethylacetate, hexane, methylethyl ketone, trichloroethylene
Solvents And Gases Nail polish remover, paint remover, paint thinner, correction fluid, and thinner, fuel gas, cigarette lighter fluid, gasoline	Acetone, ethylacetate, toluene, methylene chloride, methanol, esters, trichloroethylene, trichloroethane, propane, butane, isopropane, mixed hydrocarbons
Cleaning Agents Dry cleaning fluid, spot remover, degreaser	Xylene, petroleum distillates, chlorohydrocarbons tetrachloroethylene, tricholoroethane

CHAPTER 11: SELF-STUDY QUESTIONS

TRUE/FALSE

1. Inhalants are breathable chemical vapors that produce psychoactive effects.

2. In general, the effects of inhalants are similar to those of alcohol and other sedative-hypnotics.

3. Inhalants fall into 4 categories; solvents, gases, nitrites and sniffers.

4. The abundance of research on inhalants has produced an extensive and detailed understanding of their mechanism of action on the human body and brain.

5. Death from inhalants usually is caused by a very high concentration of fumes

6. Amyl and butyl nitrites have been associated with Kaposi's sarcoma, the most common cancer reported among AIDS patients.

7. Sustained chronic use of inhalants has not been known to cause any serious pathology.

8. Death is a rare occurrence presumably due to the short half-lives of the inhalants.

9. Elderly people are likely to abuse inhalants, in part because inhalants are readily available and inexpensive.

10. Toluene, benzene and butane are some chemicals in products where inhalants are abused.

* Answers to Self Study Tests are located on page 351

Chapter 11 Selected Reading

Anthony J.C., Warner L.A., and Kessler R.C. Comparative epidemiology of dependence on tobacco, alcohol, controlled substances, and inhalants: Basic findings from the national comorbidity survey. *Exp. Clin. Psychopharm. ,* 2, 244-268. (1994).

Bass M. Abuse of Inhalation Anesthetics. *JAMA* 1984;251:604.

Beauvais F, Wayman JC, Thurman PJ. Et al. Inhalant Abuse Among American Indian, Mexican American, and non-Latino White Adolescents. *Am J Drug Alcohol Abuse* 2002;28(1):171-187.

Epidemiology of Inhalant Abuse. National Institute on Drug Abuse website - http://www.drugabuse.gov/pdf/monographs/148.pdf

Garriott J. Death Among Inhalant Abusers. *NIDA Res Monogr* 1992;129:181-192.

Howard MO, and Jensen JM. Inhalant Use Among Antisocial Youth: Prevalence and Correlates. *Addict Behav* 1999;24:59-74.

Joseph D E, and Parker S. *Inhalants. Drugs of Abuse.* United States Drug Enforcement Administration. 2005.

Pryor, GT. Animal Research on Solvent Abuse. *NIDA Res Monogr* 1992;129;233-258.

Sharp CW, and Rosenberg NL. *Inhalants.* In: Lowinson JH, Ruiz P, Millman RB, and Langrod JG (editors), *Substance Abuse A Comprehensive Sourcebook.* Fourth Edition. Lippincott Williams & Wilkins. 2005.

CHAPTER 12: VOCABULARY LIST

Anabolic   *Refers to muscle-building*

Androgenic   *Refers to increased masculine characteristics*

Cycling   *Involves taking multiple doses of steroids over a specific period of time, stopping for a period, and starting again.*

Pyramiding   *A process in which users slowly escalate steroid abuse (increasing the number of steroids or the dose and frequency of one or more steroids used at one time), reaching a peak amount at mid-cycle and gradually tapering the dose toward the end of the cycle.*

Stacking   *When users combine several different types of steroids to maximize their effectiveness while minimizing negative effects.*

Testosterone   *The principle hormone in humans that produces male secondary sex characteristics (androgenic) and is an important hormone in maintaining adequate nitrogen balance, thus aiding in tissue healing and maintenance of muscle mass (anabolic).*

Testosterone esters *The testosterone esters all have the testosterone molecule with a carboxylic acid group (ester linkage) attached to the 17-beta hydroxyl group in common. These esters differ in structural shape and size and function only to determine the rate at which the testosterone is released from tissue.*

CHAPTER 12: STEROIDS

Steroids refer to a class of drugs that are available legally only by prescription and are used to treat conditions that occur when the body produces abnormally low amounts of testosterone, such as delayed puberty and some types of impotence. They are also prescribed to treat body wasting in patients with AIDS and other diseases that result in loss of lean muscle mass.

Anabolic and androgenic steroids are man-made substances related to male sex hormones. Anabolic refers to muscle-building (androgenic refers to increased masculine characteristics). Testosterone is the principle hormone in humans that produces male secondary sex characteristics (androgenic) and is an important hormone in maintaining adequate nitrogen balance, thus aiding in tissue healing and maintenance of muscle mass (anabolic). Testosterone has a dual action and can be described in terms of its androgenic and anabolic capacity.

Anabolic steroids are manufactured legally or illegally outside the United States and smuggled in, usually through the mail; manufactured legally and diverted to the black market; or manufactured illegally in the United States. Many substances sold as anabolic steroids are diluted, contaminated, or simply fake.

Use Patterns
Today, individuals abuse anabolic steroids to enhance performance and also to improve physical appearance. Anabolic steroids are taken orally or injected, typically in cycles of weeks or months (referred to as "cycling"), rather than continuously. Cycling involves taking multiple doses of steroids over a specific period of time, stopping for a period, and starting again. In addition, users often combine several different types of steroids to maximize their effectiveness while minimizing negative effects (referred to as "stacking"). Steroid abusers typically "stack" the drugs, meaning that they take two or more different anabolic steroids, mixing oral and/or injectable types, and sometimes even including compounds that are designed for veterinary use. Abusers think that the different steroids interact to produce an effect on muscle size that is greater than the effects of each drug individually, a theory that has not been tested scientifically. Another mode of steroid abuse is referred to as "pyramiding."

This is a process in which users slowly escalate steroid abuse (increasing the number of steroids or the dose and frequency of one or more steroids used at one time), reaching a peak amount at mid-cycle and gradually tapering the dose toward the end of the cycle. Often, steroid abusers pyramid their doses in cycles of 6 to 12 weeks. At the beginning of a cycle, the person starts with low doses of the drugs being stacked and then slowly increases the doses. In the second half of the cycle, the doses are slowly decreased to zero. This is sometimes followed by a second cycle in which the person continues to train but without drugs.

Steroid abusers believe that pyramiding allows the body time to adjust to the high doses, and the drug-free cycle allows the body's hormonal system time to recuperate. As with stacking, the perceived benefits of pyramiding and cycling have not been substantiated scientifically.

Testosterone esters have seen an increase in their propensity for abuse. The testosterone esters all have the testosterone molecule with a carboxylic acid group (ester linkage) attached to the 17-beta hydroxyl group in common. These esters differ in structural shape and size and function only to determine the rate at which the testosterone is released from tissue. Generally, the shorter the ester chain, the shorter the half-life and quicker the drug enters circulation. Longer/larger esters usually have a longer half-life and are released into the circulation more slowly. Once in the circulation, the ester is cleaved, leaving free testosterone.

Common testosterone preparations include the following:

Testosterone esters
- ✓ Testosterone propionate
- ✓ Testosterone cypionate
- ✓ Testosterone enanthate

Testosterone derivatives
- ✓ Methyltestosterone
  - Methyltestosterone is a very basic anabolic-androgenic steroid (AAS) with the only addition being a methyl group. This eliminates first pass degradation in the liver, making oral dosing possible. It also causes dose-related hepatotoxicity (liver damage).
  - Methyltestosterone exhibits really strong androgenic and estrogenic side effects and is generally a poor choice for most, if not all, uses.

- ✓ Methandrostenolone
  - Methandrostenolone was first commercially manufactured in 1960 by Ciba under the brand name Dianabol and quickly became the most used and abused steroid worldwide to date. It jokingly came to be known as "the breakfast of champions" in sports circles.
  - This drug is very anabolic with a half-life of approximately 4 hours. The methyl group added makes this anabolic-androgenic steroid an oral preparation and potentially very hepatotoxic.
  - Both Ciba and generic firms in the United States discontinued methandrostenolone in the late 1980s, but over 15 countries worldwide still produce it in generic form.

- ✓ Fluoxymesterone
  - Fluoxymesterone is a potent androgen that is produced under the brand name Halotestin, it is a very potent androgen with very little

anabolic activity. Again, the added methyl group makes oral administration possible, along with concerns for liver damage.

- This drug is not favored due to its poor anabolic effects, yet athletes still abuse it for its androgenic nature.

Nandrolone derivatives
✓ Nandrolone decanoate
- Nandrolone decanoate is 3-4 times less than that of testosterone and is one of the most widely abused AASs due to its efficacy, safety profile, and worldwide manufacture.

✓ Ethylestrenol
- Ethylestrenol was marketed in the United States under the brand name Maxibolin, but it has since been discontinued.

✓ Trenbolone
- Trenbolone is a derivative of nandrolone and is both a potent androgen and anabolic. It is comparably more androgenic than nandrolone.
- Trenbolone is a European drug with a very high abuse record. In the United States, it is used in veterinary preparations as trenbolone acetate, and as such, has found its way into the hands of those who wish to exploit its androgenic/anabolic potential.

Dihydrotestosterone derivatives
✓ Oxandrolone
- Oxandrolone is an oral preparation with a greatly increased anabolic component. This AAS is very anabolic with little androgenic effect.
- First marketed by Searle, it was discontinued in the mid 1990s. BTG remarketed this anabolic-androgenic steroid as Oxandrin, largely for the drug's use in HIV-related disease.
- Oxandrolone is one of a few agents to be routinely abused by female athletes due to its mild androgenic properties. Athletes, from weightlifters to boxers, use oxandrolone seeking to increase strength without additional weight gain.

✓ Stanozolol
- Stanozolol is an active anabolic-androgenic steroid which greatly enhances androgen receptor binding.
- Stanozolol is highly active in both androgen and anabolic sensitive tissue. It is a weaker androgen than DHT and exerts comparatively less androgenic effect.
- This anabolic-androgenic steroid is marketed in the United States and abroad as Winstrol and comes in both oral and injectable forms.

- Athletes, many in track and field, have abused it. Canadian sprinter Ben Johnson tested positive for stanozolol over a decade ago.

  ✓ Oxymetholone
  - This potent anabolic-androgenic steroid is a unique agent. It is an oral agent with greatly enhances anabolic properties. The action of this agent in androgen-sensitive tissues is much like that of DHT and is quite androgenic.
  - It is the only anabolic-androgenic steroid to date to be considered a carcinogen (*The Merck Manual of Diagnosis and Therapy,* 15th edition, 1987).
  - It is marketed in the United States as Anadrol-50 and has been abused the world over by weight lifters and strength athletes for both its strong anabolic and pronounced androgenic effects.

Effects of Steroid Use

There is increasing data about the serious health problems associated with the abuse of steroids, including both short-term and long-term side effects. Taken in combination with a program of muscle-building exercise and diet, steroids may contribute to increases in body weight and muscular strength. Steroid users subject themselves to more than 70 side effects ranging in severity from liver cancer to acne and including psychological as well as physical reactions. The liver and cardiovascular and reproductive systems are most seriously affected by steroid use.

The short-term adverse physical effects of anabolic steroid abuse are well documented. Short-term side effects include sexual and reproductive disorders, fluid retention, and severe acne. The short-term side effects in men are reversible with discontinuation of steroid use. Masculinizing effects seen in women, such as deepening of the voice, body and facial hair growth, enlarged clitoris, and baldness are not reversible and are permanent changes. The long-term adverse physical effects of anabolic steroid abuse in men and in women, other than masculinizing effects, have not been studied, and as such, are not well known.

Signs of Steroid Abuse
- Quick weight and muscle gains (when used in a weight training program)
- Aggressiveness and combativeness
- Jaundice
- Purple or red spots on the body
- Swelling of feet and lower legs
- Trembling
- Unexplained darkening of the skin
- Persistent unpleasant breath odor
- Severe acne breakouts and oily skin

Psychological effects in both sexes include very aggressive behavior known as "roid rage" and severe depression.

Physical Side Effects of Steroid Abuse	
MALES	FEMALES
Atrophy (wasting away of tissues or organs) of testicles	Menstrual irregularities
Loss of sexual drive	Infertility
Diminished or decreased sperm production	Masculinizing effects including facial hair, diminished breast size, permanently deep voice, and enlargement of the clitoris.
Breast and prostate enlargement	
Decrease hormone levels	

Health consequences include:

- In males, reduced sperm production, shrinking of the testicles, impotence, difficulty or pain in urinating, baldness, and irreversible breast enlargement (gynecomastia).
- In females, development of more masculine characteristics, such as decreased body fat and breast size, deepening of the voice, excessive growth of body hair, and loss of scalp hair, as well as clitoral enlargement.
- In adolescents of both sexes, premature termination of the adolescent growth spurt, so that for the rest of their lives, abusers remain shorter than they would have been without the drugs.
- In males and females of all ages, potentially fatal liver cysts and liver cancer; blood clotting, cholesterol changes, and hypertension, each of which can promote heart attack and stroke; and acne. Although not all scientists agree, some interpret available evidence to show that anabolic steroid abuse- - particularly in high doses -- promotes aggression that can manifest itself as fighting, physical and sexual abuse, armed robbery, and property crimes such as burglary and vandalism. Upon stopping anabolic steroids, some abusers experience symptoms of depression, fatigue, restlessness, loss of appetite, insomnia, reduced sex drive, headache, muscle and joint pain, and the desire to take more anabolic steroids.
- In injectors, infections resulting from the use of shared needles or non-sterile equipment, including HIV/AIDS, hepatitis B and C, and infective endocarditis, a potentially fatal inflammation of the inner lining of the heart. Bacterial infections can develop at the injection site, causing pain and abscess.

CHAPTER 12: SELF-STUDY QUESTIONS

TRUE/FALSE

1. Steroids are also prescribed to treat body wasting in patients with AIDS and other diseases that result in loss of lean muscle mass.

2. Testosterone is the principle hormone in humans that produces female secondary sex characteristics.

3. Anabolic refers to muscle-building and androgenic refers to increased masculine characteristics.

4. Steroid abusers typically "stack" the drugs, meaning that they take two or more different anabolic steroids

5. Another mode of steroid abuse is referred to as pyramiding which is a process where users combine three different steroids.

6. Testosterone esters have seen an increase in their propensity for abuse.

7. Steroid users subject themselves to more than 70 side effects ranging in severity from liver cancer to acne

8. The liver and cardiovascular and reproductive systems are most seriously affected by steroid use.

9. Psychological effects in both sexes include highly aggressive behavior known as "roid rage" and severe depression.

10. The long term consequences of steroid abuse are well studied and well known.

* Answers to Self Study Tests are located on page 351

Chapter 12 Selected Reading

Applegate EA, and Grivetti LE. Search for the Competitive Edge: A History of Dietary Fads and Supplements. *J Nutr* 1997;127[5 Suppl]:869S-873S.

Inaba D, Cohen W. *Uppers, Downers, All Arounders*. CNS Publications. 2000.

Connolly, S. *Steroids (Just the Facts)*. Heinemann. 2000.

Eisneberg, ER, and Galloway, GP. Anabolic-Androgenic Steroids. Lowinson, JH, Ruiz, P, Millman, RB, and Langrod, JG (editors), *Substance Abuse A Comprehensive Sourcebook*. Fourth Edition. Lippincott Williams & Wilkins. 2005.

Irving, LM, and Wall, M, Neumark-Sztainer, D and Story, M. Steroid Use Among Adolescents: Findings From Project EAT. *J Adolesc Health* 2002;30(4):243-252.

Kleiner SM. Performance-Enhancing Aids in Sport: Health Consequences and Nutritional Alternatives. *J Am Coll Nutr* 1991;10(2):163-176.

Lenehan, P. *Anabolic Steroids*. CRC. 2003.

Wilson J. Androgen Abuse By Athletes. *Endocrine Rev* 1998;9(2):181-199.

Yesalis, CE, and Cowart, VS. *The Steroids Game*. Human Kinetics Publishers. 1998.

CHAPTER 13: VOCABULARY LIST

Creatinine

Creatinine is a metabolic byproduct of protein metabolism, which normally appears in urine in relatively constant quantities over a 24-hour period with regular liquid consumption.

False Positives

Defined as a drug free sample falsely being reported as showing positive for drugs.

Gas chromatography–mass spectrometry

(GC-MS) A UTS that is able to detect small quantities of a substance and confirm the presence of a specific drug and is the most accurate, sensitive, and reliable method of testing.

Urine Toxicology Screens

(UTS) Medical testing for urinary metabolites of recreational drugs. Two types are mainly used: immunoassay and gas chromatography–mass spectrometry (GC-MS).

Immunoassays

A UTS that uses antibodies to detect the presence of specific drugs or metabolite. Immunoassay techniques are used in many home-testing kits or point-of-care screenings.

CHAPTER 13: METHODS OF DRUG TESTING

Urine, blood, hair, saliva, sweat, and nails (toenails and fingernails) are some biological specimens used to perform laboratory drug testing, and they provide different levels of specificity, sensitivity, and accuracy. Urine is most often the preferred test substance because of ease of collection. Concentrations of drugs and metabolites also tend to be high in the urine, allowing longer detection times than concentrations in the serum allow.

Two types of urine toxicology screens (UTS) are typically used; immunoassay and gas chromatography–mass spectrometry (GC-MS). Immunoassays, which use antibodies to detect the presence of specific drugs or metabolites, are the most common method for the initial screening process. Advantages of immunoassays include large-scale screening through automation and rapid detection. Forms of immunoassay techniques include cloned enzyme donor immunoassay; enzyme-multiplied immunoassay technique (EMIT), a form of enzyme immunoassay; fluorescence polarization immunoassay (FPIA); immunoturbidimetric assay; and radioimmunoassay (RIA). In addition, immunoassay techniques are used in many home-testing kits or point-of-care screenings.

The main disadvantage of immunoassays is obtaining false-positive results when detection of a drug in the same class requires a second test for confirmation. Results of immunoassays are always considered presumptive until confirmed by a laboratory-based test for the specific drug (eg, GC-MS or high-performance liquid chromatography). Yet even GC-MS can fail to identify a positive specimen (eg, hydromorphone, fentanyl) if the column is designed to detect only certain substances (eg, morphine, codeine).

Gas chromatography–mass spectrometry is considered the criterion standard for confirmatory testing. The method is able to detect small quantities of a substance and confirm the presence of a specific drug (eg, morphine in an opiate screen). It is the most accurate, sensitive, and reliable method of testing; however, the test is time-consuming, requires a high level of expertise to perform, and is costly. For these reasons, GC-MS is usually performed only after a positive result is obtained from immunoassay.

Urine Testing
Results of a urine test show the presence or absence of specific drugs or drug metabolites in the urine. Metabolites are drug residues that remain in the system for some time after the effects of the drug have worn off. A positive urine test does not necessarily mean the subject was under the influence of drugs at the time of the test. Rather, it detects and measures use of a particular drug within the previous few days. The following is a summary of the analytical methods used by laboratories to detect the presence of drugs or their metabolites in urine.

Immunoassays

These tests are most commonly used to screen samples. In the event that drugs or their metabolites are detected, then the sample is normally tested again using an even more sensitive test such as Gas Chromatography and Mass Spectometry (GCMS). Immunoassays work on the principle of antigen-antibody interaction. Antibodies are chosen which will bind selectively to drugs or their metabolites. The binding is then detected using either enzymes, radioisotopes or fluorescent compounds.

- **EMIT** (Enzyme Multiplied Immunoassay Technique) is manufactured by Syva Laboratories. It uses an enzyme as the detection mechanism. It is the cheapest, simplest to perform and the most widely used of the immunoassays. Unfortunately, it is also the easiest to fail and more worryingly, the least accurate: giving a 4-34% false positive rate.
- **RIA** (Radio Immunoassay) is manufactured by Roche Diagnostics. It is similair to EMIT but uses a radioactive isotope such as iodine instead of an enzyme. However, because it involves using radioactive substances, it is less popular than EMIT. This is a highly sensitive form of testing mainly used by the military.
- **FPI** (Fluorescence Polarization Immunoassay) is manufactured by Abbott Laboratories. Fluorescent compounds mark the selective binding of antibodies to drugs and their metabolites. It is highly sensitive and highly specific.

Thin Layer Chromatography

This procedure involves the addition of a solvent to the sample causing the drugs and their metabolites to travel up a porous strip leaving color spots behind. As each different substance travels a specific distance, the strip can then be compared with known standards. This test gives no quantitative information, it merely indicates the presence of drugs or their metabolites. Furthermore, it relies on the subjective judgement of a technician and requires considerable skill and training. It is not widely used.

Gas Chromatography and Mass Spectometry

These are the most precise tests for identifying and quantifying drugs or their metabolites in the urine. They are usually used as a confirmation test following a positive result on an Immunoassay. It involves a two step process, whereby *Gas Chromatography* separates the sample into its constituent parts and *Mass Spectometry* identifies the exact molecular structure of the compounds. The combination of Gas Chromatography and Mass Spectometry is considered to be the definitive method of establishing the presence of drugs or their metabolites in the urine. However, the equipment necessary to perform it is extremely expensive and this is reflected in the price for testing each sample. Occasionally problems do arise with poor calibration of the equipment.

Although urine is most commonly tested, occasionally laboratories use one of the following methods to detect the presence of drugs or their metabolites:

Hair Testing

Analysis of hair may provide a much longer "testing window" for the presence of drugs and drug metabolites, giving a more complete drug-use history that goes back as far as 90 days. Like urine testing, hair testing does not provide evidence of current impairment, only past use of a specific drug. Hair testing cannot be used to detect alcohol.

Perspiration Testing

Another type of drug test consists of a skin patch that measures drugs and drug metabolites in perspiration. The patch, which looks like a large adhesive bandage, is applied to the skin and worn for some length of time. A gas-permeable membrane on the patch protects the tested area from dirt and other contaminants. The sweat patch is sometimes used in the criminal justice system to monitor drug use by parolees and probationers, but so far it has not been widely used in workplaces or schools.

Saliva Testing

Traces of drugs, drug metabolites, and alcohol can be detected in oral fluids, the generic term for saliva and other material collected from the mouth. Oral fluids are easy to collect—a swab of the inner cheek is the most common way. They are harder to adulterate or substitute, and collection is less invasive than with urine or hair testing. Because drugs and drug metabolites do not remain in oral fluids as long as they do in urine, this method shows more promise in determining current use and impairment.

Alcohol Breathalyzers

Unlike urine tests, breath-alcohol tests do detect and measure current alcohol levels. The subject blows into a breath-alcohol test device, and the results are given as a number, known as the Blood Alcohol Concentration, which shows the level of alcohol in the blood at the time the test was taken. In the U.S. Department of Transportation regulations, an alcohol level of 0.04 is high enough to stop someone from performing a safety-sensitive task for that day.

Blood Testing

Although expensive and intrusive, blood testing is the most accurate confirmation of drug use. Since blood testing accurately detects the presence of the drug or its metabolites at the time of testing, the results from this type of test are the best indication of current intoxication. Blood testing for the use of drugs is primarily used in accident investigations or for health/life insurance medicals. Cannabinoids can be detected up to six hours after consumption by testing blood; after that, the metabolite concentration falls rapidly, and cannabinoids are not detectable in the blood after 22 hours.

Standard Test Panels

A standard panel typically includes amphetamine, methamphetamine, cocaine, benzodiazepines, barbiturates, phencyclidine, morphine and codeine. Special tests can include alcohol, THC and Clonazepam (Klonipin).

Urine Toxicology Screens

Urine is most commonly tested because it is the main excretory route for drugs and their metabolites. Furthermore, the drugs remain detectable for much longer and asking for a urine sample is less intrusive than a blood sample. Although drugs can be detected in saliva and perspiration, the detection time is much shorter than urine and laboratories tend not to use these tests for this reason. Finally, hair testing is uncommon because it is expensive and in any case often requires a urine test for confirmation.

Urine Creatinine

The urine creatinine level is useful, when performed with a drug screen, as an indicator of specimen validity.

Creatinine is a metabolic byproduct of protein metabolism, which normally appears in urine in relatively constant quantities over a 24-hour period with regular liquid consumption. Therefore, urine creatinine can be used as an indicator of urine water content. Greater than normal intake of water will increase the urine water content (lowering the creatinine level) consequently diluting the amount of drug in urine. Conversely, a limited intake of water can lead to an abnormally concentrated urine specimen (as occurs with dehydration) resulting in elevated creatinine levels. The urine becomes more dilute when a person drinks larger amounts of water.

Most normal urine samples will have a creatinine value between 20 and 350 mg/dl (milligrams per deciliter). A specimen with a urine creatinine level less than 20 mg/dl is considered "dilute". Among urine samples submitted for employment related drug testing, about two percent are found to be dilute. On the other hand, eight percent of those urine specimens submitted for court-directed drug testing have a creatinine level under 20 mg/dl.

A quality laboratory will measure the urine creatinine level on every specimen tested and report when the specimen is dilute. Accordingly, when the urine is more dilute, there is a lower concentration of drugs. It is recommended that negative drug test results be disqualified when the specimen has a creatinine level less than 20 mg/dl. Conversely, a positive result on a dilute specimen should not be disqualified, because this shows that the drug was in such high concentrations that it was detected even though the urine is dilute.

Urine Creatinine Interpretation

The levels at which creatinine may be considered dilute (<20 ml/dL) or abnormally dilute (<=5 mg/dL) are based on the critical points that the Substance Abuse and

Mental Health Services Administration (SAMSHA) has set as decision points for interpreting dilute or substituted urine specimens.

< 20 mg/dL **Dilute urine specimen** - most likely due to increased water intake. Can be a result of short-term water loading (flushing) in an attempt to dilute any drug below testing cutoff concentrations.

<=5 mg/dL **Abnormally dilute** - specimen showing an excessively low creatinine value. May be indication that the specimen is not consistent with normal human urine.

Note: *The above interpretations are general guidelines. Other physiological conditions may account for low creatinine concentrations such as diabetes, kidney disease or use of prescription diuretics.*

Individuals being drug tested and those responsible for urine testing programs are very aware that specimens submitted for testing are vulnerable to adulteration or tampering. Although collection procedures may be in place to ensure specimen integrity, donors have shown considerable ingenuity in their efforts to defeat the testing process. Possible methods of avoiding drug use detection include the addition of adulterants to the specimen, the substitution of someone else's urine and specimen dilution. Both specimen adulteration and specimen substitution are difficult to accomplish during an observed collection. Additionally, the presence of adulterants in a urine specimen has the same implications as the presence of drugs. As a result, the most common way to mask drug use is by "internal" dilution. This is done by excessive water consumption or by taking diuretics such as herbal teas.

Some donors deliberately drink large quantities of fluids for medical reasons or because they think it is a healthy habit. If a donor consistently provides a dilute specimen they should be reminded that it is their responsibility to provide a specimen suitable for testing and failure to do so might be considered "Refusal to Test". They should reduce their liquid consumption and limit their use of caffeine and herbal teas. Most people will comply unless they are attempting to mask their drug use.

The best way to minimize the percentage of dilute urine specimens is by using a random collection program. Unannounced specimen collection presents the donor with little time to prepare. Another good practice is to get a first morning voiding if possible, since this specimen often is more concentrated. People diluting their urine by drinking large amounts of liquids cannot continue this practice indefinitely. By increasing the frequency of collection you are likely to catch these individuals off guard.

Causes of Questionable Drug Screening Specimens

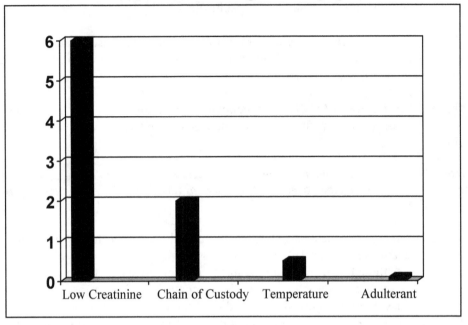

An effective additive need only fool the screening test, since the specimen would then never progress to GCMS confirmation. Some additives are more effective than others and some are more easily detected. For example, bleach, liquid soap, salt, oven cleaner, vinegar and glutaraldehyde can indeed cause a false negative EMIT screening test, but when too much is added, they also interfere with the test to the extent that the laboratory is alerted to an invalid specimen. Therefore, there is a measure of luck associated with the successful use of these products. One must use just enough additive to hide the positive result, but not so much that that the laboratory is alerted.

Observed collection provides the first line of defense against specimen tampering. Additionally, laboratories now routinely test each specimen for creatinine to identify diluted specimens. Those specimens with a low creatinine level are further tested for specific gravity. When specimen adulteration is suspected on the basis of color, odor or an EMIT screen alert, a more comprehensive battery of tests for adulterants is employed. This includes tests for oxidants, nitrites, glutaraldehyde, chromate, and surfactant (soap). As drug users expand their cover-up techniques, laboratories continue to develop more sophisticated countermeasures.

The following table describes common adulterants and the "red flags" that a laboratory can use to suspect their presence. Further procedures, such as test for nitrites, oxidants and specific gravity may be used to confirm.

Product	Adulterant	Red Flags
Bleach	Oxidant	EMIT Alert
Klear	Nitrate	GC/MS Negative
Whizzies	Nitrite	GC/MS Negative
Urine Aid	Glutaraldehyde	GC/MS Negative
Urine Luck	Chromate	GC/MS Negative
CarboClean	Diuretic (flushing)	Creatinine Low
Golden Seal	Diuretic (flushing)	Creatinine Low
Soap	Surfactant	EMIT Alert

Detectable Time Periods

It varies from person to person according to age, gender, metabolism and general state of health; also the analytical method, the type of drug, the quantity and frequency of its use influence the detection time. These drug detection times are based on urine analysis. Drug detection times for hair follicle testing tend to be higher, whereas detection times for blood, saliva and perspiration testing tend to be lower.

SUBSTANCE	APPROXIMATE DETECTION PERIOD
Alcohol (UAC)	+ = recent drinking (< 8 hours) - = no recent drinking
NOTE: Urine Alcohol Concentration (UAC): The presence of alcohol in the urine indicates alcohol intake within about the preceding 8 hours. Concentration of alcohol depends on how long the urine has been in the bladder and makes any urine quantitative measure difficult to interpret.	
Amphetamines	2-5 days
Barbiturates	Short acting 2 days, Long acting 3-4 weeks
Benzodiazepines therapeutic chronic abuse	 2 – 4 days up to 4 weeks
NOTE: Clonazepam (Klonipin) is a long half-life benzodiazepine that can be detected for approximately 3 weeks	
Cannabinoids (THC) single use moderate use (4/wk) heavy use (daily) chronic heavy use	 3 days 3 – 5 days 10 days up to 36 days
Cocaine	2-4 days
Codeine	1 - 3 days
Euphorics (MDMA)	2-4 days
Ketamine (Special K)	5-7 days
LSD	1 – 2 days (immunoassay)

Methadone	2 - 3 days
Methamphetamine	2 - 3 days
Morphine	1 - 3 days
Phencyclidine (PCP)	
single use	3 days
moderate use (4/wk)	5 – 10 days
heavy use (daily)	10 -20 days
chronic heavy use	up to 30 days
Phenobarbital	10-20 days
Propoxyphene	6 hrs - 2 days
Steroids Anabolic (oral)	14-28 days
Steroids Anabolic (parentally)	1-3 months
SOURCE: *Principles of Addiction Medicine 3rd Edition* , (Graham, A.W., Schultz, T.K., Mayo-Smith, M.F., Ries, R.K., Wilford, B.B., Eds). American Society of Addiction Medicine, 2003.	

Drug Testing - False Positives

In drug testing, a false positive is defined as a drug free sample falsely being reported as showing positive for drugs. This can occur for a number of reasons including: improper laboratory procedure, mixing up samples, incorrect paperwork and, albeit rarely, passive inhalation. But the most common cause of drug testing false positives are dilute urtine samples. Another big reason of drug testing false positives is cross reactants. A cross reactant is a substance which because of its similar chemical structure to a drug or its metabolite can cause a false positive result.

The following substances may cause cross reactivity on an Immunoassay screen but are unlikely to be mistaken on a Gas Chromatography/Mass Spectrometry test:

Ibuprofen

Ibuprofen is a common pain reliever and anti-inflammatory which even in low doses used to cause a false positive for marijuana/cannabis on the EMIT test. The EMIT has been changed to use a different enzyme to eliminate these drug test false positives. But recent evidence suggests that Ibuprofen taken in very high doses, along with other anti-inflammatories such as Naproxen will still interfere with the EMIT test.

Decongestants and Cold Remedies

Ephedrine and pseudoephedrine (and Phenylpropanolamine some time ago) are both substances found in many over-the-counter cold remedies. They can result in a drug test false positive for amphetamines on the EMIT test. Antitussives, to suppress coughs, such as dextromethorphan and perylamine may cause a drug test false positive for opiates.

Antidepressants

Aside from when this class of drugs is specifically tested for, some of them, including amitriptyline, can test positive for opiates for up to three days after use. Even quinine in tonic water may cause a positive result for opiates.

Poppy Seeds

Poppy seeds which are usually found on bread contain traces of morphine and can lead to positives for opiates. Codeine, which is found in many pain relievers, may cause a false positive for morphine or heroin because of its similar chemical structure.

Antibiotics

Certain newly developed antibiotics including amoxicillin and ampicillin have been reported to cause false positives for cocaine.

DHEA

This treatment developed for use by AIDS patients will cause a false positive for anabolic steroid use.

Enzymes

A small fraction of the population excrete large amounts of certain enzymes in their urine which may produce a positive drug test. The enzymes in question are endogenous lysozyme and malate dehydrogenate, which according to research may run as high as 10% of positive samples.

Melanin

Melanin is the pigment which protects skin and hair from UV light. It is also very similar in chemical structure to THC (Tetrahydrocannabinol, the active component in cannabis) and some data exists claiming it causes false positives for cannabis. Unfortunately, an equal amount of data suggests that there is no link whatsoever.

CHAPTER 13: SELF-STUDY QUESTIONS

TRUE/FALSE

1. *Three types of urine toxicology screens (UTS) are typically used; immunoassay, gas chromatography–mass spectrometry (GC-MS) and alcohol breathalyzers.*

2. *Gas chromatography–mass spectrometry is considered the criterion standard for confirmatory testing.*

3. *Results of a urine test show the presence or absence of specific drugs or drug metabolites in the urine.*

4. *Hair analysis may provide a much longer "testing window" for the presence of drugs and drug metabolites, giving a more complete drug-use history that goes back as far as 90 days.*

5. *Blood testing is the most accurate confirmation of drug use.*

6. *Creatinine is a metabolic byproduct of protein metabolism, which normally appears in urine in relatively constant quantities over a 24-hour period with regular liquid consumption. Therefore, urine creatinine can be used as an indicator of urine water content.*

7. *In drug testing, a false positive is defined as someone who was trying to beat the system and got caught.*

8. *The most common cause of drug testing false positives is drug switching to another similar drug tat resembles a drug of preference.*

9. *Ephedrine and pseudoephedrine are both substances found in many over-the-counter cold remedies that can result in a drug test false positive for heroin on the EMIT test.*

10. *Aside from when this class of drugs is specifically tested for, some antidepressant mediactions can test positive for opiates for up to three days after use.*

* Answers to Self Study Tests are located on page 351

Chapter 13 Selected Reading

Goldstein, G. Addiction: From Biology to Drug Policy. Oxford University Press. 2001.

Mieczkowski, T. *Drug Testing Technology: Assessment of Field Applications).* CRC. 1999.

U.S. DHHS, SAMHSA, Center for Substance Abuse Prevention (CSAP), Division of Workplace Programs (DWP). 2004. *Medical Review Officer Manual for Federal Agency Workplace Drug Testing Programs.* Rockville, Maryland.

U.S. DHHS, SAMHSA, CSAP. Guide for Drug-Free Workplace Policy Makers: Issues, Options, and Models. Rockville, Maryland. 1992.

Wong, RC and Tse, HY. *Drugs of Abuse: Body Fluid Testing.* Humana Press. 2005.

SECTION III: BEHAVIORAL PHARMACOLOGY OF PSYCHIATRIC MEDICATIONS

CHAPTER 14: VOCABULARY LIST

Agranulocytosis

An acute disease marked by high fever and a sharp drop in circulating granular white blood cells.

Akasthesia

A movement disorder characterized by a feeling of inner restlessness and a compelling need to be in constant motion. Akathisia is often a side effect of certain drugs.

Anterograde amnesia

A condition in which events that occurred after the onset of amnesia cannot be recalled and new memories cannot be formed.

Antiemetics

Drugs that are effective against vomiting and nausea. Anti-emetics are typically used to treat motion sickness, side effects of opioid analgesics, general anaesthestics and chemotherapy.

Delusions

An unshakable belief in something untrue. These irrational beliefs defy normal reasoning, and remain firm even when overwhelming proof is presented to dispute them.

Extrapyramidal Syndrome

Abnormailities of movement related to injury of to injury of motor pathways other than the pyramidal tract.

Hallucinations

False or distorted sensory experiences that appear to be real perceptions. These sensory impressions are generated by the mind rather than by any external stimuli, and may be seen, heard, felt, and even smelled or tasted.

Neuroleptic Malignant Syndrome

A rare, potentially life-threatening disorder that is usually precipitated by the use of medications that block dopamine. Most often, the drugs involved are those that treat psychosis. The syndrome results in dysfunction of the autonomic nervous system, the branch of the nervous system responsible for regulating such involuntary actions as heart rate, blood pressure, digestion, and sweating. Muscle tone, body temperature, and consciousness are also severely affected.

Neuroleptics

Tranquilizing drugs, especially one used in treating mental disorders.

Orthostatic hypotension

Also called postural hypotension — is an abnormal decrease in blood pressure that occurs when standing up from sitting or lying down. It may lead to fainting.

Psychotropic

A psychoactive drug or psychotropic substance is a drug that acts primarily upon the central nervous system where it produces an altering effect on perception, emotion, or behavior

Psychosis

A symptom or feature of mental illness typically characterized by radical changes in personality, impaired functioning, and a distorted or non-existent sense of objective reality.

Tardive dyskinesia

Tardive dyskinesia is a mostly irreversible neurological disorder of involuntary movements caused by longterm use of antipsychotic or neuroleptic drugs.

Serotonin syndrome

Aka, hyperserotonemia, it is a life-threatening drug reaction that causes the body to have too much serotonin. It most often occurs when two drugs that affect the body's level of serotonin are taken together at the same time. The drugs cause too much serotonin to be released causing restlessness, tachycardia, hypertension, hyperthermia, hallucinations, nausea and vomiting. MAOI antidepressants, dextromethorphan, meperidine, and some drugs of abuse, such as ecstasy and LSD ("acid"), have been associated with serotonin syndrome.

Schizophrenia

A psychotic disorder (or a group of disorders) marked by severely impaired thinking, emotions, and behaviors. a severe mental disorder characterized by some, but not necessarily all, of the following features: emotional blunting, intellectual *deterioration, social isolation, disorganized speech and behavior, delusions, and hallucinations.*

CHAPTER 14: MEDICATIONS FOR MENTAL HEALTH

As for any kind of medication, psychiatric medications, called *psychotropics,* do not produce the same effect in everyone. Some people may respond better to one medication than another and some may need larger dosages than others. Some people experience side effects where others do not. Age, sex, body size, body chemistry, physical illnesses and other medications are some of the factors that can influence a medication's effect. Psychotropics can increase the effectiveness of other kinds of treatment including counseling.

Psychotropic medications are generally divided into four large categories-- antipsychotics, mood-stabilizers, antidepressants, and antianxiety medications. This chapter provides an overview of each category and lists the commonly used medications.

General Precautions

- At present time, most patients are on 2 or more medications. It is important for the treating physician and psychiatrist to know all of the medications the patient is taking for optimal health care.

- Medications should never be stopped abruptly. Although the majority of these medications are not addictive, they can cause severe and serious withdrawal symptoms. Always make sure to talk with a physician before stopping any medication.

- California State regulations requires physicians to discuss with patients the medications used including their side effects, benefits and potential risks. Patients and their health care workers should become familiar with dosage, diet restrictions (if any), side effects and adverse reaction before starting these medications.

- Psychiatric medications can cause fetal defects – detected at birth. Lithium tops the list as the most dangerous. For patients taking any medication, it is important to discuss with a physician their effects during pregnancy

Schizophrenia

Many people associate schizophrenia with a disease of madness. Schizophrenia can inflict suffering for decades and 10% of the patients commit suicide. Long considered psychiatry's most challenging mysteries, it continues to perplex scientists. Most doctors view schizophrenia as a collection of disorders rather than one, yet they are not able to sort that out.

Psychotic behavior is characterized by a loss of connectedness with reality. A person may develop bizarre ideas or false beliefs about reality (*delusions*). These may be based on false perceptions of reality (*hallucinations*). These are termed a *thought disorder*. People with psychosis may hear "voices" in their heads or have strange and illogical ideas (i.e., believing that others can track their thoughts or that they are someone famous in then world).

The person may develop poor hygiene, not bathing or changing clothes, and unable to coherently communicate. They often are initially unaware that their condition is actually an illness. These behaviors are symptoms of a psychotic illness such as schizophrenia. Psychosis can also be caused by drugs (stimulants and hallucinogens), by medications (steroids) or could be part of depression. Antipsychotic medications can help these symptoms. Antipsychotic medications affect neurotransmitters) that allow communication between cells. Two such neurotransmitters, dopamine and serotonin, are thought to be associated with some of the symptoms of schizophrenia.

Schizophrenia can range in severity from the incoherent patient who remains institutionalized to a responsible productive individual who is stabilized on medication. Although much has been learned in the past 40 years, scientists still do not know what causes schizophrenia, and there is no cure. Schizophrenia strikes about 1% of the world population.

Individuals with schizophrenia are unable to think coherently anti often misinterpret the meaning of events. Consequently, they are often incapable of caring for themselves and living independently. Moreover, many live in continual fear and distress, threatened by hallucinations and plagued by paranoid delusions. The psychotic state consists of bizarre behavior, an inability to think coherently or comprehend the environment, and most importantly, an inability to recognize the presence of these abnormalities.

Many descriptions of a disorder thought to be schizophrenia have been found among civilizations predating the ancient Greeks. Physicians didn't begin to focus on schizophrenia as a distinct disorder, however, until around the 1900s when psychiatrist Emil Kraepelin coined the term *dementia praecox* to distinguish schizophrenic symptoms from depressive illness. A decade later, Swiss psychiatrist Eugen Bleuler coined the term schizophrenia. Although scientists were finally able to describe the disease, they still couldn't treat it. Dentists pulled some patients' teeth because psychiatrists thought the teeth produced a toxin that caused psychiatric symptoms. Other patients were injected with colloidal gold or deactivated horse serum, or even dropped down water wells in vain efforts to remove supposed toxins.

It wasn't until the 1930s that minor successes were first achieved. At that time, physicians began treating schizophrenic patients with electroconvulsive shock therapy. Although some improved, the changes often didn't last. The first big breakthrough in schizophrenia treatment came from an unlikely event: the French-Indochinese War in the early 1950s. Dr. Pierre Laborit, a French navy surgeon, accidentally found that *chlorpromazine,* a drug he gave wounded soldiers to control shock during surgery, also soothed them. He persuaded his colleagues to try the drug on schizophrenic patients and found it controlled thought disorders and agitation experienced by many of them. Chlorpromazine became the first antipsychotic drug used to treat schizophrenia. Laborit's discovery ushered in the use of drugs in treatment. His discovery also prompted physicians to more carefully examine the notion that schizophrenia has a biological basis, and the disease is not caused by poor toilet training, domineering mothers, or in the words of the late psychiatrist R.D. Laing, "a sane response to an insane world."

There is ample evidence that the brains of persons who have schizophrenia are, as a group, different from the brains of persons who don't have the disease. For instance, some studies using brain imaging techniques in schizophrenics show a loss of brain tissue, abnormalities in brain density, brain asymmetry, and atrophy of the cerebellum (the part of the brain involved in muscular and motor activity). Other studies have shown an excessive number of receptors for dopamine (a brain chemical involved in controlling body movements), hypoactive dopamine activity in the prefrontal cortex, abnormal electrical responses, abnormal EEGs (electroencephalograms), and abnormal eye movement in schizophrenic patients as compared to healthy controls. By all brain measures (gross pathology, neurochemistry, and microscopic pathology) it can be shown that schizophrenia ranks with multiple sclerosis, Parkinson's disease, and Alzheimer's disease as a major brain disease.

Causes of Schizophrenia

Schizophrenia seems to run in families; but how it is transmitted still remains unclear. There have been reports that obstetrical complications are associated with a higher risk of schizophrenia, and that more babies born in late winter and early spring eventually become schizophrenic. Researchers have also been intrigued by theories linking nutritional and immunological deficiencies to development of schizophrenia. It has been reported that schizophrenic patients do have immune system abnormalities, but researchers don't agree on what these include. A viral cause for the disease has also been suggested. Among babies born during the 1957 flu epidemic in Finland, a greater number developed schizophrenia than normally found in the general population. Schizophrenia is a devastating disease, but some individuals do get better. About 50% become at least moderately independent. A summary of 25 studies in which schizophrenic patients were followed for 10 years showed that 25% completely recovered (whether or not they were treated), 25% improved and were able to live a moderately independent life, 25% improved somewhat but required an extensive support network, 15% did not improve and remained hospitalized, and 10% died, usually by suicide.

The symptoms of schizophrenia are observed within a wide range of cognitive and emotional dysfunction classified as either positive or negative symptoms. *Positive symptoms* include hallucinations (primarily auditory), delusions, paranoid psychosis, bizarre behavior and thought disorders. *Negative symptoms* include flat affect (expressionless demeanor), loss of motivation, loss of interests and isolation. Alterations in brain biochemistry have been associated with some cases of positive symptoms and negative symptoms of schizophrenia. For example, theories on the biochemical basis for schizophrenia have produced some interesting causal explanations for the disorder by inferring specific alterations in certain neurotransmitter. These biochemical alterations are summarized as follows:

- Increased D2 receptor site abnormalities (positive symptoms)

- Decreased dopamine function (negative symptoms)

- Increased norepinephrine function (positive symptoms)

- Decreased serotonin function (positive symptoms)

- Decreaed glutamate (negative symptoms)

The most prominent theory of schizophrenia, one that has outlasted most others, is the dopamine hypothesis. This theory has a pharmacological foundation that tests true to research. That is, drugs that increase dopamine activity (dopamine agonists such as amphetamine, cocaine, L-dopa and methylphenidate) can produce a paranoid psychosis in normal persons. The same drugs when given to schizophrenics sometimes exacerbate the symptoms, increasing psychosis and thought disturbances. On the other hand, drugs that block certain dopamine receptors (antagonists such as neuroleptics and nalaxone) seem to ease some of the symptoms of schizophrenia. While no research can associate dopamine imbalance causes schizophrenia, there is compelling evidence for the link.

Antipsychotic Medications
Since the 1950's, antipsychotic medications have helped many patients with psychosis lead a more normal and fulfilling life by alleviating the symptoms of hallucinations (both visual and auditory) and bizarre thinking. Unfortunately, the earlier antipsychotics often produced side effects including muscle stiffness and tremor leading scientists to search for newer medicines with fewer side effects.

During the 1990s, there was the development of several new medications for schizophrenia, called atypical antipsychotics. Because they have fewer side effects than the older drugs, today they are often used as a first-line treatment. The first atypical antipsychotic, clozapine (Clozaril), was introduced in the United States in 1990 and was found to be more effective than the older medications especially for treatment-resistant schizophrenia and the risk of tardive dyskinesia was lower. However, because of the potential side effect of a serious blood disorder (agranulocytosis: the loss of the white blood cells needed for immune response), patients who are on clozapine must have a blood test every 1 or 2 weeks. Clozapine, however, continues to be the drug of choice for treatment-resistant schizophrenia patients.

Several other new antipsychotics have been developed since clozapine was introduced. The first was risperidone (Risperdal), followed by olanzapine (Zyprexa), quetiapine (Seroquel), ziprasidone (Geodon), aripiprazole (Abilify) and recently, paliperidone (Invega).

Invega is a newer atypical antipsychotic that has been approved for the treatment of schizophrenia. It is a slow-release capsule that has fewer side effects and is used once daily. It is unique in that it leaves the body through the kidneys, hence it is safe to use by patients with liver disease.

Most side effects of antipsychotic medications are mild and many will decrease or disappear after a few weeks of treatment. These include drowsiness, rapid heartbeat, and dizziness when changing position (orthostatic hypotension). Some people gain weight while taking medications. Some may develop diabetes (Type II) and can also have elevated cholesterol. Other side effects may include a decrease in sexual interest, problems with menstrual periods or skin rashes. Interestingly, some side effects can actually be useful (e.g. sedation in cases of agitation).

Long-term treatment of schizophrenia with one of the older antipsychotics may cause the side effect of tardive dyskinesia (TD). This is a condition characterized by involuntary movements, most often involving the tongue. The risk of this side effect has been reduced with the newer medications. However, there is a higher incidence of TD in women, and the risk can increase with age. Other side effects can include pseudo-Parkinson's, akasthesia and restless leg syndrome.

Antipsychotic Medications (BY GENERIC/TRADE NAME)
- aripiprazole/Abilify
- chlorpromazine/Thorazine
- chlorprothixene/Taractan
- clozapine/Clozaril
- fluphenazine/Permitil, Prolixin
- haloperidol/Haldol
- loxapine/Loxitane
- mesoridazine/Serentil
- molindone/Lidone, Moban
- olanzapine/Zyprexa
- paliperidone/Invega (new as of January 2007)

- perphenazine/Trilafon
- pimozide (for Tourette's syndrome) /Orap
- quetiapine/Seroquel
- risperidone/Risperdal
- thioridazine/Mellaril
- thiothixene/Navane
- trifluoperazine/Stelazine
- trifluopromazine/Vesprin
- ziprasidone/Geodon

Bipolar Disorder and Antimania Medications

Bipolar disorder, also known by its older name "manic depression," is a mental disorder that is characterized by constantly changing moods. A person with bipolar disorder experiences alternating "highs" (mania) and "lows" (depression). Both the manic and depressive periods can be brief, from just a few hours to a few days, or longer, lasting up to several weeks or even months. The periods of mania and depression range from person to person — many people may only experience very brief periods of these intense moods, and may not even be aware that they have bipolar disorder.

A manic episode is characterized by extreme happiness, hyperactivity, little need for sleep and racing thoughts, which may lead to rapid speech. A depressive episode is characterized by extreme sadness, a lack of energy or interest in things, an inability to enjoy normally pleasurable activities and feelings of helplessness and hopelessness. On average, someone with bipolar disorder may have up to three years of normal mood between episodes of mania or depression.

Bipolar disorder is recurrent, meaning that more than 90% of the individuals who have a single manic episode will go on to experience future episodes. Roughly 70% of manic episodes in bipolar disorder occur immediately before or after a depressive episode. Treatment seeks to reduce the feelings of mania and depression associated with the disorder, and restore balance to the person's mood.

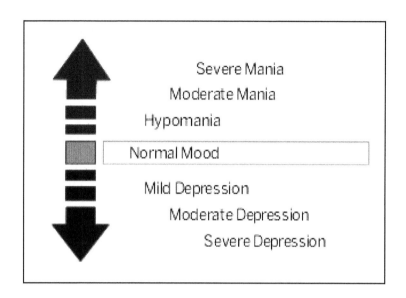

Those with bipolar disorder often describe their experience as being on an emotional roller coaster. Cycling up and down between strong emotions can keep a person from having anything approaching a "normal" life. The emotions, thoughts and behavior of a person with bipolar disorder are often experienced as beyond one's control. Friends, co-workers and family may sometimes intervene to try and help protect their interests and health. This makes the condition exhausting not only for the sufferer, but for those in contact with her or him as well.

Bipolar cycling can either be rapid, or more slowly over time. Those who experience rapid cycling can go between depression and mania as often as a few times a week (some even cycle within the same day). Most people with bipolar disorder are of the slow cycling type — they experience long periods of being up ("high" or manic phase) and of being down ("low" or depressive phase). Researchers do not yet understand why some people cycle more quickly than others.

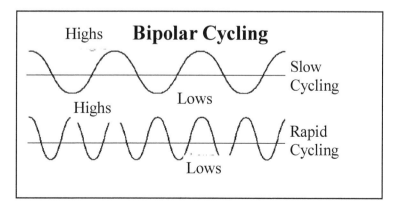

Living with bipolar disorder can be challenging in maintaining a regular lifestyle. Manic episodes can lead to family conflict or financial problems, especially when the person with bipolar disorder appears to behave erratically and irresponsibly without reason. During the manic phase, people often become impulsive and act aggressively. This can result in high-risk behavior, such as repeated intoxication, extravagant spending and risky sexual behavior.

During severe manic or depressed episodes, some people with bipolar disorder may have symptoms that overwhelm their ability to deal with everyday life, and even reality. This inability to distinguish reality from unreality results in psychotic symptoms such as hearing voices, paranoia, visual hallucinations, and false beliefs of special powers or identity. They may have distressing periods of great sadness alternating with euphoric optimism (a "natural high") and/or rage that is not typical of the person during periods of wellness. These abrupt shifts of mood interfere with reason, logic and perception to such a drastic degree that those affected may be unaware of the need for help. However, if left untreated, bipolar disorder can seriously affect nearly every aspect of a person's life.

Identifying the first episode of mania or depression and receiving early treatment is essential to managing bipolar disorder. In most cases, a depressive episode occurs before a manic episode, and many patients are treated initially as if they have major depression. Usually, the first recognized episode of bipolar disorder is a manic episode. Once a manic episode occurs, it becomes clearer that the person is suffering from an illness characterized by alternating moods. Because of this difficulty with diagnosis, family history of similar illness or episodes is particularly important. People who first seek treatment as a result of a depressed episode may continue to be treated as someone with unipolar depression until a manic episode develops. Ironically, treatment of depressed bipolar patients with antidepressants can trigger a manic episode in some patients.

The cause of bipolar disorder is not entirely known. Genetic, neurochemical and environmental factors probably interact at many levels to play a role in the onset and progression of bipolar disorder. The current thinking is that this is a predominantly biological disorder that occurs in a specific part of the brain and is due to a malfunction of the neurotransmitters. As a biological disorder, it may lie dormant and be activated spontaneously or it may be triggered by stressors in life. Although, no one is quite sure about the exact causes of bipolar disorder, researchers have found these important clues:

Genetic factors in Bipolar Disorder
- Bipolar disorder tends to be familial, meaning that it "runs in families." About half the people with bipolar disorder have a family member with a mood disorder, such as depression.
- A person who has one parent with bipolar disorder has a 15 to 25 percent chance of having the condition.

- A person who has a non-identical twin with the illness has a 25 percent chance of illness, the same risk as if both parents have bipolar disorder.
- A person who has an identical twin (having exactly the same genetic material) with bipolar disorder has an even greater risk of developing the illness about an eightfold greater risk than a nonidentical twin.

Studies of adopted twins (where a child whose biological parent had the illness is raised in an adoptive family untouched by the illness) has helped researchers learn more about the genetic causes vs. environmental and life events causes.

Neurochemical Factors in Bipolar Disorder

Bipolar disorder is primarily a biological disorder that occurs in a specific area of the brain and is due to the dysfunction of certain neurotransmitters, or chemical messengers, in the brain. These chemicals may involve neurotransmitters like norepinephrine, serotonin and probably many others. As a biological disorder, it may lie dormant and be activated on its own or it may be triggered by external factors such as psychological stress and social circumstances.

Environmental Factors in Bipolar Disorder

- A life event may trigger a mood episode in a person with a genetic disposition for bipolar disorder.
- Even without clear genetic factors, altered health habits, alcohol or drug abuse, or hormonal problems can trigger an episode.
- Among those at risk for the illness, bipolar disorder is appearing at increasingly early ages. This apparent increase in earlier occurrences may be due to underdiagnosis of the disorder in the past. This change in the age of onset may be a result of social and environmental factors that are not yet understood.
- Although substance abuse is not considered a cause of bipolar disorder, it can worsen the illness by interfering with recovery. Use of alcohol or tranquilizers may induce a more severe depressive phase.

Medication-triggered Mania

Medications such as antidepressants can trigger a manic episode in people who are susceptible to bipolar disorder. Therefore, a depressive episode must be treated carefully in those people who have had manic episodes. Because a depressive episode can turn into a manic episode when an antidepressant medication is taken, an antimanic drug is also recommended to prevent a manic episode. The antimanic drug creates a "ceiling," partially protecting the person from antidepressant-induced mania.

Certain other medications can produce a "high" that resembles mania. Appetite suppressants, for example, may trigger increased energy, decreased need for sleep and increased talkativeness. After stopping the medication, however, the person returns to his normal mood.

Substances that can cause a manic-like episode include:

- Illicit drugs such as cocaine, "designer drugs" such as Ecstasy and amphetamines.
- Excessive doses of certain over-the-counter drugs, including appetite suppressants and cold preparations.
- Nonpsychiatric medications, such as medicine for thyroid problems and corticosteroids like prednisone.
- Excessive caffeine (not moderate amounts of coffee).

If a person is vulnerable to bipolar disorder, stress, frequent use of stimulants or alcohol, and lack of sleep may prompt onset of the disorder. Certain medications also may set off a depressive or manic episode. If you have a family history of bipolar disorder, notify your physician so as to help avoid the risk of a medication-induced manic episode.

Antimania Medications

Lithium
Lithium can even out mood swings from mania to depression, and depression to mania. Lithium is not only used for manic attacks, but also as an ongoing maintenance treatment for bipolar disorder.

Regular blood tests are an important part of treatment with lithium. If too little is taken, lithium will not be effective. If too much is taken, a variety of side effects may occur. Once a person is stable, the lithium level needs to be checked every few months.

Side effects such as drowsiness, weakness, nausea, fatigue, tremor, or increased thirst, a metallic taste and increased urination can be experienced in some people taking lithium. Symptoms may disappear or decrease quickly, although hand tremor may persist. Weight gain can also occur. Because lithium may cause the thyroid gland to become under active (hypothyroidism) or sometimes enlarged (goiter), regular monitoring of thyroid function is part of the treatment.

Lithium, when combined with certain other medications, can have undesired effects. Some diuretics (substances that remove water from the body) increase the level of lithium and can cause a toxic reaction. Other diuretics, like coffee and tea, can lower the level of lithium. Signs of lithium toxicity include nausea, vomiting, diarrhea, drowsiness, mental confusion, slurred speech, blurred vision, dizziness, irregular heartbeat, and even seizures. A lithium overdose can be life threatening. However, with regular check-ups, lithium is a very safe and effective drug.

Mood Stabilizers (BY GENERIC/TRADE NAME)
- lithium carbonate/Eskalith, Lithane, Lithobid

- lithium citrate/Cibalith-S
- carbamazepine/Tegretol
- divalproex sodium (valproic acid) / Depakote
- lamotrigine/Lamictal
- topimarate/Topamax

Acute Anti-mania Medications (BY GENERIC/TRADE NAME)
- All second-generation (atypical) antipsychotics

Anticonvulsants

For some unresponsive cases, a combination of Lithium and anticonvulsants are used. In general, it is common for bilpolar patients to be on 2 or more medications. The anticonvulsant valproic acid (Depakote, divalproex sodium) is the main alternative therapy for bipolar disorder. It is as effective in non-rapid-cycling bipolar disorder as lithium but seems to be better than lithium in rapid-cycling bipolar disorder. Adverse effects can include weight gain, sedation, hair loss, headache, dizziness, anxiety, or confusion. Because in some cases valproic acid has caused liver dysfunction, liver function tests need to be performed before treatment and at intervals thereafter, particularly during the first 6 months. Other anticonvulsants used for bipolar disorder include carbamazepine (Tegretol), lamotrigine (Lamictal) and topiramate (Topamax). The atypical antipsychotics can be used as antimania drugs.

Major Depression

To describe a major depressive episode a person must either have a depressed mood or a loss of interest or pleasure in daily activities consistently for at least a 2-week period. This mood must represent a change from the person's normal mood. Social, occupational, educational or other important functioning must also be negatively impaired by the change in mood. Depressive disorders are twice as common in women as in men, although both sexes suffer its effects.

Long-term use of stimulants, such as methamphetamine and cocaine has been identified as causing or aggravating depression. Alcohol dependence frequently causes depressive symptoms as well. However psychosocial effects such as stigma, poverty and isolation associated with drug use may also be highly relevant. Depression can also co-occur with other medical disorders such as cancer, heart disease, stroke, Parkinson's disease, Alzheimer's and diabetes. In such cases, the depression is often overlooked and is not treated. Antidepressants are not stimulants, but rather reduce the symptoms of depression and help people feel the way they did before they became depressed.

Depression may be characterized by the presence of a majority of the following symptoms:

- Depressed mood most of the day, nearly every day, as indicated by either subjective report (e.g. the person feels sad or empty or appears tearful).

- Markedly diminished interest or pleasure in all, or almost all, activities most of the day, nearly every day.

- Significant weight loss when not dieting or weight gain (a change of more than 5% of body weight in a month), or decrease or increase in appetite nearly every day.

- Insomnia or hypersomnia nearly every day.

- Psychomotor agitation or retardation nearly every day.

- Fatigue or loss of energy nearly every day.

- Feelings of worthlessness or excessive or inappropriate guilt nearly every day.

- Diminished ability to think or concentrate, or indecisiveness, nearly every day.

- Recurrent thoughts of death (not just fear of dying), recurrent suicidal ideation without a specific plan, or a suicide attempt or a specific plan for committing suicide.

There are three major theories concerning depression; the catecholamine hypothesis of mood disorders, the permissive hypothesis (serotonin hypothesis) of depression and the newest theory, the stress-diathesis model of mood disorders. Each one is research-based and provides a valid and pharmacologically sound foundation in determining the basis for mood disorders. Depressive illness is more than likely a combination of these theories and not just a single explanation. However, since these explanations prove to be pharmacologically sound, (i.e. medications have shown a cause and effect relationship based on the theories), a review of each theory follows.

The most prominent biochemical theories about depression focus on the alteration of monoamine neurotransmitters (dopamine, norepinephrine, and serotonin), but particularly norepinephrine and serotonin. Medications that are clinically effective antidepressants have shown that concentration of monoamines are decreased in depressive disorders –including tricyclic antidepressants *(TCAs),* selective serotonin reuptake inhibitors *(SSRIs)* and monoamine oxidase inhibitors *(MAOIs).*

The mechanisms of action for the antidepressant medications involve prolonging the activity of monoamines in synapse (and thus functioning as agonist_drugs). Studies to date have proposed that there is a decrease in the activity of the NE -5-HT component in depression and an increase in the NE-DA component in mania.

The catecholamine hypothesis states that depression stems from a deficiency of norepinephrine (NE) in certain brain areas, and that mania arises from an overabundance of NE. The link between NE depletion and depression has gained tremendous experimental support. Studies have in fact directly linked low levels of NE to depression. In addition, postmortem studies show increased densities of certain NE receptors in the cortex of suicide victims. It has been well established that when monoamine agonist drugs are given to depressed patients, the symptoms of depression subside. Conversely, when non-depressed individuals are given monoamine antagonist drugs, significant depression will ultimately set in.

Corroborating these drug-induced behavioral states are HVA (dopamine metabolites) and MHPG (norepinephrine metabolites). That is, these metabolites increase during monoamine agonist actions and decrease during monoamine antagonist actions. A recent discovery supporting the catecholamine hypothesis is that new drugs selectively able to block NE reuptake, (increasing NE levels in synapse) are effective antidepressants for many people.

The research concerning NE and depression is valid and reliable. However, during the 1990s, research in the function of serotonin (5-HT) began to take the forefront over dopamine and norepinephrine research that had previously held much of the research interest.

The permissive hypothesis shows that depleted 5-HT levels in the brain causes depression. According to this theory, 5-HT depletion in synapse is caused by "permitting" (promoting) a drop in NE levels; 5-HT circuit defects could certainly hinder NE signaling. 5-HT-producing nuerons project from the raphe nuclei to neurons in diverse areas of the CNS, including those that secrete or control NE. 5-HT depletion might also contribute to depression by affecting other neurons as well, since 5-HT neurons extend into brain regions affected by depression, including the amygdala, hypothalamus and cortical areas.

Supporting this theory are findings of low levels of 5-HT metabolites and by-products within the cerebrospinal fluid in depressed people, and especially suicidal patients. Also supporting this theory is the discovery of upregulated 5-HT Type2 receptors and NE receptors in brain tissues of depressed patients. As you recall from the chapter on neurotransmitters, upregulation suggests a neuroadaptive response to low levels of neurotransmitters in synapse. Further evidence for this theory comes from the efficacy of drugs that block presynaptic reuptake, transported from removing 5-HT out of the synapse (i.e. SSRIs like Prozac, Paxil and Zoloft).

The other theory that explains depression is the *Stress-Diathesis Model of Mood Disorders.* This theory emphasizes the role of hormone abnormalities in depression, rather than the neurotransmitters 5-HT or NE. The model recognizes the interaction of stress and innate predisposition (diathesis) causing depression. Basically, this theory links depression to a dysregulation of the hypothalamic-pituitaryadrenal axis (HPA), the system that manages the body's response to stress. The hypothalamus, as you recall, releases peptides (small chains of amino acids) that act on the pituitary, directing its release of various hormones into the blood, and controlling the release of other hormones from target glands. In addition to hormonal function, they also feed back to the pituitary and hypothalamus, where they alter their signaling to maintain balance.

The Stress-Diathesis Model of Mood Disorders has uncovered profound evidence to show that the HPA axis does not respond well in depressed individuals. When the body detects a threat to its homeostasis, the hypothalamus increases release of *corticotropin-releasing factor* (CRF) which then triggers the pituitary to release *ACTH* (adrenocorticotropic hormone). ACTH then chemically signals the adrenal gland to release cortisol. This cascade of events not only prepares the body for the fight-or-flight response, but also suppresses other biological processes that might distract from dealing with the stress. Cortisol is stimulated and delivers glucose and energy to the muscles. CRF depresses the appetite for food and sex, and elevates alertness. Together, this biochemical signaling prepares the individual for confronting stressful situations (real or imagined).

Chronic activation of the HPA axis seems to produce an array of illnesses, in particular depression. In fact, the link between HPA axis hyperactivity and depression is one of the most replicated findings in behavioral neuroscience. Several studies have shown CRF concentrations in cerebrospinal fluid to be elevated in depressed patients compared with control groups or individuals with other psychiatric disorders. Further, postmortem brain tissue studies of depressed patients have shown exaggerated CRF-producing neurons in the hypothalamus and in the expression of the CRF gene (resulting in an increase in CRF synthesis). The elevation of CRF is reduced with anti-depressants, and sometimes even with electro-convulsive therapy. Discoveries of these hormonal abnormalities and depression also suggest a partial scenario for people who have endured a traumatic childhood and became depressed later in life.

Antidepressant Medications
The choice of an antidepressant is based on the individual's symptoms. Some people notice improvement in the first couple of weeks; but usually the medication must be taken regularly for at least 6 - 8 weeks before the full antidepressant effect occurs.

To give a medication enough time to be effective and to prevent a relapse of the depression once the patient is responding to an antidepressant, the medication is continued for 6 to 12 months. When a medication can be discontinued, a withdrawal schedule should be developed to taper off the medication slowly (generally up to 3 – 4 months). People who have had two or more depressive episodes in the past may need to take antidepressants for life.

From the 1960s through the 1980s, tricyclic antidepressants (named for their chemical structure) were the treatment of choice for major depression. Most of these medications affected two chemical neurotransmitters, norepinephrine and serotonin.

Though the tricyclics (TCs) are as effective in treating depression as the newer antidepressants, their side effects are usually more profound. Overdoses on TCs can be fatal due to toxic effects on the heart. Other antidepressants introduced during this period were monoamine oxidase inhibitors (MAOIs). MAOIs are effective for some people with major depression who do not respond to other medications. They are also effective for the treatment of panic disorder and bipolar depression. The MAOIs approved for the treatment of depression are phenelzine (Nardil), tranylcypromine (Parnate), and isocarboxazid (Marplan). Because substances in certain foods and beverages can cause toxic interactions when combined, people taking MAOIs must adhere to a very strict diet.

Since the 1990s, there have been newer antidepressants with fewer side effects than the older ones. Some of these medications target the neurotransmitter, serotonin, and are called selective serotonin reuptake inhibitors (SSRIs). These include fluoxetine (Prozac), sertraline (Zoloft), fluvoxamine (Luvox), paroxetine (Paxil), and escitalopram (Lexapro). During the later 1990s, even newer medications were introduced that, like the tricyclics, targeted both norepinephrine and serotonin but have fewer side effects. These newer medications include venlafaxine (Effexor) and nefazadone (Serzone). Other new antidepressants chemically unrelated to the other medications are the sedating mirtazepine (Remeron) and the more activating bupropion (Wellbutrin). Wellbutrin has not been associated with weight gain or sexual dysfunction but is not used for people with, or who are at risk for, a seizure disorder. Cymbalta (duloxetine) was introduced in 2004.

Side Effects of Antidepressant Medications
Antidepressants may cause mild, and often temporary, side effects. Typically, these are not very serious. The most common side effects of tricyclic antidepressants include symptoms of:
  • Dry mouth

- Constipation
- Bladder problems--emptying the bladder completely may be difficult, and the urine stream may not be as strong as usual.
- Sexual problems--sexual functioning may be impaired
- Blurred vision
- Dizziness
- Increased heart rate--pulse rate is often elevated.
- Drowsiness - persisting during daytime hours

The newer antidepressants, including the SSRIs, have different types of side effects including symptoms of:
- Sexual problems--fairly common, but reversible, in both men and women.
- Headache--this will usually go away after a short time.
- Nausea--may occur after a dose, but it will disappear quickly.
- Nervousness and insomnia (trouble falling asleep or waking often during the night)--these may occur during the first few weeks; dosage reductions or time will usually resolve them.
- Agitation (feeling jittery)
- Sleep changes

Antidepressants (BY GENERIC/TRADE NAME)
- amitriptyline/Elavil
- amoxapine/Asendin
- bupropion/Wellbutrin
- citalopram (SSRI) / Celexa
- clomipramine/Anafranil
- desipramine/Norpramin, Pertofrane
- doxepin/Adapin, Sinequan
- escitalopram (SSRI) / Lexapro
- fluvoxamine (SSRI) / Luvox
- duloxetine/Cymbalta
- fluoxetine (SSRI) / Prozac
- imipramine/Tofranil
- isocarboxazid (MAOI) / Marplan
- maprotiline/Ludiomil
- mirtazapine/Remeron
- nefazodone/Serzone
- nortriptyline/Aventyl, Pamelor
- paroxetine (SSRI) / Paxil
- phenelzine (MAOI) / Nardil
- protriptyline/Vivactil
- selegeline (MAOI) / Emsam
- sertraline (SSRI) / Zoloft

- tranylcypromine (MAOI) / Parnate
- trazodone/Desyrel
- trimipramine/Surmontil
- venlafaxine/Effexor

Any of these side effects can be amplified when an SSRI is combined with other medications that affect the same neurotransmitter serotonin. In the most extreme cases, such a combination of medications (e.g., an SSRI and an MAOI) may result in a potentially serious, sometimes even fatal, condition called the serotonin syndrome, characterized by fever, confusion, muscle rigidity, and cardiac, liver, or kidney problems.

Medications of any kind, whether prescribed, over-the-counter, or even some of the herbal supplements should not be mixed together because of possible serious toxic reactions. Some drugs, although safe when taken alone, can cause severe side effects if taken with other drugs. Alcohol (wine, beer, and hard liquor) or street drugs may reduce the effectiveness of antidepressants and their use need to be avoided by anyone taking antidepressants. Trazedone and Doxepin are commonly used as sleep aides, whether alone or in combination with other medications.

Emsam (selegeline) is an MAOI that has a very low side effect profile due to its transdermal route of administration. A daily skin patch of 6 mg does not require the dietary restriction that is required of the other MAOI antidepressant medications.

Anxiety Disorders
Unlike fear, which is a response to a realistic immediate danger, anxiety is a fearful response occurring in the absence of a specific danger, or it can be anticipatory anxiety. According to the National Institute of Health, anxiety disorders are the most common form of mental disorder in the population with a one-year prevalence of 9.7%. Patients experiencing anxiety may present with complaints of excessive fear or worry, or repetitive, intrusive thoughts including worrying about the future, health or relationships. These people find it hard to relax, concentrate and sleep with physical symptoms such as heart palpitations, tension and muscle pain, sweating, hyperventilation, dizziness, faintness, headaches, nausea, indigestion and loss of sexual interest. In these disorders the symptoms associated with anxiety are accompanied by changes in thoughts, emotions and behavior that substantially interfere with the person's usual ability to live and work.

Anxiety usually begins in early adulthood and can be triggered by a series of life events. Anxiety disorders can be complicated by self-medication with alcohol and other substances. Similarly substance abuse may be complicated by the development of anxiety symptoms. Anxiety is common in withdrawal from alcohol, benzodiazepines, and opioids and is also common during intoxication with stimulants, marijuana and hallucinogens and, at times, can be very difficult to distinguish primary symptoms of anxiety from those caused by substabnce abuse.

The failure to recognize and treat anxiety can lead to worsening of substance use and associated problems vice versa.

Anxiety Subtypes

There are a number of anxiety subtypes including:

- **Panic disorder**, where a person suffers recurrent panic attacks that cause significant distress or disability. Panic attacks involve an abrupt onset of intense fear.

- **Obsessive-Compulsive disorder**, where a person experiences constant unwanted thoughts and conducts elaborate rituals in an attempt to control or banish these.

- **Social Phobia**, where a person experiences fear that others will judge everything they do in a negative way, particularly when in the presence of unfamiliar people or under specific scrutiny.

- **Posttraumatic Stress Disorder**, where a person experiences flashbacks, intrusive thoughts or nightmares for years following major traumas like assault, war, torture, rape, vehicle accidents, and fires. Posttraumatic stress disorder is usually presented with anxiety and hyper arousal.

Antianxiety Medications

Antianxiety medications include the benzodiazepines, which can relieve symptoms within a relatively short time. They have few side effects but can include drowsiness and loss of coordination; fatigue and mental slowing or confusion. These effects make it dangerous for people taking benzodiazepines to drive or operate machinery. Also, falling is common and potentially dangerous for the elderly. Both antidepressants and antianxiety medications are used to treat anxiety disorders. The activity of most antidepressants provides effectiveness in anxiety disorders as well as depression. The first medication specifically approved for use in the treatment of OCD was the tricyclic antidepressant clomipramine (Anafranil).

The SSRIs, fluoxetine (Prozac), fluvoxamine (Luvox), paroxetine (Paxil), and sertraline (Zoloft) have now been approved for use with OCD. Paroxetine has also been approved for social anxiety disorder (social phobia), GAD, and panic disorder; and sertraline is approved for panic disorder and PTSD. Venlafaxine (Effexor) has been approved for GAD.

Abstinence from alcohol and opioids is advised when taking benzodiazepines because the interaction between benzodiazepines and these other drugs can lead to serious and possibly life-threatening complications, including respiratory failure (breathing stops). People taking benzodiazepines for weeks or months may develop tolerance for and dependence on these drugs. Abuse and withdrawal reactions are also possible.

A withdrawal reaction may occur if benzodiazepine treatment is stopped abruptly. Symptoms may include anxiety, shakiness, headache, dizziness, sleeplessness, loss of appetite, or in extreme cases, seizures. A withdrawal reaction may be mistaken for a return of the anxiety because many of the symptoms are similar. After a person has taken benzodiazepines for an extended period of time, the dosage is gradually reduced before it is stopped completely.

Commonly used benzodiazepines include clonazepam (Klonopin), alprazolam (Xanax), diazepam (Valium), lorazepam (Ativan) and chlordiazepoxide (Libirum). The only medication specifically for anxiety disorders other than the benzodiazepines is buspirone (BuSpar). Unlike the benzodiazepines, buspirone must be taken consistently for at least 2 weeks to achieve an antianxiety effect and therefore cannot be used on an "as-needed" basis.

Beta-blockers, medications often used to treat heart conditions and high blood pressure, are sometimes also used to control *performance anxiety* when the individual must face a specific stressful situation. Propranolol (Inderal, Inderide) and Clonidine is a commonly used beta-blocker.

Antianxiety Medications (BY GENERIC/TRADE NAME)

(All of these antianxiety medications, except buspirone, are benzodiazepines)
- alprazolam/Xanax
- buspirone/BuSpar
- chlordiazepoxide/Librax, Libritabs, Librium
- clonazepam/Klonopin
- clorazepate/Tranxene
- diazepam/Valium
- halazepam/Paxipam
- lorazepam/Ativan
- oxazepam/Serax
- prazepam/Centrax

A Note about ADHD and Its Treatment

Although ADHD is present at time of birth, it is commonly diagnosed at age 5 years and later. This condition is characterized by inattention (also poor focusing and concentration), hyperactivity (more common in males), impulsivity, and poor academic performance (in spite of high intelligence potential). About one half of patients with ADHD have learning disabilities. In recent years, there has been more emphasis placed on adult type of ADHD (present since birth).

Medication used to treat ADHD include:
Stimulants:
- methylphenidate/Ritalin

- dextroamphetamine/Dexedrine
- dextraoamphetamine/levoamphetamine/Adderall
- methylphenidate HCl/Concerta

In cases of drug addicted persons with ADHD, stimulants are not used, partly due to their high potential for abuse.

In 2003, a medication called *Strattera* (a norpepinerphine reuptake inhibitor), was the first non-stimulant drug approved for use in children and adults with ADHD. Common side effects are weight loss, retarded growth (in children), decreased sleep, agitation and headache. A second-line of treatment for ADHD is the use of Wellbutrin (for persons with chemical dependency disorders and patients who do not respond to stimulant medications). Wellbutrin is an antidepressant (see antidepressant section).

NOTE: The Food and Drug Administration (FDA) is increasingly publicizing the dangers of stimulants due to sudden death and psychiatric complications. It is advisable for patients on these medications to get an EKG to help rule out congenital heart disease that is unknown to these patients.

CHAPTER 14: SELF-STUDY QUESTIONS

TRUE/FALSE

1. *Psychotropic medications tend to produce the same effect in most people.*

2. *Although much has been learned in the past 40 years, scientists still do not know what causes schizophrenia, and there is no cure.*

3. *The symptoms of schizophrenia are observed within a wide range of cognitive and emotional dysfunction classified as either upregulated or downregulated symptoms.*

4. *Most side effects of antipsychotic medications are mild and many will decrease or disappear after a few weeks of treatment.*

5. *Bipolar disorder, also known by its older name "manic depression," is a mental disorder that is characterized by constantly changing moods.*

6. *All second-generation (atypical) antipsychotics can be used as acute anti-mania medications.*

7. *The most prominent biochemical theory about depression focuses on the alteration of the neurotransmitter acetylcholine.*

8. *Since the 1990s, there have been newer antidepressants with fewer side effects than the older ones. Some of these medications target the neurotransmitter, serotonin, and are called selective serotonin reuptake inhibitors (SSRIs).*

9. *Antianxiety medications include the benzodiazepines, which can relieve symptoms within a relatively short time.*

10. *Both antidepressants, antianxiety and stimulant medications are used to treat anxiety disorders.*

* Answers to Self Study Tests are located on page 351

Chapter 14 Selected Reading

American Psychiatric Association (1996) Diagnostic and Statistical Manual of Mental Disorders (4th Edition)

Blader, J.C.,G. A. Carlson, *Biological Psychiatry*, 15 July 2007.

Bressert, S. PsychCentral website - http://psychcentral.com/. Accessed June 2008.

Dennison, SJ. Substance Abuse Disorders in Individuals with Co-Occurring Psychiatric Disorders.Lowinson, JH, Ruiz, P, Millman, RB, and Langrod, JG (editors). In: *Substance Abuse A Comprehensive Sourcebook*. 4th Edition. Lippincott Williams & Wilkins. 2005.

Department of Health and Human Services. 1999. Mental Health: A Report of the Surgeon General. Rockville, MD: Department of Health and Human Services, Substance Abuse and Mental Health Services Administration, National Institute of Mental Health.

Hyman SE, Rudorfer MV. Depressive and bipolar mood disorders. In: Dale DC, Federman DD, eds. *Scientific American. Medicine. Vol. 3.* New York: Healtheon/WebMD Corp., 2000; Sect. 13, Subsect. II, p. 1.

Huxley NA, Parikh SV, Baldessarini RJ. Effectiveness of psychosocial treatments in bipolar disorder: state of the evidence. *Harvard Review of Psychiatry,* 2000; 8(3): 126-40.

Moreno, C, *et al.*, *Archives of General Psychiatry*, September 2007.

Mueser KT, Goodman LB, Trumbetta SL, Rosenberg SD, Osher FC, Vidaver R, Auciello P, Foy DW. Trauma and posttraumatic stress disorder in severe mental illness. *Journal of Consulting and Clinical Psychology,* 1998; 66(3): 493-9.

National Institute of Drug Abuse website at www.drugabuse.gov.

National Institute of Health (NIH)

National Institute of Mental Health website at www.nimh.nih.gov

Physicians' Desk Reference Drug Guide for Mental Health Professionals, 1st Edition. Montavale, NJ: Medical Economics Data Production Co. 2002.

Sachs GS, Printz DJ, Kahn DA, Carpenter D, Docherty JP. The expert consensus guideline series: medication treatment of bipolar disorder 2000. *Postgraduate Medicine,* 2000; Spec No:1-104.

Soares JC, Mann JJ. The functional neuroanatomy of mood disorders. *Journal of Psychiatric Research,* 1997; 31(4): 393-432.

Strakowski SM, DelBello MP. The co-occurrence of bipolar and substance use disorders. *Clinical Psychology Review,* 2000; 20(2): 191-206.

Thase ME, Sachs GS. Bipolar depression: pharmacotherapy and related therapeutic strategies. *Biological Psychiatry,* 2000; 48(6): 558-72.

CHAPTER 15: VOCABULARY LIST

CAGE
A brief alcohol assessment tool. *C*ut down on drinking unsuccessfully, *A*nnoyed by people concerned azbouty the person;s drinking, *G*uilt about the growing problems caused by drinking, and the need for an *E*ye opener drink after sleeping to calm the nerves.

CAGE-AID
CAGE questions *A*dapted to *I*nclude *D*rugs

Comorbidity
The presence of one or more disorders in addition to a primary disease or disorder.

Dual Diagnosis
The term used to describe the comorbid condition of a person considered to be suffering from a mental illness and a substance abuse problem.

Sequential treatment
A treatment method that has serial or nonsimultaneous treatment participation in both mental health and addiction treatment settings.

Parallel treatment
A treatment approach that has simultaneous treatment involvement in both mental health and addiction treatment settings

Integrated treatment
A treatment approach that combines elements of both mental health and addiction treatment into a unified and comprehensive treatment program for patients with dual disorders.

CHAPTER 15: A REVIEW OF CO-OCCURRING DISORDERS

A person who has both substance abuse and psychiatric problems is said to have a dual diagnosis, sometimes also called, co-occurring disorders, or dual disorders.Mental disorders and substance use occur together very frequently and interact negatively on one another. To recover fully, the person needs treatment for both problems and their management requires a long-term perspective.

Prevalence

An estimated 17.6 million American adults (8.5 percent) meet standard diagnostic criteria for an alcohol use disorder and approximately 4.2 million (2 percent) meet criteria for a drug use disorder. Overall, about one-tenth (9.4 percent) of American adults, or 19.4 million persons, meet clinical criteria for a substance use disorder — either an alcohol or drug use disorder or both — according to results from the 2001-2002 National *Epidemiologic Survey on Alcohol and Related Conditions (NESARC) reported in the current Archives of General Psychiatry*, Volume 61, August 2004.

Conducted by the National Institute on Alcohol Abuse and Alcoholism, National Institutes of Health, the NESARC is a representative survey of the U.S. civilian noninstitutionalized population aged 18 years and older. With more than 43,000 adult Americans participating, the NESARC is the largest study ever conducted of the co-occurrence of psychiatric disorders among U.S. adults.

Results from the NESARC show that 19.2 million adults (9.2 percent) meet diagnostic criteria for independent mood disorders (including major depression, dysthymia, manic disorder, and hypomania) and 23 million (11.08 percent) meet criteria for independent anxiety disorders (including panic disorder, generalized anxiety disorder, and specific and social phobias).

The NESARC is the first national epidemiologic survey to use the Diagnostic and Statistical Manual of Mental Disorders-Fourth Edition (DSM-IV) definitions of independent mood and anxiety disorders to examine the comorbidity, or co-occurrence, of mental health disorders. Independent mood and anxiety disorders exclude transient cases of these disorders that result from alcohol and/or drug withdrawal or intoxication, conditions that usually improve rapidly without treatment once substance use ceases. The distinction is important because the diagnosis of current mood and anxiety disorders among active substance abusers is complicated by the fact that many symptoms of intoxication and withdrawal from alcohol and other substances resemble the symptoms of mood and anxiety disorders and thus, the additional psychiatric disorder may be overlooked.

The NESARC results show substantial comorbidity between substance use disorders and independent mood and anxiety disorders is pervasive in the U.S. general population: About 20 percent of persons with a current (at the time of the survey or within the past year) substance use disorder experience a mood or anxiety disorder within the same time period. Similarly, about 20 percent of persons with a current mood or anxiety disorder experience a current substance use disorder.

NESARC results also indicate high rates of comorbidity among persons who sought treatment for mood, anxiety, or substance use disorders. The high rates of comorbidity among treated persons suggest that primary care physicians, mental health specialists, and alcohol and drug abuse specialists should assess patients for multiple mental health disorders, the authors conclude.

The other major report on co-occurring disorders is published in the *Journal of the American Medical Association (JAMA)*. This research states that:

- Of all people diagnosed as mentally ill, 29% currently abuse either alcohol or drugs and 60% will abuse either alcohol or other drugs some time during their lifetime.
- Roughly 50 percent of individuals with severe mental disorders are affected by substance abuse.
- Adults with a substance use disorder in 2002 were almost three times as likely to have serious mental illness (20.4 percent) as those who did not have a substance use disorder (7.0 percent), according to a 2003 report from the Substance Abuse and Mental Health Services Administration (SAMHSA).
- 37% of alcohol abusers and 53% of drug abusers also have at least one serious mental illness.

Additionally, The National Institute of Mental Health has sponsored two of the research studies on the groups most commonly affected by substance abuse.

- 10 million Americans are affected by a dual-diagnosis disorder each year
- 56% of individuals with a bipolar disorder (Manic depressive illness) abuse substances
- 47% of individuals with a schizophrenic disorder abuse substances
- 32% of individuals with a mood disorder other than bipolar abuse substances
- 27% of individuals with an anxiety disorder abuse substances

These large percentages look very different from an overall 15% of substance abuse disorders in the general population.

A central question about dual diagnosis is which came fist – the substance abuse or the psychiatric disorder? Research has shown that it can go either way. Often the psychiatric problem develops first. In an attempt to feel calmer, more energized and alert, or more joyful, a person with emotional problems may use drugs or drink to self medicate. Frequent self-medication may eventually lead to a dependency on alcohol or drugs. If it does, the person then suffers from not just one problem, but two. In adolescents, however, drug or alcohol abuse may merge and continue into adulthood, which may contribute to the development of emotional difficulties or psychiatric disorders.

In other cases, alcohol or drug dependency is the primary condition. A person whose substance abuse problem has become severe may develop symptoms of a psychiatric disorder including episodes of depression, anger, hallucinations, or suicide attempts. In terms of treatment for dual diagnosis, people have asked which diagnosis should be treated first. It is often difficult to separate what symptoms belong to which diagnosis. Since many symptoms of substance abuse mimic or mask other psychiatric conditions, the person must go through withdrawal from alcohol and/or other drugs before the clinician can accurately assess whether there is a psychiatric problem also.

That being said, research has concluded that both problems should be treated simultaneously or in an integrated fashion. For any substance abuser, however, the first step in treatment must be detoxification -- a period of time during which the body is allowed to cleanse itself of alcohol or drugs. For opioid addiction, it may be best to get the addicted patient stabilized on methadone so that the withdrawal and craving aspects can be suspended. Some persons with co-existing psychiatric problems will need mental health evaluation and treatment to get through detoxification or stabilization.

Mood Disorders
The term mood disorders covers up to 70-75% of all psychiatric presentations. This includes all types of depression, bipolar disorder and the related anxiety and psychosis. They cause major financial burden on the economy due to loss of productivity, lower immunity and predisposition to health problems. Suicide and hospital stays cost huge sums of money. The focus nowadays is to get these patients well fast and achieve remission.

The most common diagnosis is Major Depression, with or without psychotic features. Although the symptoms and presentation varies for different individuals, lack of pleasure, sad mood, and lack of motivation top the list. Suicidal ideation may be present with or without history of attempts.

Although there is a notion that addicts "treat themselves" with street drugs, it is not clear whether addicts carry a diagnosis of major depression more than the general population. Typically addicts carry the burden of financial, legal and custody problems, more than the average person. It may be argued that they are more disposed to "situational depression" given how chaotic their lives may be. It is also true that once an addict stops using stimulants, e.g. amphetamines, it seems that they are more predisposed to weight gain, sleep problems, poor concentration and attention. These cluster of symptoms are commonly referred to as vegetative symptoms of depression.

It seems that major depression rarely exists in a pure form. Anxiety and related disorders are seen up to 90% of the cases. There is a debate whether these co-existing conditions are a cause of, a result of, or just a related condition to depression. Common one is agoraphobia, generalized anxiety disorder, panic attacks and post-traumatic stress disorder.

In the last decade, there has been more emphasis on bipolar (manic-depressive) disorder, and the fact that a patient can present with psychosis as part of their manic-hypomanic states. Good psychiatric skills are needed to decide what cause of psychosis is being faced with. Bipolar disorder encompasses a wide variety of symptoms, with life-long disabilities. Symptoms can be treated in an outpatient setting, but more serious presentations may require hospitalizations and even residential placements.

Depression and Substance Use
People can develop co-existing depression and substance use problems for a variety of reasons. The question about which came first is vexed but should not delay treatment of either disorder. Preferably the substance use should be ceased but this is not always possible. People self medicate with a variety of drugs to alleviate the symptoms of the depression. The effect that the drugs have depends on the drug itself, the particular individual's response to the drug, the duration of the drug use and the particulars of the mental disorder, in this case depression.

Long-term use of stimulants, such as amphetamines and MDMA has been identified as producing depletion of neurotransmitters, thus causing or aggravating depression. Alcohol dependence frequently causes depressive symptoms. However psychosocial effects such as stigma, poverty and isolation associated with drug use may also be highly relevant.

CLINICAL ISSUES WITH CANNABIS, HALLUCINOGENS AND DEPRESSION

Effect of Substance on Mental Disorder.
- Some people may use cannabis to self manage their depressive symptoms.
- However the sedative effect of cannabis may exacerbate depression.
- Amotivational syndrome (associated with long term heavy usage) may simulate the cognitive and psychomotor features of depression.
- Long-term heavy use also thought to cause a depression like syndrome.
- Cannabis may mask appetite loss, thus concealing the extent of vegetative changes in more severe depression.
- Drug interaction with therapeutic agents. Cannabis will augment the sedative effect of benzodiazepines and tricyclic antidepressants.
- Cannabis has been reported to cause mania with fluoxetine. Confusion, depersonalization, psychosis and hypomania have also been reported with concurrent use of cannabis and SSRIs. LSD may induce a serotonin syndrome with SSRIs.

CLINICAL ISSUES WITH ALCOHOL AND DEPRESSION

<u>Effect of Substance on Mental Disorder</u>
Depression is a common feature of alcohol dependence. In many instances the depression will resolve if the alcohol is ceased. In addition the depressant effect of alcohol will exacerbate a clinical depressive disorder. In fact chronic heavy use has been shown to induce a depression-like condition that is difficult to distinguish from major depressive disorder itself. Similarly a depression like set of symptoms may emerge during or after alcohol withdrawal.

DRUG INTERACTIONS:
Alcohol induced sedation will exacerbate the effects of benzodiazepines, tricyclic antidepressants, nefazodone and mirtazepine. Chronic alcohol use has a variable effect on the metabolism of some antidepressants. Does not interact with imipramine, diazepam or disulfiram. Naltrexone will have a blocking effect on opiates used as analgesics.

CLINICAL ISSUES WITH DEPRESSION AND OPIATE USE

<u>Effect of Opioids on Mental Disorder</u>
Opioids' depressive effects will exacerbate depressive disorders. Again the euphoric effects may assist with some of the more negative cognitive symptoms of depression. Some depression resolves once patients are stabilized on methadone.

DRUG INTERACTIONS:
Opioids will exacerbate the effects of the sedative antidepressants, especially the tricyclics. Fluoxetine, fluvoxamine, paroxetine and nefazodone potently inhibit some of the CYP 450 systems in the liver; these enzyme systems metabolize several opioids including methadone. Fluvoxamine has been associated with methadone toxicity, and then when ceased, opioid withdrawal has developed. Citalopram and sertraline are less likely to have this effect. Carbamazepine (used as a mood stabilizer) will induce the metabolism of methadone and reduce levels. Sodium valproate does not have this effect.

CLINICAL ISSUES WITH DEPRESSION AND STIMULANT USE

<u>Effect of Substance on Mental Disorder</u>
Depression is a common feature of the cycle of dependence in stimulant users. People with depression sometimes use stimulants to self-treat the lack of energy associated with the depression. However tolerance to this effect develops quite quickly. There is a risk that stimulants might provide the severely psycho-motor retarded depressed person with the ability to self harm. Depression is exacerbated when the stimulant effect wears off. Stimulant effect on sleep may worsen sleep wake cycle disturbances associated with depression. NOTE: Depression is common in the months following cessation of stimulants, particularly methamphetamine.

<u>Interactions Between Stimulants And Antidepressants:</u>
Irreversible monoamine oxidase inhibitors (i.e. pheneizine) should not be prescribed if stimulants

are used. Some stimulants inhibit the metabolism of tri- and tetra-cyclic antidepressants. If the clinician is aware of stimulant use then other anti-depressants are probable better choices. Most antidepressants as well as cocaine both lower seizure thresholds. Increased seizures have been reported. Serotonin syndrome may occur with cocaine or MDMA/ecstasy and SSRIs and patients should be warned about this. MDMA metabolized through CYP 2D6. This is inhibited by fluoxetine, paroxetine and norfluoxetine.

CLINICAL ISSUES IN DEPRESSION AND BENZODIAZEPINE USE

Effect of Substance on Mental Disorder

Benzodiazepines can relieve some of the symptoms of depression such as insomnia and agitation. However their sedative and depressive actions exacerbate the more negative symptoms of depression such as lack of energy, negative cognitions and anhedonia. Sleep quality is impaired by benzodiazepines with suppression of REM sleep. Adverse reactions to the benzodiazepine. For example paradoxical reactions such as aggression.

DRUG INTERACTIONS:
Benzodiazepines will exacerbate the sedative effect of the tricyclic and other antidepressants. Disulfiram will increase the plasma concentrations of diazepam. The addition of nefazodone, fluoxetine and fluvoxamine will increase the levels of alprazolam, midazolam and triazolam potentially to toxic levels.

Anxiety Disorders
Generalized anxiety disorder can be difficult to diagnose due to its prevalence and co-existence with other psychiatric conditions. Rapid heart beat, sweaty palms, and feeling of losing one's mind and losing control are very common. PTSD (post-traumatic stress disorder) became widely known as a result of traumatic exposure during the Vietnam War, and later subsequent wars. Currently it is used to describe the after effects of any exposure to a serious trauma, including child abuse, sexual exploitation and even time in locked up in prison. The hallmark of this condition is hyper arousal, i.e., an increase symptoms anxiety, feelings of worthlessness and has pending doom. Depression is almost always present, but can be masked by frank anxiety and restless. Other anxiety disorders can also present in the same individual. Adults and children respond best to antidepressants in combination with support, group and individual therapy.

Adult ADHD, although it has its roots in early childhood, is a rather common (10-15%) presentation in amphetamine abusers/addicts. Amphetamines, like the stimulants physicians use for the treatment of this disorder, help improve attention, focus, memory and a general feeling of well-being. With treatment, patients are more productive, finish projects and their organizational skills improve. In children, the most prescribed medication is Ritalin. Although it is not an amphetamine, its stimulant action is very similar to amphetamine. Due to its addiction potential, its use in addicts is somewhat controversial. Dexedrine and Adderall are amphetamine-based products; hence their use should be closely monitored. Non-stimulant medications are Strattera and Wellbutrin which are alternatives in addicts. All of these medications can curb the appetite and cause weight loss and insomnia.

Obsessive-compulsive disorder is the compulsive need to repeat thoughts and actions to help control anxiety and a sense of loss of control. This condition is underreported due to the embarrassment of the patient, but usually admitted to upon inquiry. Depression can result from this condition due to its limiting and isolating results, but minor forms exists in successful and well-know individuals. Medication and behavioral techniques alone are equally effective, but best results are achieved when combined.

CLINICAL ISSUES WITH ANXIETY DISORDERS AND CANNABIS/HALLUCINOGENS

Effect of Substance on Mental Disorder
Cannabis and the other hallucinogens can induce anxiety in susceptible people. This occurs during intoxication and when high doses have been used, for some time afterwards when drug levels have dropped. Some people use cannabis to help them cope with the symptoms of an anxiety disorder that is not being properly managed.

DRUG INTERACTION WITH THERAPEUTIC AGENTS:
Cannabis will augment the sedative effect of benzodiazepines and tricyclic antidepressants. It has also been reported to cause mania with fluoxetine. Confusion, depersonalisation, psychosis and hypomania have also been reported with concurrent use of cannabis and SSRIs. LSD may induce a serotonin syndrome with SSRIs.

CLINICAL ISSUES WITH ALCOHOL AND ANXIETY DISORDERS

Effect of Substance on Mental Disorder
Alcohol has long been used to self medicate for symptoms of anxiety disorders. The effect is sustained although tolerance occurs. When alcohol levels drop then there is a reappearance of the anxiety symptoms given the appropriate environment.

DRUG INTERACTIONS:
Alcohol will enhance the sedation that occurs with tricyclic antidepressants, some of which are still used for severe anxiety disorders. Nefazodone has caused liver toxicity so its use with people with established liver disease is best avoided.

CLINICAL ISSUES ANXIETY DISORDERS AND OPIATE USE

Effect of Substance on Mental Disorder
Opioids can have a positive effect on some Symptoms of anxiety through their soporific and sedative effects and euphoria. However withdrawal effects can exacerbate and be exacerbated by anxiety disorders.

DRUG INTERACTIONS: REACTIONS:

Benzodiazepines are often used in the management of anxiety despite problems with tolerance and dependence. Benzodiazepines and opioids used together increase the risk of fatal opiate overdose. Similarly the use of methadone and benzodiazepines increases the risk of sedation. Fluoxetine, fluvoxamine, paroxetine and nefazodone potently inhibit some of the cytochrome systems in the liver; these enzyme systems metabolise several opioids including methadone and buprenorphine. Citalopram and sertraline have less risk of this effect.

CLINICAL ISSUES ANXIETY DISORDERS AND STIMULANT USE

Effect of Substance on Mental Disorder

Stimulants generally make the symptoms of anxiety disorders worse. Chronic amphetamine, and cocaine use can precipitate anxiety states and panic attacks. High dose use can precipitate obsessive cognitions and compulsive behavior.

DRUG INTERACTIONS:

Irreversible monoamine oxidase inhibitors (tranylcypramine or phenylzine) should not be prescribed if stimulants are used. Some stimulants inhibit the metabolism of tri- and tetra-cyclic antidepressants. If the clinician is aware of stimulant use then other anti-depressants are probably better choices. Serotonin syndrome may occur with cocaine, amphetamines or MDMA/ecstasy and SSRIs. Paroxetine, fluoxetine and norfluoxetine and nefazodone potently inhibit CYP 2D6 which metabolizes cocaine and MDMA. This may result in elevated levels of these latter substances.

CLINICAL ISSUES WITH BENZODIAZEPINES AND ANXIETY DISORDERS

Effect of Substance on Mental Disorder

Benzodiazepines are very effective for treating the acute symptoms of anxiety. However tolerance and dependence develop within a short period of time. If short acting benzodiazepines are used (eg alprazolam, oxazepam, temazepam) rapidly fluctuating blood drug levels may exacerbate the symptoms of the anxiety disorder.

DRUG INTERACTIONS:

Benzodiazepines will exacerbate the sedative effect of the tricyclic and other antidepressants. Disulfiram will increase the plasma concentrations of diazepam. The addition of nefazodone, fluoxetine and fluvoxamine will increase the levels of diazepam, alprazolam, midazolam and triazolam potentially to toxic levels.

Psychotic Disorders

Psychosis is a very common presentation in this population. This may include paranoid ideation, delusions and even frank hallucination. Patients may not understand the seriousness of psychosis, and the evaluator has to ask specific questions about hearing voices, seeing things, confusion, and thinking problems. If anger and impulsivity compound psychosis, disastrous results may affect such patients for the rest of their lives. In most situations, hallucinations require immediate if not urgent evaluation and intervention.

The person experiencing psychosis in the context of concurrent illicit drug use presents a problem that is challenging for the diagnostic and clinical skills of the counselor. The psychoses are characterized by a loss of connectedness with reality. A person may develop false ideas or beliefs about reality (delusions). These may be based on false perceptions of reality (hallucinations). These are termed thought disorder. Examples are tangential thinking, loose associations between words and thoughts, and incoherence. Psychosis is commonly seen with depression, although it can present itself as "drug induced" psychosis, which improves fast. Visual hallucinations are more common with drug induced psychosis and mania, and auditory hallucinations are more common in schizophrenia.

There are two broad classes of functional psychotic disorders, schizophrenia and bipolar disorder. Generally schizophrenia is a chronic condition with exacerbations, but always with some background symptoms, while bipolar disorder is generally an intermittent condition with full recovery in between episodes. There is considerable overlap between the two conditions and "fluidity of diagnosis". Schizophrenia itself has so called "negative symptoms" such as social withdrawal and lack of energy and motivation that are similar to those found in depression. While the clinician may realize that the psychosis could be drug-induced and is cautious in the prescription of antipsychotics or sedatives to control the symptoms, they may be under pressure to respond to the manifestation of bizarre or potentially destructive thinking or behavior. On the other hand alterations to the way the person behaves and thinks may be subtle in their early stages when early intervention may be most appropriate.

Comorbidity with psychosis
It is important to differentiate between three different phenomena with regard to psychosis and substance use:
- First, people can suffer from an acute psychotic episode in response to substance use, in particular cannabis and the stimulants.
- Secondly these substances can precipitate a psychotic disorder in predisposed individuals.
- Thirdly use of substances can exacerbate the symptoms in people with a chronic psychotic disorder. Use of these drugs will often exacerbate their condition and make rehabilitation much more difficult.

NOTE: People with psychosis tend to use a broad range of substances for a variety of reasons.

CLINICAL ISSUES IN THE MANAGEMENT OF PSYCHOSIS AND CANNABIS/HALLUCINOGENS.

Effect of Substance on Mental Disorder
As mentioned above cannabis and other hallucinogens certainly can precipitate acute psychotic episodes both in people with established psychotic disorders and in those who do not. Psychotic episodes tend to occur more frequently at high doses and in the person who is using them for the

first time. Many people using these drugs realize early on that the drug makes them "a bit paranoid" and make the decision not to use them again.

In some people regular cannabis use may augment metabolism of anti-psychotic agents and lessen side effects, thus reinforcing the use of the cannabis. A similar interaction is thought to underlie the high rates of cigarette usage amongst people with psychotic disorders.

DRUG INTERACTIONS: Most of the active ingredients of cannabis are metabolized through the hepatic CYP 450 system. The sedative effect of cannabis will augment similar side-effects of the antipsychotics. Cigarette smoking will induce the metabolism of the typical anti-psychotics and reduce plasma levels. It is unclear whether chronic cannabis consumption does the same.

CLINICAL ISSUES WITH ALCOHOL AND PSYCHOSIS

Effect of Substance on Mental Disorder
Long term effects on the course of schizophrenia unclear. However alcohol has the potential for making an already disordered lifestyle even more disordered. Relapse rates are higher for those people with schizophrenia and harmful alcohol use. Alcohol tends to make the negative symptoms of schizophrenia worse. It probably has little effect on the positive symptoms.

DRUG INTERACTIONS:
Alcohol will exacerbate the sedative effects of many of the anti-psychotics and cause additional psychomotor incoordination. Alcohol exacerbates the orthostatic hypotension problems associated with many of the anti-psychotics.

CLINICAL ISSUES WITH SCHIZOPHRENIA AND OPIATE USE

Effect of Substance on Mental Disorder
As mentioned above the effects of opioids tend to be sedative and do not assist with self-management of the negative symptoms of schizophrenia. However the euphoric response from the opioids may alleviate the depression and isolation that is often associated with psychotic illness. Opioid use is associated with poorer outcomes for the psychotic disorder.

DRUG INTERACTIONS:
Opioids (including methadone and buprenorphine) have an additional sedative effect to that of the anti-psychotics. Care with driving and machinery. No significant pharmacokinetic interactions between methadone or buprenorphine and anti-psychotics. No interactions between naltrexone and antipsychotics.

MAJOR CLINICAL ISSUES WITH PSYCHOSIS AND STIMULANT USE

Effect of Substance on Mental Disorder
Stimulants certainly can precipitate acute psychotic episodes both in people with established psychotic disorders and in those who do not. Psychotic episodes tend to occur more frequently at high doses and in the person who is using them for the first time.

Psychotic symptoms are very common in those with stimulant dependence. Many people using these drugs realize early on that the drug makes them "a bit paranoid" and make the decision not to use them again. Generally outcomes for people with schizophrenia using stimulants are not as good as for those who do not use cannabis. Occasional use of low dose stimulants is unlikely to induce an acute psychotic episode in most people.

DRUG INTERACTIONS:
Stimulants generally do not interfere with anti-psychotics.

CLINICAL ISSUES WITH PSYCHOSIS AND BENZODIAZEPINE USE

Effect of Substance on Mental Disorder
Benzodiazepines can be used for the management of the acute agitation and anxiety associated with an acute psychotic state. They are used by patients to self manage positive psychotic symptoms. May exacerbate negative symptoms such as depression and psychomotor retardation as well as slowing of cognitive behaviors.

DRUG INTERACTIONS:
Benzodiazepines will increase the sedative effects of the antipsychotics. This is sometimes used to assist with management of acute episodes. Benzodiazepines may induce delirium, severe sedation and respiratory collapse when used with clozapine.

General Clinical Management
Management should be based on the patient's "readiness for change". This *readiness for change* might be different for the management of the substance use than it is for the mental disorder. Management should aim to increase the patient's awareness of the negative effect that the substance use and the mental disorder are having on each other.. Management should involve family or other care givers where appropriate.

Specific management
Detoxification should be offered as a first step to enable engagement in long-term approaches and decision-making. Specific management steps should include where appropriate:

- information provision;
- structured problem solving;
- motivational interviewing;
- brief behavioral or cognitive approaches.

Personality Disorders
Personality disorders, also know as character disorders, are common among this population. Sometimes these disorders are referred to as "Axis II" diagnosis, referring to the DSM IV manual. Although it is hard to treat these disorders (e.g. antisocial and borderline), it is important to treat the accompanying symptoms of depression, anxiety, panic, obsessive-compulsive, and sleep problems. Treating these

symptoms improves the odds for these patients to stay clean, and rely less on street drugs. Acting-out is common with this diagnosis, and the treating physician or therapist should be careful in preventing these patients from accusing them of improper or unprofessional conduct. They seem to always complain about their lives, and how the system and provider are not helping them enough or correctly.

General Assessment Issues
Irrespective of the treatment or intervention setting, and notwithstanding the crisis that may have initiated the treatment contact, all treatment contacts with patients who may have dual disorders should include a basic screening for psychiatric and substance abuse disorders. With respect to both psychiatric and substance abuse disorders, the assessment process should be sensitive to biological, psychological, and social issues.

Full assessments of patients with dual disorders should be performed by clinicians who have certified training in the areas that they assess. However, clinicians who are not certified can learn to perform screening tests. Assessments of patients who may have dual disorders should include at least a brief mental status exam (MSE) to assess for the presence and severity of psychiatric problems, as well as a screening for substance abuse disorders.

The "ABC" model is a simple screening technique for the presence of psychiatric disorders.

ABC Model for Psychiatric Screening
- Appearance, alertness, affect, and anxiety:
  Appearance:
  General appearance, hygiene, and dress.
  Alertness:
  What is the level of consciousness?
  Affect:
  Elation or depression: gestures, facial expression, and speech.
  Anxiety:
  Is the individual nervous, phobic, or panicky?
- Behavior:
  Movements:
  Rate (Hyperactive, hypoactive, abrupt, or constant?).
  Organization:
  Coherent and goal-oriented?
  Purpose:
  Bizarre, stereotypical, dangerous, or impulsive?
  Speech:
  Rate, organization, coherence, and content.
- Cognition:
  Orientation:

Person, place, time, and condition.
Calculation:
Memory and simple tasks.
Reasoning:
Insight, judgment, problem solving.
Coherence:
Incoherent ideas, delusions, and hallucinations?

The CAGE questionnaire and the CAGE questionnaire modified for other drugs (CAGEAID) are rapid and accurate screening tools for substance abuse disorders. The substances used most often by patients with dual disorders are the same as those used by society in general: alcohol, marijuana, cocaine, and more rarely, opioids. It is recommended that all front-line AOD and mental health staff receive detailed training in the use of a mental status exam and substance abuse screening tests.

CAGE

1. Have you ever felt you should **c**ut down, on your drinking?

2. Have people **a**nnoyed you by criticizing your drinking?

3. Have you ever felt bad or **g**uilty about your drinking?

4. Have you ever had a drink first thing in the morning to steady your nerves or to get rid of a hangover (**e**ye opener)?

Scoring: Item responses on the CAGE are scored 0 for "no" and 1 for "yes" answers, with a higher score an indication of alcohol problems. A total score of 2 or greater is considered clinically significant.

The normal cutoff for the CAGE is two positive answers, however, the Consensus Panel recommends that the primary care clinicians lower the threshold to one positive answer to cast a wider net and identify more patients who may have substance abuse disorders. A number of other screening tools are available.

CAGE Questions Adapted to Include Drugs (CAGE-AID)
1. Have you ever felt you ought to cut down on your drinking or drug use?

2. Have people annoyed you by criticizing your drinking or drug use?

3. Have you felt bad or guilty about your drinking or drug use?

4. Have you ever had a drink or used drugs first thing in the morning to steady your nerves or to get rid of a hangover (eye-opener)?

Treatment Considerations
Integrated dual disorders treatment has been shown to work effectively for both disorders. People with dual disorders have a better chance of recovery from both

disorders when their mental health practitioners provide combined mental health and substance abuse treatments. Dual disorders are common with more than half of all adults with severe mental illness are further impaired by substance use disorders (abuse or dependence related to alcohol or other drugs). People with dual disorders are at high risk for many additional problems such as symptomatic relapses, hospitalizations, financial problems, family problems, homelessness, suicide, violence, sexual and physical victimization, incarceration, serious medical illnesses, such as HIV and hepatitis B and C, and early death.

As the mental health and substance abuse treatment fields have become increasingly aware of the existence of patients with dual disorders, various attempts have been made to adapt treatment to the special needs of these patients. These attempts have reflected philosophical differences about the nature of dual disorders, as well as differing opinions regarding the best way to treat them. These attempts also reflect the limitations of available resources, as well as differences in treatment responses for different types and severities of dual disorders. Three approaches have been taken to treatment.

The first and historically most common model of dual disorder treatment is sequential treatment. In this model of treatment, the patient is treated by one system (addiction or mental health) and then by the other. Indeed, some clinicians believe that addiction treatment must always be initiated first, and that the individual must be in a stage of abstinent recovery from addiction before treatment for the psychiatric disorder can begin. On the other hand, other clinicians believe that treatment for the psychiatric disorder should begin prior to the initiation of abstinence and addiction treatment. Still other clinicians believe that symptom severity at the time of entry to treatment should dictate whether the individual is treated in a mental health setting or an addiction treatment setting or that the disorder that emerged first should be treated first.

The term sequential treatment describes the serial or nonsimultaneous participation in both mental health and addiction treatment settings. For example, a person with dual disorders may receive treatment at a community mental health center program during occasional periods of depression and attend a local substance abuse treatment program following infrequent alcoholic binges. Systems that have developed serial treatment approaches generally incorporate one of the above orientations toward the treatment of patients with dual disorders.

A related approach involves parallel treatment: the simultaneous involvement of the patient in both mental health and addiction treatment settings. For example, an individual may participate in substance abuse education and drug refusal classes at an addiction treatment program, participate in a 12-step group such as AA, and attend group therapy and medication education classes at a mental health center. Both parallel and sequential treatments involve the utilization of existing treatment programs and settings. Thus, mental health treatment is provided by mental health clinicians, and addiction treatment is provided by addiction treatment clinicians. Coordination between settings is quite variable.

A third model, called integrated treatment, is an approach that combines elements of both mental health and addiction treatment into a unified and comprehensive treatment program for patients with dual disorders. Ideally, integrated treatment involves clinicians cross-trained in both mental health and addiction, as well as a unified case management approach, making it possible to monitor and treat patients through various psychiatric and substance abuse crises.

There are advantages and disadvantages in sequential, parallel, and integrated treatment approaches. Differences in dual disorder combinations, symptom severity, and degree of impairment greatly affect the appropriateness of a treatment model for a specific individual. For example, sequential and parallel treatment may be most appropriate for patients who have a very severe problem with one disorder, but a mild problem with the other. However, patients with dual disorders who obtain treatment from two separate systems frequently receive conflicting therapeutic messages; in addition, financial coverage and even confidentiality laws vary between the two systems.

Integrated treatment places the burden of treatment continuity on a case manager who is expert in both psychiatric and substance abuse disorders. Further, integrated treatment involves simultaneous treatment of both disorders in a setting designed to accommodate both problems.

Basic components of integrated dual disorders treatment
Providing effective integrated dual disorders treatment involves the following:

- *Knowledge about alcohol and drug use, as well as mental illnesses*
  Clinicians know the effects of alcohol and drugs and their interactions with mental illness.
- *Integrated services*
  Clinicians provide services for both mental illness and substance use at the same time.
- *Stage-wise treatment*
  People go through a process over time to recover and different services are helpful at different stages of recovery.
- *Assessment*
  Consumers collaborate with clinicians to develop an individualized treatment plan for both substance use disorder and mental illness.
- *Motivational treatment*
  Clinicians use specific listening and counseling skills to help consumers develop awareness, hopefulness, and motivation for recovery. This is important for consumers who are demoralized and not ready for substance abuse treatment.

- *Substance abuse counseling*
  Substance abuse counseling helps people with dual disorders to develop the skills and find the supports needed to pursue recovery from substance use disorder.

CHAPTER 15: SELF-STUDY QUESTIONS

TRUE/FALSE

1. *A person who has both substance abuse and psychiatric problems is said to have a dual sicknesses.*

2. *Overall, about one-tenth (9.4 percent) of American adults, or 19.4 million persons, meet clinical criteria for a substance use disorder.*

3. *According to the National Institute of Mental Health 10 million Americans are affected by a dual-diagnosis disorder each year.*

4. *It is generally accepted that mental illness is the primary condition in dual disorders.*

5. *Research has concluded that both problems of mental illness and substance abuse should be treated simultaneously or in an integrated fashion.*

6. *Stimulants certainly can precipitate acute psychotic episodes both in people with established psychotic disorders and in those who do not.*

7. *Alcohol will exacerbate the sedative effects of many of the anti-psychotics and cause additional psychomotor incoordination.*

8. *Assessments of patients who may have dual disorders should include at least a brief mental status exam (MSE)sess for the presence and severity of psychiatric problems, but no screening for substance abuse disorders is needed since the MSE is sufficient.*

9. *The CAGE and CAGEAID questionnaires are rapid and accurate screening tools for HIV-AIDS.*

10. *Integrated treatment places the burden of treatment continuity on a case manager who is expert in both psychiatric and substance abuse disorders.*

* Answers to Self Study Tests are located on page 351

Chapter 15 Selected Reading

American Psychiatric Association, *Diagnostic and Statistical Manual of Mental Disorders,* 4th Edition *(DSM-IV),* Washington, D.C., 1994.

Bridget F. Grant; Frederick S. Stinson; Deborah A. Dawson; S. Patricia Chou; Mary C. Dufour; Wilson Compton; Roger P. Pickering; Kenneth Kaplan. Prevalence and Co-occurrence of Substance Use Disorders and Independent Mood and Anxiety Disorders: Results From the National Epidemiologic Survey on Alcohol and Related Conditions. Arch Gen Psychiatry, Aug 2004; 61: 807 - 816.

Chouljian JL, Shumway M, Balancio E, et al. Substance Abuse Among Schizophrenic Outpatient Prevalence, Course, and Relation to Functional Status. Am Clin Psychiatry. 1995;7(1):19-24.

Dennison, SJ. Substance Abuse Disorders in Individuals with Co-Occurring Psychiatric Disorde Lowinson, JH, Ruiz, P, Millman, RB, and Langrod, JG (editors). In: *Substance Abuse A Comprehensive Sourcebook.* 4th Edition. Lippincott Williams & Wilkins. 2005.

Drake, R. E., Essock, S. M., Shaner, A., Carey, K. B., Minkoff, K., Kola, L., Lynde, D.,
Osher, F. C., Clark, R. E., & Richards, L. (2001). Implementing dual diagnosis services for clients with severe mental illness. *Psychiatric Services, 52,* 469-476.

Dual Diagnosis-The Problem (2005) from
http://alcoholism.about.com/cs/dual/a/aa981209.htm

Erickson, C.K. and Wilcox, R.E.: Neurobiological Causes of Addiction, *J. Soc. Work Pract. Addict .* 1 :7-22 (2001).

Foundations Associates (2004) from http://www.dualdiagnosis.org/index.php?id=9

Hasin D.S., Hatzenbueler M., Smith S., Grant B.F., Co-occurring DSM-IV drug abuse in DSM-IV drug dependence: Results from the National Epidemiologic Survey on Alcohol and Related Conditions. *Drug Alc. Depend.* 80: 117-123. (2005).

Mueser, K. T., Bellack, A. S., & Blanchard, J. J. (1992) Comorbidity of schizophrenia and substance abuse: Implications for treatment. *Journal of Consulting and Clinical Psychology, 60,* 845-856.Nolen-Hoeksema, S. (2004). *Abnormal psychology.* (3rd ed.). New York: McGraw Hill.

Phillips, P, and Labrow, J. (2004). *Understanding Dual Diagnosis.* from http://www.mind.org.uk/Information/Booklets/Understanding/Understanding+dual+d iagnosis.htm

Regier, D. A., Farmer, M. E., Rae, D. S., et al., Comorbidity of mental disorders with alcohol and other drug abuse, *JAMA* 264(19):2511-2518 (1990).

Ridenour, T.A., Maldonado-Molina, M., Compton, W.M., Spitznagel, E.L., Cottler, L.B., Factors associated with the transition from abuse to dependence among substance abusers: Implications for a measure of addictive liability. *Drug Alc. Depend.* 80: 1-14 (2005).

Sciacca K. On Co-Occurring Addictive and Mental Disorders: A Brief History of the Origins of Dual Diagnosis Treatment and Program Development (an uninvited response). Am J Orthopsychhiatry. 1996;66:3.

Stinson, F.S., Grant, B.F., Dawson, D.A., Ruan, W.J., Huang, B., Saha, T., Comorbidity between DSM-IV alcohol and specific drug use disorders in the United States: Results from the National Epidemiologic Survey on Alcohol and Related Conditions. *Drug Alc. Depend.* 80: 105-116 (2005).

Tohen M, Zarate CAJ. Bipolar Disorder and Comorbid Substance Use Disorder. In: Goldberg JF, Harrow M, eds. Bipolar Disorders: Clinical Course and Outcome. American Psychiatric Press. 1999:171-184.

APPENDIX SECTION

- Principles of Drug Addiction Treatment: A Research-Based Guide (NIDA)

- Drug Use and Infectious Diseases

- Hepatitis C

- HIV – AIDS

- Glossary

Principles of Drug Addiction Treatment
Research-Based Principles of Drug Addiction Treatment

To share the results of an extensive body of research and foster more widespread use of scientifically based treatment components, the National Institute on Drug Abuse (NIDA) prepared the information below. This research-based information summarizes the basic overarching principles that characterize effective drug addiction treatment. The section that follows, *Frequently Asked Questions about Drug Addiction Treatment,* elaborates on these principles.

1. **No single treatment is appropriate for all individuals.** Matching treatment settings, interventions, and services to each individual's particular problems and needs is critical to his or her ultimate success in returning to productive functioning in the family, workplace, and society.

2. **Treatment needs to be readily available.** Because individuals who are addicted to drugs may be uncertain about entering treatment, taking advantage of opportunities when they are ready for treatment is crucial. Potential treatment applicants can be lost if treatment is not immediately available or is not readily accessible.

3. **Effective treatment attends to multiple needs of the individual, not just his or her drug use.** To be effective, treatment must address the individual's drug use and any associated medical, psychological, social, vocational, and legal problems.

4. **An individual's treatment and services plan must be assessed continually and modified as necessary to ensure that the plan meets the person's changing needs.** A patient may require varying combinations of services and treatment components during the course of treatment and recovery. In addition to counseling or psychotherapy, a patient at times may require medication, other medical services, family therapy, parenting instruction, vocational rehabilitation, and social and legal services. It is critical that the treatment approach be appropriate to the individual's age, gender, ethnicity, and culture.

5. **Remaining in treatment for an adequate period of time is critical for treatment effectiveness.** The appropriate duration for an individual depends on his or her problems and needs. Research indicates that for most patients, the threshold of significant improvement is reached at about 3 months in treatment. After this threshold is reached, additional treatment can produce further progress toward recovery. Because people often leave treatment prematurely, programs should include strategies to engage and keep patients in treatment.

6. **Counseling (individual and/or group) and other behavioral therapies are critical components of effective treatment for addiction.** In therapy, patients address issues of motivation, build skills to resist drug use, replace drug-using activities with constructive and rewarding nondrug-using activities, and improve problem-solving abilities. Behavioral therapy also facilitates interpersonal relationships and the individual's ability to function in the family and community.

7. **Medications are an important element of treatment for many patients, especially when combined with counseling and other behavioral therapies.** Methadone and buprenorphine are very effective in helping individuals addicted to heroin or other opiates stabilize their lives and reduce their illicit drug use. Naltrexone is also an effective medication for some opiate addicts and some patients with co-occurring alcohol dependence. For persons addicted to nicotine, a nicotine replacement product (such as patches or gum) or an oral medication (such as bupropion, Zyban or Chantix) can be an effective component of treatment. For patients with mental disorders, both behavioral treatments and medications can be critically important.

8. **Addicted or drug-abusing individuals with coexisting mental disorders should have both disorders treated in an integrated way.** Because addictive disorders and mental disorders often occur in the same individual, patients presenting for either condition should be assessed and treated for the co-occurrence of the other type of disorder.

9. **Medical detoxification is only the first stage of addiction treatment and by itself does little to change long-term drug use.** Medical detoxification safely manages the acute physical symptoms of withdrawal associated with stopping drug use. While detoxification alone is rarely sufficient to help addicts achieve long-term abstinence, for some individuals it is a strongly indicated precursor to effective drug addiction treatment.

10. **Treatment does not need to be voluntary to be effective.** Strong motivation can facilitate the treatment process. Sanctions or enticements in the family, employment setting, or criminal justice system can increase significantly both treatment entry and retention rates and the success of drug treatment interventions.

11. **Possible drug use during treatment must be monitored continuously.** Lapses to drug use can occur during treatment. The objective monitoring of a patient's drug and alcohol use during treatment, such as through urinalysis or other tests, can help the patient withstand urges to use drugs. Such monitoring also can provide early evidence of drug use so that the individual's treatment plan can be adjusted. Feedback to patients who test positive for illicit drug use is an important element of monitoring.

12. **Treatment programs should provide assessment for HIV/AIDS, hepatitis B and C, tuberculosis and other infectious diseases, and counseling to help patients modify or change behaviors that place themselves or others at risk of infection.** Counseling can help patients avoid high-risk behavior. Counseling also can help people who are already infected manage their illness.

13. **Recovery from drug addiction can be a long-term process and frequently requires multiple episodes of treatment.** As with other chronic illnesses, relapses to drug use can occur during or after successful treatment episodes. Addicted individuals may require prolonged treatment and multiple episodes of treatment to achieve long-term abstinence and fully restored functioning. Participation in self-help support programs during and following treatment often is helpful in maintaining abstinence.

FREQUENTLY ASKED QUESTIONS
About Drug Addiction Treatment

1. **What is drug addiction treatment?**

   There are many addictive drugs, and treatments for specific drugs can differ. Treatment also varies depending on the characteristics of the patient. Problems associated with an individual's drug addiction can vary significantly. People who are addicted to drugs come from all walks of life. Many suffer from mental health, occupational, health, or social problems that make their addictive disorders much more difficult to treat. Even if there are few associated problems, the severity of addiction itself ranges widely among people.

   A variety of scientifically based approaches to drug addiction treatment exists. Drug addiction treatment can include behavioral therapy (such as counseling, cognitive therapy, or psychotherapy), medications, or their combination. Behavioral therapies offer people strategies for coping with their drug cravings, teach them ways to avoid drugs and prevent relapse, and help them deal with relapse if it occurs. When a person's drug-related behavior places him or her at higher risk for AIDS or other infectious diseases, behavioral therapies can help to reduce the risk of disease transmission.

2. **Why can't drug addicts quit on their own?**

   Nearly all addicted individuals believe in the beginning that they can stop using drugs on their own, and most try to stop without treatment. However, most of these attempts result in failure to achieve long-term abstinence. Research has shown that long-term drug use results in significant changes in brain function that persist long after the individual stops using drugs. These drug-induced changes in brain function may have many behavioral consequences, including the compulsion to use drugs despite adverse consequences in the defining characteristic of addiction.

   Understanding that addiction has such an important biological component may help explain an individual's difficulty in achieving and maintaining abstinence without treatment. Psychological stress from work or family problems, social cues (such as meeting individuals from one's drug-using past), or the environment (such as encountering streets, objects, or even smells associated with drug use) can interact with biological factors to hinder attainment of sustained abstinence and make relapse more likely. Research studies indicate that even the most severely addicted individuals can participate actively in treatment and that active participation is essential to good outcomes.

3. **How effective is drug addiction treatment?**

   In addition to stopping drug use, the goal of treatment is to return the individual to productive functioning in the family, workplace, and community. Measures of effectiveness typically include levels of criminal behavior, family functioning, employability, and medical condition. Overall, treatment of addiction is as successful as treatment of other chronic diseases, such as diabetes, hypertension, and asthma.

The treatment of addiction is as successful as treatment of other chronic diseases such as diabetes, hypertension, and asthma.

   According to several studies, drug treatment reduces drug use by 40 to 60 percent and significantly decreases criminal activity during and after treatment. For example, a study of therapeutic community treatment for drug offenders demonstrated that arrests for violent and nonviolent criminal acts were reduced by 40 percent or more. Methadone treatment has been shown to decrease criminal behavior by as much as 50 percent. Research shows that drug addiction treatment reduces the risk of HIV infection and that interventions to prevent HIV are much less costly than treating HIV-related illnesses. Treatment can improve the prospects for employment, with gains of up to 40 percent after treatment.

4. **How long does drug addiction treatment usually last?**

   Individuals progress through drug addiction treatment at various speeds, so there is no predetermined length of treatment. However, research has shown unequivocally that good outcomes are contingent on adequate lengths of treatment. Generally, for residential or outpatient treatment, participation for less than 90 days is of limited or no effectiveness, and treatments lasting significantly longer often are indicated. For methadone maintenance, 12 months of treatment is the minimum, and some opiate-addicted individuals will continue to benefit from methadone maintenance treatment over a period of years. Many people who enter treatment drop out before receiving all the benefits that treatment can provide. Successful outcomes may require more than one treatment experience. Many addicted individuals have multiple episodes of treatment, often with a cumulative impact.

5. **What helps people stay in treatment?**

   Since successful outcomes often depend upon retaining the person long enough to gain the full benefits of treatment, strategies for keeping an individual in the program are critical. Whether a patient stays in treatment depends on factors associated with both the individual and the program. Individual factors related to engagement and retention include motivation to change drug-using behavior, degree of support from family and friends, and whether there is pressure to stay in treatment from the criminal justice system, child protection services, employers, or the family. Within the program, successful counselors are able to establish a positive, therapeutic relationship with the patient. The counselor should ensure that a treatment plan is established and followed so that the individual knows what to expect during treatment. Medical, psychiatric, and social services should be available.

Since some individual problems (such as serious mental illness, severe cocaine or crack use, and criminal involvement) increase the likelihood of a patient dropping out, intensive treatment with a range of components may be required to retain patients who have these problems. The provider then should ensure a transition to continuing care or "aftercare" following the patient's completion of formal treatment.

6. **Is the use of medications like methadone simply replacing one drug addiction with another?**
No. As used in maintenance treatment, methadone and buprenorphine are not heroin substitutes. They are safe and extrmeley effective medications for opiate addiction that are administered by mouth in regular, fixed doses. Their pharmacological effects are markedly different from those of heroin.

7. **What Role Can The Criminal Justice System Play In The Treatment Of Drug Addiction?**
Increasingly, research is demonstrating that treatment for drug-addicted offenders during and after incarceration can have a significant beneficial effect upon future drug use, criminal behavior, and social functioning. The case for integrating drug addiction treatment approaches with the criminal justice system is compelling. Combining prison- and community-based treatment for drug-addicted offenders reduces the risk of both recidivism to drug-related criminal behavior and relapse to drug use. For example, a recent study found that prisoners who participated in a therapeutic treatment program in the Delaware State Prison and continued to receive treatment in a work-release program after prison were 70 percent less likely than nonparticipants to return to drug use and incur rearrest.

The most effective models integrate criminal justice and drug treatment systems and services. Treatment and criminal justice personnel work together on plans and implementation of screening, placement, testing, monitoring, and supervision, as well as on the systematic use of sanctions and rewards for drug abusers in the criminal justice system. Treatment for incarcerated drug abusers must include continuing care, monitoring, and supervision after release and during parole.

8. **How does drug addiction treatment help reduce the spread of HIV/AIDS and other infectious diseases?**

Many drug addicts, such as heroin or cocaine addicts and particularly injection drug users, are at increased risk for HIV/AIDS as well as other infectious diseases like hepatitis, tuberculosis, and sexually transmitted infections. For these individuals and the community at large, drug addiction treatment is disease prevention.

Drug injectors who do not enter treatment are up to six times more likely to become infected with HIV than injectors who enter and remain in treatment. Drug users who enter and continue in treatment reduce activities that can spread disease, such as sharing injection equipment and engaging in unprotected sexual activity. Participation in treatment also presents opportunities for screening, counseling, and referral for additional services. The best drug abuse treatment programs provide HIV counseling and offer HIV testing to their patients.

9. **Where Do 12-Step or Self-Help Programs Fit Into Drug Addiction Treatment?**
Self-help groups can complement and extend the effects of professional treatment. The most prominent self-help groups are those affiliated with Alcoholics Anonymous (AA), Narcotics Anonymous (NA), and Cocaine Anonymous (CA), all of which are based on the 12-step model, and Smart Recovery. Most drug addiction treatment programs encourage patients to participate in a self-help group during and after formal treatment.

10. **Is Drug Addiction Treatment Worth Its Cost?**
Drug addiction treatment is cost-effective in reducing drug use and its associated health and social costs. Treatment is less expensive than alternatives, such as not treating addicts or simply incarcerating addicts. For example, the average cost for 1 full year of methadone maintenance treatment is approximately $4,700 per patient, whereas 1 full year of imprisonment costs approximately $18,400 per person.

According to several conservative estimates, every $1 invested in addiction treatment programs yields a return of between $4 and $7 in reduced drug-related crime, criminal justice costs, and theft alone. When savings related to health care are included, total savings can exceed costs by a ratio of 12 to 1. Major savings to the individual and society also come from significant drops in interpersonal conflicts, improvements in workplace productivity, and reductions in drug-related accidents.

Source

Principles of Drug Addiction Treatment: A Research-based Guide (NCADI publication BKD347). Copies of the booklet can be obtained from the National Clearinghouse for Alcohol and Drug Information, PO Box 2245, Rockville, MD 20847. 1-800-729-6686

Selected Websites

Addiction Research at Brookhaven: www.bnl.gov/CTN/addiction.asp

American Society of Addiction Medicine: www.asam.org

Association for Medical Education and Research in Substance Abuse: www.amersa.org

National Institute of Drug Abuse. www.drugabuse.gov

Substance Abuse and Mental Health Services Administration: www.samhsa.gov

The Science of Addiction (NIDA): www.drugabuse.gov/scienceofaddiction/

The Science of Addictions and Addictions Treatment: www.addictionscience.net

Drug Use and Infectious Diseases

The use of illicit drugs is associated with the transmission of HIV/AIDS and other infectious diseases, such as hepatitis B and C and tuberculosis. Furthermore, drug use can result in many other health problems. With the establishment of NIDA's new Center for AIDS and Other Medical Consequences of Drug Abuse, NIDA has the unique opportunity to assess both short- and long-term medical consequences associated with drug use. It has long been known that injection drug use is related to a significant percentage of new AIDS cases each year. More recently, research has indicated that hepatitis C is spreading rapidly among injection drug users, with current estimates indicating infection rates of 65 to 90 percent among this population.

Since AIDS was first identified in 1981, more than 1 million Americans have become infected with HIV. According to the Centers for Disease Control and Prevention, drug use remains the second most common mode of exposure among AIDS cases nationwide. Through June 1997, injection-related AIDS cases accounted for 32 percent of total diagnoses.

Overall and in each age group surveyed, respondents who had used illicit drugs in the past year were more likely than those who had not to have had a blood test for HIV. In addition, illicit drug users were more likely than nonusers to be sexually active and to have had two or more sexual partners within the past year. At the same time, those illicit drug users who reported having two or more sexual partners within the past year were less likely to say that they always used a condom.

Selected Reading

Des Jarlais, D.C.; Marmor, M.; Paone, D.; et al. HIV incidence among injecting drug users in New York City syringe-exchange programmes. *Lancet* 348:987-991, 1996.

Paone, D.; Des Jarlais, D.; Clark, J.; et al. Update: Syringe-exchange programs-- United States, 1996. *Morbidity and Mortality Weekly Report* 46(24):565-568, 1997.

Brook, D.W.; Brook, J.S.; Whiteman, M.; et al. Needle-sharing: A longitudinal study of psychosocial risk and protective factors. *American Journal on Addictions* 5(3):209-219, 1996.

Garfein, R.; Vlahov, D.; Galai, N.; et al. Viral infections in short-term drug users. *American Journal of Public Health* 86:655-661, 1996.

Hershow, R.C.; Riester, K.A.; Lew, J.; et al. Increased vertical transmission of human immunodeficiency virus from hepatitis C virus-coinfected mothers. Women and Infants Transmission Study. *Journal of Infectious Diseases* 176:414- 420, 1997.

Management of hepatitis C.; *NIH Consensus Statement Online,* March 24-26. 15(3): 1-41, 1997.

HEPATITIS C VIRUS

The use of illicit drugs is associated with the transmission of hepatitis. It has long been known that injection drug use is related to a significant percentage of new AIDS cases each year. More recently, research has indicated that hepatitis is spreading rapidly among injection drug users, with current estimates indicating infection rates of 65 to 90 percent among this population.

Hepatitis is an inflammation of the liver causing soreness and swelling. Hepatitis C (HCV) is one of the viruses (A, B, C, D, and E), which together account for the vast majority of cases of viral hepatitis. It is an enveloped RNA virus in the *flaviviridae* family which appears to have a narrow host range. Humans and chimpanzees are the only known species susceptible to infection, with both species developing similar disease. Hepatitis can be caused by many things including a lack of blood supply to the liver, toxic exposure, autoimmune disorders, injuries to the liver, and some medicines. However, hepatitis is most commonly caused by a virus and most infections are due to illegal injection drug use.

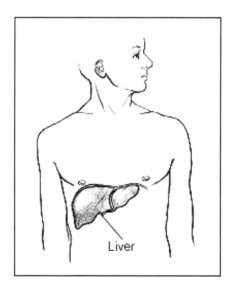

Hepatitis C (HCV) is the most common chronic blood-borne infection in the United States. Approximately 4 million Americans have been infected with the hepatitis C virus (HCV). And epidemiologic studies show that HCV is now endemic among injection drug users (IDUs), the result of risk behaviors such as sharing of syringes and other paraphernalia. In contrast to the epidemiological trends of hepatitis B virus (HBV), the proportion of reported HCV cases acquired through intravenous drug use remains high (12 percent versus 36 percent, respectively). The risk of acquiring HCV through intravenous drug use also increases as the duration and frequency of drug use increases. Intravenous drug users contract both HBV and HCV by sharing contaminated needles. Studies have shown that intravenous drug users are at high risk to acquire HBV and HCV, as seroprevalence rates range from 65 to 90 percent.

In fact, over the past decade injection drug use has become the major mode of HCV transmission in the United States. Research shows that over 60 percent of IDUs who had been injecting for 1 year or less are likely to already be infected with the virus. Overall prevalence of HCV is 76.5 percent among IDUs who had been injecting drugs for 6 years or less. Thus, HCV is a serious medical consequence of drug abuse that needs to be considered when providing care to drug abusers.

An important feature of HCV is the relative mutability of its genome, which in turn is probably related to the high propensity (80%) of inducing chronic infection. HCV is clustered into several distinct genotypes which may be important in determining the severity of the disease and the response to treatment. The mutagenic nature of HCV is probably the reason why there are vaccines for hepatitis A and hepatitis B, but not for HCV.

Hepatitis C can't be spread unless a person has direct contact with infected blood. This means a person who has hepatitis C can't pass the virus to others through casual contact such as sneezing, coughing, shaking hands, hugging, kissing, sharing eating utensils or drinking glasses, swimming in a pool, or using public toilets. Most people who are infected with hepatitis C don't have any symptoms for years. However, hepatitis C is a chronic illness (it doesn't go away). If you have hepatitis C, you need to be watched carefully by a doctor because it can lead to cirrhosis (a liver disease) and liver cancer.

HCV is a major cause of acute hepatitis and chronic liver disease, including cirrhosis and liver cancer. HCV is usually spread through direct contact with the blood of a person who has the disease. Many times, the cause of hepatitis C is never found. Sharing razors or toothbrushes can transmit the hepatitis C virus. It can be transmitted by needles used for tattooing or body piercing. It can even be passed from a mother to her unborn baby.

Clinical Features of Acute Infection
The incubation period of HCV infection before the onset of clinical symptoms ranges from 15 to 150 days. In acute infections, the most common symptoms are fatigue and jaundice; however, the majority of cases (between 60% and 70%), even those that develop chronic infection, are asymptomatic.

Diagnostic tests commercially available today are based on Enzyme immunosorbant assays (EIA) for the detection of HCV specific antibodies. EIAs can detect more than 95% of chronically infected patients but can detect only 50% to 70% of acute infections. A recombinant immunoblot assay (RIBA) that identifies antibodies which react with individual HCV antigens is often used as a supplemental test for confirmation of a positive EIA result. Testing for HCV circulating by amplification tests RNA (e.g. polymerase chain reaction or PCR, branched DNA assay) is also being utilized for confirmation of serological results as well as for assessing the effectiveness of antiviral therapy. A positive result indicates the presence of active infection and a potential for spread of the infection and or/the development of chronic liver disease.

Treatment

Good health habits are essential for those who have hepatitis C, especially avoidance of alcohol and other medications and drugs that are hepatotoxic. Although there is no cure for HCV, many people can benefit from treatment.

Antiviral drugs such as interferon taken alone or in combination with ribavirin, are used for the treatment of persons with chronic hepatitis C. Treatment with interferon alone is effective in about 10% to 20% of patients. Interferon combined with ribavirin is effective in about 30% to 50% of patients. Ribavirin does not appear to be effective when used alone. Standard drug therapy available include the following:

- peginterferon alfa-2b (brand name: PEG-Intron)
- peginterferon alfa-2a (brand name: Pegasys)

These medicines are given as a weekly injection.

Other medicines available to treat HCV include:
- interferon alfa-2a (brand name:Roferon-A)
- interferon alfa-2b (brand name: Intron A)
- interferon alfacon-1 (brand name: Infergen)
- interferon alfa-2b plus ribavirin (brand name: Rebetron)

These medicines are given as an injection every day, every other day or 3 times a week, for several months or longer. The length of treatment depends on how severe the infection is.

Prevention

Although there are vaccines for other forms of hepatitis, none exists to protect against HCV. However, prevention of illegal drug injection would eliminate the greatest risk factor for HCV infection. Therefore, drug addiction treatment can play a major role in reducing HCV transmission. Research shows that drug users who enter and remain in treatment reduce high-risk activities, such as sharing needles and other drug injection paraphernalia, that are responsible for spreading HCV. AIDS outreach and HIV prevention programs for out-of-treatment drug users that reduce HIV risk also reduce the risk of HCV transmission.

Research is in progress but the high mutability of the HCV genome complicates vaccine development. Lack of knowledge of any protective immune response following HCV infection also impedes vaccine research. It is not known whether the immune system is able to eliminate the virus. Some studies, however, have shown the presence of virus--neutralizing antibodies in patients with HCV infection.

In the absence of a vaccine, all precautions to prevent infection must be taken including:

- Screening and testing of blood and organ donors;
- Virus inactivation of plasma derived products;
- Implementation and maintenance of infection control practices in health care settings, including appropriate sterilization of medical and dental equipment;
- Promotion of behavior change among the general public and health care workers to reduce overuse of injections and to use safe injection practices; and risk reduction counseling for persons with high-risk drug and sexual practices.

Alcohol and Hepatitis C

Alcohol is a potent toxin to the liver, even in people without HCV infection. Regardless of the level of alcohol use, people with HCV are at risk for cirrhosis of the liver. Hepatitis C impairs the liver's natural function of breaking down alcohol and removing toxic by-products. As a result, the toxins in alcohol are not removed completely and remain within the body, creating a greater toxic environment. People with HCV should avoid alcohol use altogether.

Based on the data, for every 100 people infected with HCV, statistically 15 people get rid of the virus through their own immune system. 85 will develop chronic or long-term infection. Of these 85 remaining people, 66 will get only minor liver damage. However, 17 will develop cirrhosis and may have symptoms of advanced liver disease and 2 will progress to develop liver cancer. While 17% and 2% are low numbers statistically, this makes prevention even more important. Learning to live a "hepatoenhancing" lifestyle is obviously extremely important for persons infected with HCV.

QUICK VIEW OF VIRAL HEPATITIS TYPES

Viral Hepatitis A (HAV)

HAV is a liver disease caused by the hepatitis A virus. Hepatitis A can affect anyone. In the United States, hepatitis A can occur in situations ranging from isolated cases of disease to widespread epidemics. It does not lead to chronic infection.

Transmission: Ingestion of fecal matter, even in microscopic amounts, from close person-to-person contact or ingestion of contaminated food or drinks. Good personal hygiene and proper sanitation can help prevent hepatitis A. Vaccines are also available for long-term prevention of hepatitis A virus infection in persons 12 months of age and older. Immune globulin is available for short-term prevention of hepatitis A virus infection in individuals of all ages.

Symptoms: Adults will have signs and symptoms more often than children. Jaundice, fatigue, abdominal pain, fever, loss of appetite, nausea and diarrhea. There is no chronic (long-term) infection. Once you have had hepatitis A, you cannot get it again. About 15% of people infected with HAV will have prolonged or relapsing symptoms over a 6-9 month period.

Vaccination: Hepatitis A vaccination is recommended for all children starting at age 1 year, travelers to certain countries, and others at risk.

Viral Hepatitis B (HBV)

HBV is a liver disease caused by the hepatitis B virus (HBV). It ranges in severity from a mild illness, lasting a few weeks (acute), to a serious long-term (chronic) illness. HBV can cause lifelong infection, cirrhosis (scarring) of the liver, liver cancer, liver failure, and death. Hepatitis B vaccine is available for all age groups to prevent hepatitis B virus infection.

Transmission: Transmission occurs when blood from an infected person enters the body of a person who is not infected. HBV is spread through having sex with an infected person without using a condom (the efficacy of latex condoms in preventing infection with HBV is unknown, but their proper use might reduce transmission), by sharing drugs, needles when injecting drugs, through needle sticks or sharps exposures on the job, or from an infected mother to her baby during birth. Persons at risk for HBV infection might also be at risk for infection with hepatitis C virus (HCV) or HIV.

Symptoms: About 30% of persons have no signs or symptoms. Signs and symptoms are less common in children than adults and include jaundice, fatigue, abdominal pain, loss of appetite, nausea, vomiting, and joint pain.

Vaccination: Hepatitis B vaccination is recommended for all infants, older children and adolescents who were not vaccinated previously, and adults at risk for HBV infection.

Viral Hepatitis C (HCV)

Transmission: Occurs when blood from an infected person enters the body of a person who is not infected. HCV is spread through sharing needles when injecting drugs, through needle sticks or sharps exposures on the job, or from an infected mother to her baby during birth. Most infections are due to illegal injection drug use.

Symptoms: 80% of persons have no signs or symptoms.

Long-Term Effects: Chronic infection: 55%-85% of infected persons. Chronic liver disease: 70% of chronically infected persons. Deaths from chronic liver disease: 1%-5% of infected persons may die. HCV is the leading indication for liver transplant.

Recommendations for testing based on risk for HCV infection: Persons at risk for HCV infection might also be at risk for infection with hepatitis B virus (HBV) or HIV.

Recommendations for Testing Based on Risk for HCV Infection

PERSONS	RISK OF INFECTION	TESTING RECOMMENDED
Injecting drug users	High	Yes
Recipients of clotting factors made before 1987	High	Yes
Hemodialysis patients	Intermediate	Yes
Recipients of blood and/or solid organs before 1992	Intermediate	Yes
People with undiagnosed liver problems	Intermediate	Yes
Infants born to infected mothers	Intermediate	After 12-18 mos. old
Healthcare/public safety workers	Low	Only after known exposure
People having sex with multiple partners	Low	No*
People having sex with an infected steady partner	Low	No*
*Anyone who wants to get tested should ask their doctor.		

Treatment: HCV positive persons should be evaluated by their doctor for liver disease. Interferon and ribavirin are two drugs licensed for the treatment of persons with chronic hepatitis C. Interferon can be taken alone or in combination with ribavirin. Combination therapy, using pegylated interferon and ribavirin, is currently the treatment of choice. Combination therapy can get rid of the virus in up to 5 out of

10 persons for genotype 1 and in up to 8 out of 10 persons for genotype 2 and 3. Drinking alcohol can make your liver disease worse.

Selected Links
American Liver Foundation
http://www.liverfoundation.org
75 Maiden Lane, Suite 603
New York, NY 10038-4810
800-GO-LIVER

Hepatitis C: Part II. Prevention Counseling and Medical Evaluation
by LA Moyer, R.N., EE Mast, M.D., M.P.H., and MJ Alter, Ph.D.
(*American Family Physician* January 15, 1999, http://www.aafp.org/afp/990115ap/349.html)

HIV Infection and AIDS: An Overview

AIDS was first reported in the United States in 1981 and has since become a major worldwide epidemic. AIDS is caused by the human immunodeficiency virus (HIV) . By killing or damaging cells of the body's immune system, HIV progressively destroys the body's ability to fight infections and certain cancers. People diagnosed with AIDS may get life-threatening diseases called opportunistic infections. These infections are caused by microbes such as viruses or bacteria that usually do not make healthy people sick.

Since 1981, more than 980,000 cases of AIDS have been reported in the United States to the Centers for Disease Control and Prevention (CDC). According to CDC, more than 1,000,000 Americans may be infected with HIV, one-quarter of whom are unaware of their infection. The epidemic is growing most rapidly among minority populations and is a leading killer of African-American males ages 25 to 44. According, AIDS affects nearly seven times more African Americans and three times more Hispanics than whites. In recent years, an increasing number of African-American women and children are being affected by HIV/AIDS.

Transmission
HIV is spread most often through unprotected sex with an infected partner. The virus can enter the body through the lining of the vagina, vulva, penis, rectum, or mouth during sex.

Risky behavior
HIV can infect anyone who practices risky behaviors such as
- Sharing drug needles or syringes
- Having sexual contact, including oral sexual contact, with an infected person without using a condom
- Having sexual contact with someone whose HIV status is unknown

Infected blood

HIV also is spread through contact with infected blood. Before donated blood was screened for evidence of HIV infection and before heat-treating techniques to destroy HIV in blood products were introduced, HIV was transmitted through transfusions of contaminated blood or blood components. Today, because of blood screening and heat treatment, the risk of getting HIV from blood transfusions is extremely small.

Contaminated needles

HIV is often spread among injection drug users when they share needles or syringes contaminated with very small quantities of blood from someone infected with the virus. It is rare for a patient to be the source of HIV transmitted to a healthcare provider or vice versa by accidental sticks with contaminated needles or other medical instruments.

Mother to child

Women can transmit HIV to their babies during pregnancy or birth. Approximately one-quarter to one-third of all untreated pregnant women infected with HIV will pass the infection to their babies. HIV also can be spread to babies through the breast milk of mothers infected with the virus. If the mother takes certain drugs during pregnancy, she can significantly reduce the chances that her baby will get infected with HIV. If healthcare providers treat HIV-infected pregnant women and deliver their babies by cesarean section, the chances of the baby being infected can be reduced to a rate of 1 percent. HIV infection of newborns has been almost eradicated in the United States because of appropriate treatment.

A study sponsored by the National Institute of Allergy and Infectious Diseases (NIAID) in Uganda found a highly effective and safe drug for preventing transmission of HIV from an infected mother to her newborn. Independent studies have also confirmed this finding. This regimen is more affordable and practical than any other examined to date. Results from the study show that a single oral dose of the antiretroviral drug nevirapine (NVP) given to an HIV-infected woman in labor and another to her baby within 3 days of birth reduces the transmission rate of HIV by half compared with a similar short course of AZT (azidothymidine).

Saliva

Although researchers have found HIV in the saliva of infected people, there is no evidence that the virus is spread by contact with saliva. Laboratory studies reveal that saliva has natural properties that limit the power of HIV to infect, and the amount of virus in saliva appears to be very low. Research studies of people infected with HIV have found no evidence that the virus is spread to others through saliva by kissing. The lining of the mouth, however, can be infected by HIV, and instances of HIV transmission through oral intercourse have been reported. Scientists have found no evidence that HIV is spread through sweat, tears, urine, or feces.

Casual contact
Studies of families of HIV-infected people have shown clearly that HIV is not spread through casual contact such as the sharing of food utensils, towels and bedding, swimming pools, telephones, or toilet seats.
NOTE: HIV is not spread by biting insects such as mosquitoes or bedbugs.

*Sexually transmitted **infections***
People with a <u>sexually transmitted infection</u>, such as syphilis, genital herpes, chlamydia, gonorrhea, or bacterial vaginosis, may be more susceptible to getting HIV infection during sex with infected partners.

Symptoms

Early symptoms
Many people will not have any symptoms when they first become infected with HIV. They may, however, have a flu-like illness within a month or two after exposure to the virus. This illness may include
- Fever
- Headache
- Tiredness
- Enlarged lymph nodes (glands of the immune system easily felt in the neck and groin)

These symptoms usually disappear within a week to a month and are often mistaken for those of another viral infection. During this period, people are very infectious, and HIV is present in large quantities in genital fluids.

Later symptoms
More persistent or severe symptoms may not appear for 10 years or more after HIV first enters the body in adults, or within 2 years in children born with HIV infection. This period of asymptomatic infection varies greatly in each person. Some people may begin to have symptoms within a few months, while others may be symptom-free for more than 10 years.

Even during the asymptomatic period, the virus is actively multiplying, infecting, and killing cells of the immune system. The virus can also hide within infected cells and be inactive. The most obvious effect of HIV infection is a decline in the number of CD4 positive T (CD4+) cells found in the blood-the immune system's key infection fighters. The virus slowly disables or destroys these cells without causing symptoms.

As the immune system becomes more debilitated, a variety of complications start to take over. For many people, the first signs of infection are large lymph nodes, or swollen glands that may be enlarged for more than 3 months. Other symptoms often experienced months to years before the onset of AIDS include
- Lack of energy

- Weight loss
- Frequent fevers and sweats
- Persistent or frequent yeast infections (oral or vaginal)
- Persistent skin rashes or flaky skin
- Pelvic inflammatory disease in women that does not respond to treatment
- Short-term memory loss

Some people develop frequent and severe herpes infections that cause mouth, genital, or anal sores, or a painful nerve disease called shingles. Children may grow slowly or get sick a frequently.

Acquired Immunodeficiency Syndrome (AIDS)
AIDS is the name given to the later stages of an HIV infection.

Symptoms of opportunistic infections common in people with AIDS include
- Coughing and shortness of breath
- Seizures and lack of coordination
- Difficult or painful swallowing
- Mental symptoms such as confusion and forgetfulness
- Severe and persistent diarrhea
- Fever
- Vision loss
- Nausea, abdominal cramps, and vomiting
- Weight loss and extreme fatigue
- Severe headaches
- Coma

Children with AIDS may get the same opportunistic infections as do adults with the disease. In addition, they also may have severe forms of the typically common childhood bacterial infections, such as conjunctivitis (pink eye), ear infections, and tonsillitis.

People with AIDS are also particularly prone to developing various cancers, especially those caused by viruses such as Kaposi's sarcoma and cervical cancer, or cancers of the immune system known as lymphomas. These cancers are usually more aggressive and difficult to treat in people with AIDS. Signs of Kaposi's sarcoma in light-skinned people are round brown, reddish, or purple spots that develop in the skin or in the mouth. In dark-skinned people, the spots are more pigmented.

During the course of HIV infection, most people experience a gradual decline in the number of CD4+ T cells, although some may have abrupt and dramatic drops in their CD4+ T-cell counts. A person with CD4+ T cells above 200 may experience some of the early symptoms of HIV disease. Others may have no symptoms even though their CD4+ T-cell count is below 200. Many people are so debilitated by the symptoms of AIDS that they cannot hold a steady job or do household chores. Other people with

AIDS may experience phases of intense life-threatening illness followed by phases in which they function normally.

A small number of people first infected with HIV 10 or more years ago have not developed symptoms of AIDS. Scientists are trying to determine what factors may account for the lack of progression to AIDS in some people, such as

- Whether their immune systems have particular characteristics
- Whether they were infected with a less aggressive strain of the virus
- If their genes may protect them from the effects of HIV

Scientists hope that understanding the body's natural method of controlling infection may lead to ideas for protective HIV vaccines and use of vaccines to prevent the disease from progressing.

About T-Cells

A T-cell is a type of lymphocyte which is a type of white blood cell. About 15 to 40 percent of white blood cells are lymphocytes
. And they are some of the most important cells in the immune system giving protection from viral infections; helping other cells fight bacterial and fungal infections; producing antibodies; fighting cancers; and coordinating the activities of other cells in the immune system.

The two main types of lymphocytes are B-cells and T-cells. B-cells are created and mature in bone marrow, while T-cells are created in bone marrow, but mature in the thymus gland (T for thymus). B-cells produce antibodies. Antibodies help the body destroy abnormal cells and infective organisms such as bacteria, viruses, and fungi.

T-cells are divided into three groups:

- **Helper T-Cells** (also called T4 or CD4+ cells) help other cells destroy infective organisms.

- **Suppressor T-Cells** (also called T8 or CD8+ cells) suppress the activity of other lymphocytes so they don't destroy normal tissue.

- **Killer T-Cells** (also called cytotoxic T lymphocytes, or CTLs, and are another kind of T8 or CD8+ cell) recognize and destroy abnormal or infected cells.

The normal T4 count is somewhere between 500 and 1500 cells per cubic millimeter of blood (a drop, more or less). In the absence of anti-HIV treatment, the T4 cell count decreases, on average, about 50 to 100 cells each year. AIDS-related diseases (opportunistic infections) such as pneumocystis carinii pneuomonia (PCP) can occur if the T4 count falls below 200. And, a large number of other infections can occur if it drops below 50 to 100 cells. Because of this, drugs to prevent these infections (prophylactic treatment) are started once the T4 cell count falls below certain levels, such as 200 in the case of PCP.

Diagnosis

Because early HIV infection often causes no symptoms, a healthcare provider usually can diagnose it by testing blood for the presence of antibodies (disease-fighting proteins) to HIV. HIV antibodies generally do not reach noticeable levels in the blood for 1 to 3 months after infection. It may take the antibodies as long as 6 months to be produced in quantities large enough to show up in standard blood tests. Hence, to determine whether a person has been recently infected (acute infection), a healthcare provider can screen blood for the presence of HIV genetic material. Direct screening of HIV is extremely critical in order to prevent transmission of HIV from recently infected individuals.

Anyone who has been exposed to the virus should get an HIV test as soon as the immune system is likely to develop antibodies to the virus-within 6 weeks to 12 months after possible exposure to the virus. By getting tested early, a healthcare provider can give advice to an infected person about when to start treatment to help the immune system combat HIV and help prevent the emergence of certain opportunistic infections (see section on treatment). Early testing also alerts an infect person to avoid high-risk behaviors that could spread the virus to others. Most healthcare providers can do HIV testing and will usually offer counseling at the same time. Of course, testing can be done anonymously at many sites if a person is concerned about confidentiality.

Healthcare providers diagnose HIV infection by using two different types of antibody tests: ELISA (enzyme-linked immunosorbent assay) and Western blot. If a person is highly likely to be infected with HIV but has tested negative for both tests, a healthcare provider may request additional tests. A person also may be told to repeat antibody testing at a later date, when antibodies to HIV are more likely to have developed.

Babies born to mothers infected with HIV may or may not be infected with the virus, but all carry their mothers' antibodies to HIV for several months. If these babies lack symptoms, healthcare providers cannot make a definitive diagnosis of HIV infection using standard antibody tests. Instead, they are using new technologies to detect HIV and more accurately determine HIV infection in infants between ages 3 months and 15 months. Researchers are evaluating a number of blood tests to determine which ones are best for diagnosing HIV infection in babies younger than 3 months.

Treatment

When AIDS first surfaced in the United States, there were no drugs to combat the underlying immune deficiency and few treatments existed for the opportunistic diseases that resulted. Researchers, however, have developed drugs to fight both HIV infection and its associated infections and cancers.

Integrase Inhibitors

In order for HIV to successfully take over a CD4 cell's machinery so that it can produce new viruses, HIV's RNA is converted into DNA by the reverse transcriptase enzyme (nucleotide/nucleoside reverse transcriptase inhibitors can block this process). After the "reverse transcription" of RNA into DNA is complete, HIV's DNA must then be incorporated into the CD4 cell's DNA. This is known as integration. As their name implies, integrase inhibitors work by blocking this process.

Integrase inhibitors offer a lot of hope for HIV-positive people, especially those who have developed HIV resistance to drugs that target HIV's two other major enzymes: reverse transcriptase and protease. Protease inhibitors, interrupt the virus from making copies of itself at a later step in its life cycle.

Reverse transcriptase (RT) inhibitors, interrupts an early stage of the virus making copies of itself. Nucleoside/nucleotide RT inhibitors are faulty DNA building blocks. When these faulty pieces are incorporated into the HIV DNA (during the process when the HIV RNA is converted to HIV DNA), the DNA chain cannot be completed, thereby blocking HIV from replicating in a cell. Non-nucleoside RT inhibitors bind to reverse transcriptase, interfering with its ability to convert the HIV RNA into HIV DNA. This class of drugs may slow the spread of HIV in the body and delay the start of opportunistic infections.

There is another class of drugs, known at fusion inhibitors, to treat HIV infection. Fuzeon (enfuvirtide or T-20), the first approved fusion inhibitor, works by interfering with the ability of HIV-1 to enter into cells by blocking the merging of the virus with the cell membranes. This inhibition blocks HIV's ability to enter and infect the human immune cells. Fuzeon is designed for use in combination with other anti-HIV treatments. It reduces the level of HIV infection in the blood and may be effective against HIV that has become resistant to current antiviral treatment schedules.

Because HIV can become resistant to any of these drugs, healthcare providers must use a combination treatment to effectively suppress the virus. When multiple drugs (three or more) are used in combination, it is referred to as highly active antiretroviral therapy, (HAART) , and can be used by people who are newly infected with HIV as well as people with AIDS. Recently, FDA approved the first one-a-day three drug-combination pill called Atripla.

Researchers have credited HAART as being a major factor in significantly reducing the number of deaths from AIDS in this country. While HAART is not a cure for AIDS, it has greatly improved the health of many people with AIDS and it reduces the amount of virus circulating in the blood to nearly undetectable levels. Researchers, however, have shown that HIV remains present in hiding places, such as the lymph nodes, brain, testes, and retina of the eye, even in people who have been treated.

Side effects

Despite the beneficial effects of HAART, there are side effects associated with the use of antiviral drugs that can be severe. Some of the nucleoside RT inhibitors may cause a decrease of red or white blood cells, especially when taken in the later stages of the disease. Some may also cause inflammation of the pancreas and painful nerve damage. There have been reports of complications and other severe reactions, including death, to some of the antiretroviral nucleoside analogs when used alone or in combination. Therefore, health experts recommend that anyone on antiretroviral therapy be routinely seen and followed by their healthcare provider.

The most common side effects associated with protease inhibitors include nausea, diarrhea, and other gastrointestinal symptoms. In addition, protease inhibitors can interact with other drugs resulting in serious side effects. Fuzeon may also cause severe allergic reactions such as pneumonia, trouble breathing, chills and fever, skin rash, blood in urine, vomiting, and low blood pressure. Local skin reactions are also possible since it is given as an injection underneath the skin. People taking HIV drugs should contact their healthcare providers immediately if they have any of these symptoms.

Opportunistic infections

A number of available drugs help treat opportunistic infections. These drugs include

- Foscarnet and ganciclovir to treat <u>CMV (cytomegalovirus)</u> eye infections
- Fluconazole to treat yeast and other fungal infections
- TMP/SMX (trimethoprim/sulfamethoxazole) or pentamidine to treat PCP (Pneumocystis carinii pneumonia)

Cancers

Healthcare providers use radiation, chemotherapy, or injections of alpha interferon-a genetically engineered protein that occurs naturally in the human body-to treat Kaposi's sarcoma or other <u>cancers</u> associated with HIV infection.

Prevention

Because there is no vaccine for HIV, the only way people can prevent infection with the virus is to avoid behaviors putting them at risk of infection, such as sharing needles and having unprotected sex. Many people infected with HIV have no symptoms. Therefore, there is no way of knowing with certainty whether a sexual partner is infected unless he or she has repeatedly tested negative for the virus and has not engaged in any risky behavior. Abstaining from having sex or use male latex condoms or female polyurethane condoms may offer partial protection, during oral, anal, or vaginal sex. Only water-based lubricants should be used with male latex condoms.

Although some laboratory evidence shows that spermicides can kill HIV, researchers have not found that these products can prevent a person from getting HIV. Recently, NIAID-supported two studies that found adult male medical circumcision reduces a man's risk of acquiring HIV infection by approximately 50 percent. The studies, conducted in Uganda and Kenya, pertain only to heterosexual transmission. As with most prevention strategies, adult male medical circumcision is not completely effective at preventing HIV transmission. Circumcision will be most effective when it is part of a more complete prevention strategy including the ABCs (Abstinence, Be Faithful, Use Condoms) of HIV prevention.

Selected Links

AIDS*info*
P.O. Box 6303
Rockville, MD 20849-6303
1-800-HIV-0440 (1-800-448-0440) or 301-519-0459
1-888-480-3739 (TTY/TDD)

National Institutes of Health HIV vaccine clinical trials
1-866-833-LIFE (1-866-833-5433).

National Institutes of Health HIV/AIDS clinical trials
1-800-243-7644

GLOSSARY

Absorption | The process of entry into the blood after a drug is administered.

Acetaldehyde | The first metabolite of alcohol during biotransformation; causes highly toxic reaction if it accumulates in the body.

Acetylcholine | (ACh) A neurotransmitter released at neuromuscular junctions and selected CNS synapses; involved with memory and movement.

Acetylcholinesterase | (AChE) An enzyme that degrades acetylcholine.

Action potential | Discrete electrical signal that propagates down the axon of the cell to the axon .endings.

Adenylate cyclase | A catalytic enzyme that facilitates the conversion of ATP to cAMP (see "second messenger").

Adiponectin | Hormone secreted by adipose (fatty) tissue that seems to be involved in energy homeostasis; it enhances insulin sensitivity and glucose tolerance, as well as oxidation of fatty acids in muscle. Its blood concentration is reduced in obese people and those with Type II diabetes.

Agonist | A substance that mimics a neurotransmitter at synapse.

Akathesia | A movement disorder sometimes as a side effect of antipsychotic medication.

Alcohol | The first enzyme that converts alcohol into acetaldehyde.
dehyrogenase

Analgesic | A drug that suppresses pain sensation.

Anandamide | An identified endogenous cannabinoid substance that binds to an endogenous THC receptor.

Antagonist | A substance that blocks the effects of a neurotransmitter at synapse.

Anticholinergic | A substance that inhibits or blocks the effects of ACh, causing dry mouth, urinary retention, blurred vision, dilated pupils and delirium.

Antiemetic	A substance that prevents nausea and vomiting.
Anxiety	Commonly experienced apprehension, tension or uneasiness from anticipated danger, the source of which is unknown or unrecognized.
Anxiolytics	A substance that treats the symptoms of anxiety; usually relating to the benzodiazepine drugs (like Valium).
Arrhythmia	An irregular (not rhythmic) heart beat.
Astrocytes	Glial cells that support neurons by filtering fluids for the blood brain barrier.
Ataxia	A decrease in movement and loss of muscle coordination.
Autonomic nervous system	One of the two main subdivisions of the peripheral nervous system that mediates the sympathetic fight-flight response and parasympathetic feed-breed response.
Autoreceptor	A protein receptor on the presynpatic membrance that assists in regulating transmitter substance release.
Axon	The part of the neuron that transmits electrical impulses from the cell body to the axon endings for neurotransmitter release; axons can be myelinated to help facilitate the nerve impulse.
Axon Endings	Also called terminal endings, they lie at the end of the axon and form presynaptic membrane where neurotransmitters are released.
BAL	(Blood Alcohol Level) A measure of the amount of alcohol in the blood expressed as either percentage or in mgs per100ml of blood.
Barbiturates	A class of sedative-hypnotic drugs that inhibit neural activity.
Basal ganglia	Deep lying structures in both cerebral hemispheres, including the substantia nigra; involved in regulation of movement.

Benzodiazepines	A class of anti-anxiety drugs and muscle relaxants.
Bipolar Disorder	A psychiatric condition marked by severe mood swings that cycle between mania (hyperactivity) and depression.
Blood-Brain-Barrier	The combination of specialized capillaries and glial cells that restrict drug entry into the brain.
Calcium	(Ca+) An essential element to nervous system function; Ca+ plays a critical role in metabolic processes in neurons and also neurotransmitter release.
Cannabinoids	Also, called phytocannabinoids, are those compounds commonly found in the marijuana plant of which there are over 60.
Cannabinoid receptors	The chemistry of the ES is the endocannabinoids where they are released into synapse and bind to and activate distinct cannabinoid receptor. To date, 2 types of cannabinoid receptors have been identified; CB1 and CB2. CB1 receptors are found primarily in the brain and the CB2 receptors are located mainly in immune cells and in peripheral tissues of the body in adipocytes (or "fat cells") that are associated with lipid and glucose metabolism.
Catecholamine	A class of neurotransmitters within the nervous system, including epinephrine, norepinephrine and dopamine.
COMT	Catechol-O-methyl transferase. The enzyme that degrades the catecholamines.
cAMP	Cyclic adenosine monophosphate. A second messenger in neurotransmission that also increases glucose production in cells.
Cell Body	The metabolic center of the neuron also called the soma.
CNS	The Central Nervous System. One of two anatomical divisions of the nervous system; includes the brain and the spinal cord.
Cerebellum	The structure located within the hindbrain that controls motor coordination and balance.
Channel	(Ion Channel) A membrane spanning protein that mediates

the flow of ions into and out of cells.

Chloride	(C1-) An essential element in the nervous system; influx of Cl- is a common inhibitory mechanism.
Cirrhosis	A potentially fatal disease marked by hardening of the liver commonly as a result of chronic alcohol intake.
Cognition	The processing of information by the brain; specifically perception, reasoning and memory.
Comorbid	Two diverse syndromes coexisting simultaneously; for example, a person who is inflicted with both mental illness and substance abuse.
Compulsion	An insistent, intrusive and unwanted action that is repeated over and over.
Cerebral cortex	One of the major components of the cerebral hemispheres that is divided into four lobes.
Corticotropin-releasing factor	(CRF) A hormone produced by the brain that controls cortisol levels; elevated levels are associated with depression.
Cross tolerance	Tolerance developed with one drug that will also prevent actions from other drugs in the same class.
Delirium tremons	(DTs) A stage of alcohol withdrawal characterized by tremors, hallucinations and disorientation; only seen in a small percentage of alcoholics.
Delusion	A belief that is clearly implausible but compelling; false or imaginary perception that may be central to a person's life.
Dendrites	Extensions from the cell body of a neuron that receives information from other neurons.
Dependence	A state where tolerance to the effects of a drug takes place after repeat drug administration, and where there is withdrawal upon cessation of use.
Depolarized	State of a neuron after it has been discharge, in response to the polarized ion-charge that was generated.

Dopamine	(DA) One of the monoamine neurotransmitters involved in movement, pleasure, and the brain's reward circuit.
Dose-response curve	A way of expressing the relationship between the effects of a drug and the amount required to obtain the level of effect.
DNA	(deoxyribonucleic acid) Contained within the chromosomes in the cell nucleus, contains information for protein synthesis.
Dynorphin	One of the endogenous opioids.
Dysphoria	Displeasure, unhappiness, depression and emotional pain, that may usually be long-lasting yet not severe.
Endocannabinoids	Endocannabinoid, is a word condensed from two other words; endogenous: from within, and cannabinoid: substances resembling the components within the C. sativa plant. The two major endocannabinoids are arachidonoyl ethanolamide (anandamide) and 2-arachidonoyl glycerol (2-AG).
Endocannabinoid system	(ES) is a physiological system consisting of cannabinoid receptors and corresponding chemical messengers that is believed to play an important role in regulating body weight, glucose and lipid metabolism, pain, movement, cognitive functioning and addiction.
Endoplasmic reticulum	The area in the cell body that manufactures peptides, proteins and neurotransmitters.
Endorphin	One of the endogenous opioids.
Enkephalin	Another of the endogenous opioids.
Enzyme	A type of protein that accelerates a chemical reaction, and usually controls metabolism.
Epinephrine	An excitatory neurotransmitter.
EPS	(Extrapyramidal Syndrome) The movement disorder that is associated with aging, use of antipsychotics, meperidine analog MPTP, etc; characterized by tremors, weakness, impaired motor coordination, stooped posture and disinterest.

Extrapyramidal System	A functional system of motor neurons controlling gait, posture and fine movements; the substantia nigra is part of this system.
Fetal alcohol syndrome	(FAS) Mental retardation and deformity in infants caused by the mother's consumption of alcohol during pregnancy and thus exposing the fetus to the drug's toxic effects.
G-protein	A membrane protein that acts as a second messenger in neurotransmission.
GABA	(Gamma amino-butyric acid) A neurotransmitter with CNS inhibitory function.
Gene	The fundamental physical and functional unit of heredity.
Glial Cells	Cells in the nervous system that provide structural support for neurons.
Glutamate	An excitatory neurotransmitter.
Half-life	The amount of time required for the body to metabolize and rid half of the circulating drug.
Hallucination	A perception without an objective basis; an imaginary voice, vision, smell or taste, or cross-over sensation of these.
Hippocampus	A structure within the limbic system involved with aspects of memory storage.
Hypertension	Abnormal and dangerously high blood pressure.
Hypnotic	A substance that induces sleep or a state of unconsciousness.
Hypothalamus	A structure of the brain that regulates autonomic, endocrine and visceral functions.
HVA	(Homovanillic acid) An end product of dopamine metabolism.
Indoleamine	A class of monoamines, which includes serotonin.
Kinase	(Protein) An enzyme that uses ATP to catalyze the phosphorylation of other proteins and thereby modifying their functions.

Korsakoff's Psychosis	A disorder caused y chronic and excessive alcohol consumption and characterized by memory loss and confusion.
L-DOPA	A precursor to the catecholamines.
Ligand	A substance that acts in the same manner as a neurotransmitter.
Limbic System	The system in the forebrain that plays a critic role in learning, memory and emotions.
Lipid	Another name for fat; fatty cellular tissue.
Lipid solubility	The ability of a drug to dissolve in fat.
Lipophilic	Having an affinity for, tending to combine with, or capable of dissolving in lipids.
Medial Forebrain Bundle	(MFB) A neural system involving the nucleus accumbens and associated with pleasure and positive reinforcement.
Medulla	A structure in the hindbrain that aids the autonomic process of digestion, breathing and control of heart rate.
MCLP	(Mesocorticolimbic Pathway) A dopamine system running though the ventral tegmental area and the nucleus accumbens liked to behavioral reward.
Metabolic Syndrome	The Metabolic Syndrome is a cluster of conditions that occur together, increasing your risk of heart disease, stroke and diabetes. The main features of metabolic syndrome include insulin resistance, hypertension (high blood pressure, cholesterol abnormalities, and an increased risk for clotting. Patients are most often overweight or obese.
Metabolic tolerance	Tolerance that is a result of increased metabolism of the drug.
Metabolism	A biological process that transforms chemicals into states that are either beneficial to the body or less toxic than their original form, in preparation to be eliminated; mostly conducted in the liver.
Metabolite	A generally water-soluble by-product after biotransformation

by the liver.

Mitochondria	Intracellular structures that provide energy by high energy bonds such as ATP.
Monoamines	The group of neurotransmitters comprised of a single amino acid, including epinephrine, norephinephrine, dopamine and serotonin.
Monamine oxidase	(MAO) The enzyme that destroys monoamines in synapse
Muscarinic receptor	A receptor in the ACh system that can be activated by muscarine or blocked by atrpoine.
Mydriasis	Prolonged abnormal dilatation of the pupil of the eye caused by disease or a drug.
Myelin	The lipid covering along axons that increases the speed of the nerve signal.
Neuron	One of two major classes of cells in the nervous system, besides glial cells; actively communicate and process neurological information.
Neurotransmitters	Specialized chemical messengers produced and released by neurons to communicate with other neurons.
Neuroleptics	Also called antipsychotics or major tranquilizers, these are used primarily to cause a reduction in the symptoms of psychosis, particularly schizophrenia.
Norepinephrine	One of the excitatory neurotransmitter substances in the nervous system
Nucleus accumbens	An area within the MFB which plays an important role in the mediation of positive reinforcement (pleasure center).
Obsession	An irrational thought, image or idea that is irresistible and recurrent.
OCD	Obsessive-Compusive Disorder. A mental disorder characterized by recurrent and persistent thoughts, images or ideas perceived by the patient as intrusive and senseless (obsessions) and by stereotypic, repetitive, purposeful actions perceived as unnecessary (compulsions).

Opioids	All members of the class of compounds that act similarly to morphine, producing analgesia, sedation and drive reduction.
Parasympathetic nervous system	The division of the autonomic nervous system that generates rest, digestion, heart rate and blood pressure.
Parenteral	A route of administration that avoids the "enterals" or digestive tract; includes methods such as injection and inhalation.
Parkinson's disease	A movement disorder that involves degeneration of dopamine-containing neurons within the substantia nigra.
Peptides	A chain of amino acids linked together in a specific order to form a compound (like endorphins).
Peripheral nervous system	One of two anatomical divisions of the nervous system; includes the external neurons and axons of the skeletal and autonomic nervous systems.
pH factor	The relative acidity or base of a biological fluid, where acidic solutions have a pH between 0 and 7, and alkaline solutions have a pH between 7 and 14.
Placebo	A procedure (or substance) that is inert and contains nobiological activity for any given condition.
Psychosis	A mental state characterized by extreme impairment of perception of reality including hallucinations, delusions, incoherence and bizarre behavior; prominent feature of schizophrenia
Psychotomimetic	A drug that produces effects that mimic psychosis.
Pyrolysis	Decomposition or transformation of a compound caused by heat.
Raphe nuclei	A hindbrain structure that regulates sleep.
Receptor	Protein embedded in the postsynaptic membrane that binds to one or two specific neurotransmitters; thereby turning a particular biological mechanism on or off; generally found in the dendrites and cell body of neurons.
Reuptake	Removal of the neurotransmitter from synapse by the

presynaptic membrane retracting its chemical release.

Reverse tolerance	(Sensitization) Occurs when there is an increase in response to a drug after repeated administration.
Serotonin	(5-HT) A neurotransmitter substance classified as an indoleamine within the monamine group.
Schizophrenia	A mental disorder consisting of positive symptoms (hallucinations, illogical thought and impulsivity), and negative symptoms (blunt emotions, apathy and withdrawal); positive symptoms associated with psychosis.
Second messenger	A substance released inside a neuron in response to a neurotransmitter at a receptor site. A second messenger causes a change in the conductance of the postsynaptic membrane.
Somatic nervous system	The division of the peripheral nervous system made of nerves that control voluntary muscles.
SSRI	(Selective Serotonin Reuptake Inhibitors) A class of antidpressants that block the withdrawal of certain neurotransmitters in synapse, thus increasing the neurotransmitters' presence.
Sympathetic Nervous System	The division of the autonomic nervous system that mediates the fight-flight-fright response.
Sympathomimetics	A class of drugs that mimic the effects of arousal and other sympathetic responses.
Synapse	The area of communication between neurons where neurotransmitters are released from one neuron to another.
Tachycardia	Abnormally rapid heart rate.
Tardive dyskinesia	An irreversible movement disorder often caused by continuous use anti-psychotic medications.
Therpeutic index	(TI) An indicator for a drug's safety calculated by dividing the effective dose (ED) by the lethal dose (LD).
Titration	Adjusting the dose of a drug to obtain or maintain a particular effect.

Tolerance	The decrease in potency of a drug with repeated administration; an adaptive process where the intensity of a drug's effects are reduced.
VTA	(Ventral tegmental area) An area of the brain that mediates pleasure and constitutes a part of the brain's reward circuitry; opioid and dopamine receptors are found in high density in the VTA. The organs located inside the body cavity (heart, kidney, etc.)
Viscera	The organs located inside the body cavity (heart, kidney, etc.)
Wernicke's syndrome	Thiamine (Vitamin B-1) deficiency induced brain damage common to many alcoholics which causes Korsakoff's psychosis.
Withdrawal	The physiological symptoms that occur when some drugs are abruptly discontinued after repeat administration. Symptoms of withdrawal are usually opposite to the drug's effects.

ANSWER KEY TO THE SELF-STUDY QUESTIONS

Chapter One:
1. True   2. True   3. False   4. True   5. False   6. True   7. False   8. True   9. True   10. True

Chapter Two:
1. False   2. False   3. False   4. True   5. True   6. True   7. True   8. True   9. False   10. True

 Chapter Three:
1. True   2. True   3. True   4. True   5. False   6. True   7. True   8. False   9. True   10. True

Chapter Four:
1. True   2. True   3. False   4. True   5. True   6. True   7. True   8. False   9. True   10. True

Chapter Five:
1. True   2. True   3. True   4. False   5. True   6. False   7. True   8. True   9. True   10. True

Chapter Six:
1. True   2. True   3. True   4. False   5. False   6. False   7. True   8. True   9. True   10. True

Chapter Seven:
1. False   2. True   3. True   4. True   5. True   6. True   7. False   8. True   9. True   10. False

Chapter Eight:
1. True   2. False   3. True   4. True   5. False   6. True   7. True   8. False   9. True   10. True

Chapter Nine:
1. True   2. False   3. True   4. True   5. True   6. True   7. True   8. True   9. True   10. True

Chapter Ten:
1. True   2. False   3. True   4. False   5. False   6. True   7. True   8. True   9. False   10. True

Chapter Eleven:
1. True   2. True   3. False   4. False   5. True   6. True   7. False   8. True   9. False   10. True

Chapter Twelve:
1. True   2. False   3. True   4. True   5. False   6. True   7. True   8. True   9. True   10. False

Chapter Thirteen:
1. False   2. True   3. True   4. True   5. True   6. True   7. False   8. False   9. False   10. True

Chapter 14:
1. False   2. True   3. False   4. True   5. True   6. True   7. False   8. True   9. True   10. False

Chapter 15:
1. False   2. True   3. True   4. False   5. True   6. True   7. True   8. False   9. False   10. True

INDEX

mixed-function enzymatic oxidizing system, 22
monoamine oxidase, 149, 151
monoamine oxidase inhibitors, 276, 279, 295
mood disorders, 293
mood stabilizer, 295
mood-stabilizers, 265
morphine, 122, 169, 170, 177, 178, 192, 247
myelin, 59
Naltrexone, 138
ndocannabinoids, 192
ndogenous cannabinoid system., 191
negative reinforcement, 104
negative symptoms, 268
nerve impulse, 60
neuron, 57, 173
neurons, 277
neurotransmitter, 57, 60
neurotransmitters, 58, 62, 63, 66, 67, 68, 77, 78, 84, 91, 92, 103, 149, 177, 194, 266, 272, 273, 276, 277, 294
neurotransmitters., 80
nicotine, 103, 111
nitric oxide, 91
nociception, 171
norepinephrine, 81, 149, 273, 279
nucleus accumbens, 49, 80, 105, 106, 114, 122, 156, 160, 204
occipital lobe, 51
pain, 170, 171, 173, 179
Papaver somniferum., 169
parallel treatment, 304
parasympathetic nervous system, 42
parietal lobe, 50
passive transport, 20
peripheral nervous system, 41, 83, 91
permissive hypothesis, 276
pharmacokinetics, 14, 16
pharmacology, 11, 15
phencyclidine, 220
Physostigma venenosum, 220

phytocannabinoids, 191
placebo, 16
pons, 45
positive reinforcement, 104
positive symptoms, 268
postsynaptic, 69
postsynaptic membrane, 62
potency, 16
prefrontal cortex, 267
presynaptic membrane, 62
Principles of Drug Addiction Treatment, 313
Protease inhibitors, 337
psilocybin, 217, 222
pyramiding, 237
receptor sites, 64, 68
resting potential, 60
reticular formation, 45
Reverse transcriptase (RT) inhibitors, 337
roid rage, 241
saltatory conduction, 59
Salvia Divinorum, 222
schizophrenia, 80, 265, 299
scopolamine, 219
selective serotonin reuptake inhibitors, 276, 279
sensitization, 110, 221
sequential treatment, 304
serotonin, 68, 83, 84, 123, 130, 133, 149, 152, 193, 216, 266, 273, 279, 281
serotonin syndrome, 84, 281
solubility, 18, 19, 22
soma, 58
stabilization, 182
stacking, 237
steady state, 15, 25
steroids, 48, 237, 240
stress-diathesis model of mood disorders, 276
Substance P, 92
substantia nigra, 81
substantia nigras, 92
sympathetic nervous system, 42, 81

354

CPSIA information can be obtained
at www.ICGtesting.com
Printed in the USA
LVHW050100021222
734348LV00005B/381

9 781440 472923